Occupational Therapy in Mental Health

Considerations for Advanced Practice

Edited by Marian Kavanaugh Scheinholtz, MS, OT/L

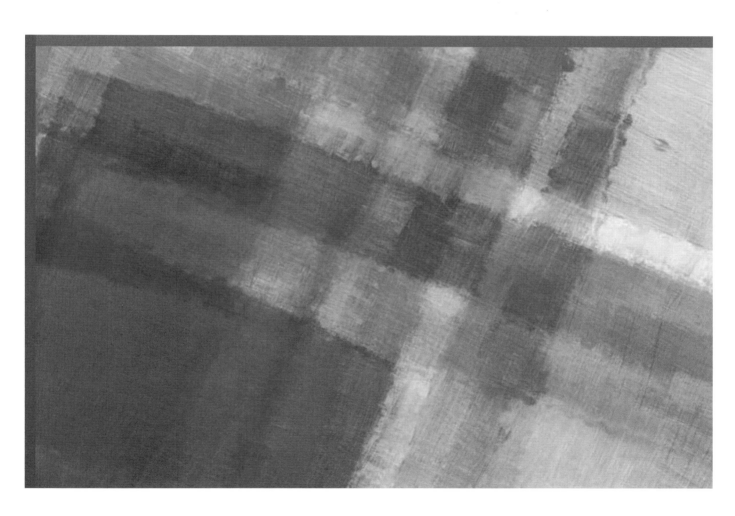

AOTA PRESS
The American
Occupational Therapy
Association, Inc.

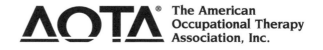

AOTA® The American Occupational Therapy Association, Inc.

Centennial Vision

We envision that occupational therapy is a powerful, widely recognized, science-driven, and evidence-based profession with a globally connected and diverse workforce meeting society's occupational needs.

Vision Statement

The American Occupational Therapy Association advances occupational therapy as the pre-eminent profession in promoting the health, productivity, and quality of life of individuals and society through the therapeutic application of occupation.

Mission Statement

The American Occupational Therapy Association advances the quality, availability, use, and support of occupational therapy through standard-setting, advocacy, education, and research on behalf of its members and the public.

AOTA Staff

Frederick P. Somers, *Executive Director*
Christopher M. Bluhm, *Chief Operating Officer*
Maureen Freda Peterson, *Chief Professional Affairs Officer*

Chris Davis, *Director, AOTA Press*
Sarah D. Hertfelder, *Continuing Education Program Manager*
Caroline Polk, *Project Manager*
Linda Weidemann, *Wolf Creek Publishing Services, Compositor*

Beth Ledford, *Director, Marketing*
Emily Zhang, *Technology Marketing Specialist*
Jennifer Folden, *Marketing Specialist*

The American Occupational Therapy Association, Inc.
4720 Montgomery Lane
Bethesda, MD 20814
Phone: 301-652-AOTA (2682)
TDD: 800-377-8555
Fax: 301-652-7711
www.aota.org
To order: 877-404-AOTA (2682)

Disclaimers

This publication is designed to provide accurate and authoritative information in regard to the subject matter covered. It is sold or distributed with the understanding that the publisher is not engaged in rendering legal, accounting, or other professional service. If legal advice or other expert assistance is required, the services of a competent professional person should be sought.
— *From the Declaration of Principles jointly adopted by the American Bar Association and a Committee of Publishers and Associations*

It is the objective of the American Occupational Therapy Association to be a forum for free expression and interchange of ideas. The opinions expressed by the contributors to this work are their own and not necessarily those of the American Occupational Therapy Association.

ISBN-13: 978-1-56900-274-2
ISBN-10: 1-56900-274-2
Library of Congress Control No.: 2010903787

Contents

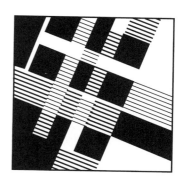

Dedication

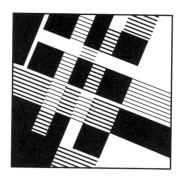

In recognition of their journey of recovery, I dedicate this text to everyone whose life has been touched by mental illness and to their supporters. And with gratitude, I further dedicate it to my family, friends, and mentors whose love and support have enabled me to go forward each day and to achieve what has sometimes seemed impossible—most especially, to Dolly, Jim, Fred, and Doug.

Acknowledgments

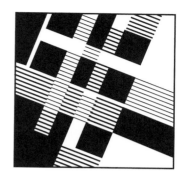

Many thanks to the authors of this publication, whose time, effort, commitment, and wealth of experience have been essential to its production.

Special thanks to Sarah Hertfelder for her professional and personal support of the editor, authors, and others who were involved in the development and completion of this project.

Thanks to the American Occupational Therapy Association Board of Directors and staff for recognizing the need for this project and providing the support to accomplish it.

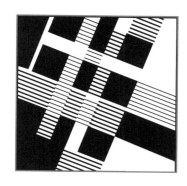

About the Editor

Marian Kavanaugh Scheinholtz, MS, OT/L, is public health advisor in the Community Support Programs Branch of the Division of Service and Systems Improvement of the Center for Mental Health Services, Substance Abuse and Mental Health Services Administration (SAMHSA). In this capacity, she administers the Older Adult Mental Health grant program, the development of evidence-based practice toolkits, and the Mental Health Transformation State Incentive grant for the state of Missouri. She is also assisting in the development of the Primary Care and Behavioral Healthcare Integration initiative.

Before joining SAMHSA, Scheinholtz was mental health program manager for the American Occupational Therapy Association (AOTA) for 12 years. While at AOTA, Scheinholtz initiated and managed national occupational therapy mental health programs and represented AOTA to accrediting agencies, including the Joint Commission, the Commission on Accreditation of Rehabilitation Facilities, and the National Committee for Quality Assurance. In addition, she supported the AOTA international program and activities and the multicultural and diversity program, and she led efforts to develop evidence-based practice guidelines on occupational therapy interventions for autism and serious mental illness.

Scheinholtz's clinical practice preceded her AOTA tenure; it included directing two psychosocial rehabilitation community-based programs for people with serious mental illness and serving as occupational therapist for the National Institute of Mental Health research program for people with schizophrenia.

Scheinholtz is a graduate of the Virginia Commonwealth University/Medical College of Virginia occupational therapy program and has a bachelor's degree in psychology from the University of Pittsburgh. She is a person with lived experience who is an advocate for consumers of mental health services. She has also written and presented on consumers as providers in national and international forums.

About the Authors

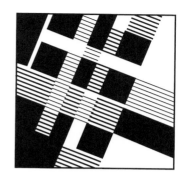

Onda Bennett, PhD, OTR/L, is interim dean of university programs and associate professor in the Department of Occupational Therapy at Eastern Kentucky University (EKU). In addition, she holds a graduate faculty position at the University of Kentucky Rehabilitation Science Doctoral Program. Bennett's clinical background has been primarily in designing and implementing community-based mental health programs. During her clinical career, she facilitated the development of a continuum of rehabilitation day programs for western New York, receiving the New York State Occupational Therapy Award for Outstanding Practice in Mental Health. For the past 20 years, she has held administrative and teaching positions in higher education. Her research and teaching have focused on evidence-based practice in occupational therapy, community mental health, and pedagogy in higher education.

In addition to managing university programs, Bennett leads a nationally recognized program at EKU that is designed to transform the university's efforts to enhance students' critical and creative thinking. Bennett continues to work with students at the doctoral and master's levels on evidence-based practice in mental health and education.

Katherine A. Burson, MS, OTR/L, CPRP, is the director of rehabilitation services for the Illinois Department of Human Services Division of Mental Health. A graduate of Washington University in St. Louis, she has worked in mental health practice for more than 25 years as an occupational therapist, educator, consultant, supervisor, and administrator in private for-profit, not-for-profit, and government settings.

Burson has partnered with others to develop and implement a variety of innovative rehabilitation initiatives that bring science into service and help better meet the participation needs of society. Among them are programs to allow elderly people at risk for institutionalization to regain their ability to participate in desired roles and remain in their homes, people with long hospitalizations to successfully return to their communities in their desired roles, and people desiring career advancement to succeed in college.

Burson has contributed to several grant-funded initiatives to integrate workforce, education, and human services systems to improve employment and postsecondary education outcomes for people with psychiatric conditions. Since 2005, she has led the Division of Mental Health's effort to make the evidence-based Individual Placement and Support model of supported employment widely available in Illinois by partnering with a broad coalition of stakeholders. The result has been an exponential increase in service capacity, doubling yearly for 4 consecutive years, and the work continues. In October 2008, the Illinois Chapter of the National Alliance on Mental Illness (NAMI) recognized Burson as a "Friend of NAMI Illinois" for this work.

A frequent speaker at occupational therapy conferences and former member of the Mental Health Standing Committee, Burson chaired the American Occupational Therapy Association's (AOTA's) ad hoc group to identify the core knowledge and skills necessary for entry-level occupational therapy practice in mental health.

Elizabeth Cara, PhD, OTR/L, is professor of occupational therapy at San Jose State University in California. She has 19 years of experience in occupational therapy education. Before entering academia, she worked for 15 years as an occupational therapist in mental health settings.

Cara teaches research and advanced clinical practice courses and has taught a variety of courses on fieldwork. She developed an innovative online group fieldwork course and has published and presented extensively on fieldwork and other topics. She is the lead editor and coauthor of the popular text *Psychosocial Occupational Therapy: A Clinical Practice.*

Roxanne Castaneda, MS, OTR/L, is in private practice focusing on people with mental illness, mental retardation with severe and challenging reputations, and forensic involvement. Her work focuses on community transition and negotiation with support systems and the judiciary and emphasizes successful community integration.

Castaneda has served as the assistant statewide forensic coordinator, developmental disabilities for the state of Maryland; director of community forensic evaluation and resource development for the Maryland Department of Health and Mental Hygiene; and director of community forensic services for the Massachusetts Department of Mental Health. She has been part-time faculty at the Towson University Occupational Therapy and Occupational Science Department since 1989.

Castaneda received her occupational therapy degree from the University of the Philippines and her graduate degree in applied behavioral sciences with a concentration in organization development from Johns Hopkins University. She was an invited participant at the Senior Executive Training for the Kennedy School of Government, Harvard University. She is on the Maryland Occupational Therapy Association's Roster of Merit and a recipient of AOTA's Recognition of Achievement Award.

Tina Champagne, MEd, OTR/L, CCAP, is the occupational therapy program director for the Center for Human Development in Springfield, Massachusetts; an adjunct professor for American International College's occupational therapy department; and an independent consultant. She has conducted research and published on the topic of sensory processing and sensory modulation in mental health. She is on the faculty of the National Executive Training Institute for the National Association of State Mental Health Program Directors, works closely on many projects with the

Massachusetts State Department of Mental Health, and has presented for numerous occupational therapy and mental health organizations on national and international levels.

Champagne received the 2008 Massachusetts State Department of Mental Health Commissioner's Distinguished Service award and a State Senate citation for innovations in implementing sensory approaches for prevention and crisis deescalation purposes, supporting the national trauma-informed, recovery-focused, and restraint and seclusion reduction initiatives. She is the chair of AOTA's Mental Health Special Interest Section (MHSIS).

Mariana D'Amico, EdD, OTR/L, BCP, is an assistant professor in the Schools of Allied Health Sciences and Graduate Studies at the Medical College of Georgia. She has extensive clinical and teaching experience. Courses taught include Pediatric Assessment and Intervention, Contemporary Practice, Mental Health Programming, Vision Rehabilitation, Applied Concepts of Wellness and Illness, and School System Practice.

D'Amico's research interests focus on coping and adaptation across the lifespan, leadership, sensory processing, quality of life, and occupational performance outcomes. She serves on the review boards of the *American Journal of Occupational Therapy* and the *International Journal of Rehabilitation Research*. She was a State of Georgia Governor's Teaching Fellow for academic year 2008–2009.

Robert W. Gibson, PhD, OTR/L, is an associate professor in the Department of Occupational Therapy, Schools of Allied Health Sciences and Graduate Studies at the Medical College of Georgia. Gibson teaches evidence-based practice, research design, and mental health courses in the occupational therapy curriculum.

In addition to being an occupational therapist, Gibson is a medical anthropologist. Gibson's areas of research include efficacy of occupational therapy mental health practice, health disparities, sickle cell disease, health care transition, and qualitative research methods. Gibson is a member of the Sickle Cell Center at the Medical College of Georgia, serves as a member of the Southeast Newborn Screening and Genetics Collaborative and the AOTA Transition Task Force, and reviews for the *American Journal of Occupational Therapy* and *Pediatrics*. Gibson was a State of Georgia Governor's Teaching Fellow during the 2007–2008 academic year.

Karla W. Gray, OTR/L, LICSW, graduated from the University of Puget Sound (Washington) in 1971 with a degree in occupational therapy and obtained a master of social work degree in 1988. She is licensed in both professions in Washington State. Gray has worked extensively with people who have mental illness, their families, and the systems designed to support the consumer in managing the effects of the illnesses. She has served as the AOTA MHSIS newsletter editor, AOTA representative to the Joint Commission Behavioral Health Professional and Technical Advisory Committee, and a member of AOTA ad hoc committees. She has also held several positions within the Washington Occupational Therapy Association.

Gray has presented and published works on a variety of topics, including group therapy, occupational therapy in partial hospitalization, the occupation of caregiving, successful voting with mental illness, and management issues. She is an active member of NAMI.

Susan Haiman, MPS, CPRP, OTR/L, FAOTA, has been a mental health practitioner and educator for more than 35 years. She has lectured widely on a variety of topics, including occupational therapy with adolescents, community-based programs, and models for private practice. Her interests include a grant-funded program using occupational therapy models to teach life skills to incarcerated women with mental illness. She has served as chair of the AOTA MHSIS, is in private practice, and is an associate professor of occupational therapy at Philadelphia University.

Lynn Jaffe, ScD, OTR/L, is an associate professor in the Department of Occupational Therapy, Schools of Allied Health Sciences and Graduate Studies, Medical College of Georgia, where her primary teaching responsibilities are in the research sequence. Statewide, Jaffe is a collaborator with Project SCEIs (Skilled Credentialed Early Interventionists), through which she develops and monitors Web-based courses for the Georgia Department of Community Health, Division of Public Health, Babies Can't Wait unit. She serves on the review board for the *American Journal of Occupational Therapy*. Jaffe was a State of Georgia Governor's Teaching Fellow during the 2002–2003 academic year.

Linda T. Learnard, OTR/L, has more than 35 years of experience in occupational therapy practice. She has worked primarily in areas of mental health and community practice but has provided services across all disability areas. Learnard has owned and operated her private practice for more than 20 years, providing services to state vocational rehabilitation and adult protective services as well as to the Maine state departments of mental health, developmental disabilities, and corrections. Ongoing services are also provided to community mental health agencies, community support, and residential programs.

Dana W. Logsdon, MS, OTR/L, is the occupational and physical therapy coordinator for Fayette County Public Schools in Lexington, Kentucky. She completed her master's of science in occupational therapy at Eastern Kentucky University in May 2007. In partial fulfillment of requirements for her master's degree, Logsdon worked on an AOTA–sponsored Evidence-Based Literature Review of Occupational Therapy Interventions in Mental Health, focusing on participation in paid and unpaid employment. She continued to complete this project following graduation. A Critically Appraised Topic on the subject is available to AOTA members on the association's Web site.

Lisa Mahaffey, MS, OTR/L, is an assistant professor at Midwestern University. Her 25-year history as an occupational therapy clinician has always been in mental health. She has worked in a variety of settings, including inpatient and outpatient mental health programs with adults, adolescents, children, and geriatrics. She has also worked with adults with chronic illness in community settings and with children in a therapeutic day school. Mahaffey's most recent clinical position required that she develop and manage a therapeutic program for older adults with mental illness, including people with dementia.

Mahaffey served as the chair of the AOTA MHSIS from 2006 to 2009 and is on the board of directors for the Illinois Occupational Therapy Association. She regularly speaks to care providers and family members in Chicago-area organizations about understanding and responding effectively to the behaviors of people with dementia and keeping them engaged in occupation and socially connected.

M. Beth Merryman, PhD, OTR/L, received a BS in occupational therapy from the Ohio State University, an MS in health science from Towson University, and a PhD in policy sciences from University of Maryland–Baltimore County. She is an associate professor in the Department of Occupational Therapy and Occupational Science at Towson University. Her teaching and research focus on supports and barriers to recovery as well as system and policy issues related to meaningful daily life for people with disabilities, particularly those with serious mental illnesses. She is a leader in a variety of advocacy activities related to community mental health and disability awareness, including serving on the board of directors of a community mental health center, as the faculty advisor for the Active Minds club on the Towson campus, with NAMI as a trainer for the Hearing Voices That Are Distressing workshops, and campus disability-related events.

Sarah Nielsen, MMGT, OTR/L, has been employed with the Trinity Child Adolescent Partial Hospitalization Program in Minot, North Dakota, for the past 9 years. She serves children ages 5 to 17 who struggle with emotional and behavioral difficulties. Nielsen is responsible for occupational therapy assessment, group and individual intervention, behavioral planning, coordination of school services, and transition planning for students. She also provides behavioral and self-regulation education to school systems, special education units, family services agencies, and community organizations.

Nielsen is also an adjunct faculty member of the University of North Dakota Occupational Therapy Program, where she teaches an online course on psychosocial aspects of children, adolescents, and young adults as well as the online Introduction to Occupational Therapy course.

Deborah B. Pitts, MBA, OTR/L, CPRP, BCMH, is a clinical faculty member of the University of Southern California Department of Occupational Science and Occupational Therapy. She has developed expertise in the philosophy and practice of psychiatric rehabilitation. She weaves her expertise in the areas of schizophrenia, psychosocial rehabilitation, and community support programs into her interest in how occupation influences the lived experience of recovery for people with psychiatric disabilities.

Pitts has provided consultation to local and statewide providers of community-based psychiatric rehabilitation services. She also has conducted numerous workshops and published in the occupational therapy and psychiatric rehabilitation journals and textbooks, including serving as co-editor for a special edition of the *Psychiatric Rehabilitation Journal* (Winter 2009) focused on occupational therapy contributions to psychiatric rehabilitation.

Pitts served as AOTA's MHSIS chairperson from 2003 to 2006 and as a Professional Development Liaison from 2006 to 2009. She chaired the work group that developed the competencies for AOTA's Board Certification in Mental Health and serves as the mental health representative for the Board for Advanced and Specialty Certification. She chaired or served as a member of recent AOTA ad hoc work groups that have focused on mental health practice issues.

Pitts has been active in advocating for increasing the presence of occupational therapy practitioners in California's public mental health system, including the development of an occupational therapy educators consortium and of a white paper and presentation to the California Mental Health Planning Council on the role and value of occupational therapy practitioners in public mental health.

Janie B. Scott, MA, OT/L, FAOTA, is a part-time lecturer in Towson University's Occupational Therapy/Occupational Science Department and is an occupational therapy and aging-in-place consultant. She is an expert witness for the Office of Medicare Hearing and Appeals and is engaged in a grant on falls prevention.

Additionally, Scott was AOTA's Practice Department director and ethics officer. Her publication topics include occupational therapy consultation, ethics, autism spectrum disorders, community rehabilitation, older drivers, and multicultural issues. Her "Everyday Ethics" column was regularly published in *OT Practice* and on the AOTA Web site.

Scott's volunteer experiences include several positions with the Maryland Occupational Therapy Association, AOTA, and the Homes for Life Coalition of Howard County, Maryland.

Margaret (Peggy) Swarbrick, PhD, OTR, CPRP, is director of the Institute for Wellness and Recovery Initiatives, Collaborative Support Programs of New Jersey (a large statewide agency run by people living with mental illness in collaboration with professionals), and a part-time assistant clinical professor in the Department of Psychiatric Rehabilitation and Counseling Professions at the University of Medicine and Dentistry of New Jersey (UMDNJ) School of Health-Related Professions (SHRP). Swarbrick has worked for many years as an occupational therapist in a variety of settings providing wellness and recovery-focused services. She has published extensively and has lectured nationally and internationally on issues such as wellness, employment, asset-building programs, and peer-delivered self-help models.

Swarbrick earned a doctorate in occupational therapy from New York University and completed a postdoctoral fellowship in advanced training and research from the National Institute on Disability and Rehabilitation Research at the Department of Psychiatric Rehabilitation and Counseling Professions, UMDNJ–SHRP.

Diane B. Tewfik, MA, OTR/L, is a cofounder of the Mental Health Task Force of the Metropolitan New York District of the New York State Occupational Therapy Association, a group dedicated to revitalizing mental health in occupational therapy. As an educator and a practitioner, she has presented locally, nationally, and internationally and is widely published on topics related to mental health and mental health services. In 2003, she received AOTA's Recognition of Achievement Award for Preserving Mental Health in Occupational Therapy. She is currently a consultant at Palladia, Inc., a substance abuse treatment center in New York City.

Renee Watling, PhD, OTR/L, has been a pediatric occupational therapist in Washington State since 1992 and has worked in clinic, school, and private practice settings. Watling has lectured extensively at state, regional, and national conferences on the topics of sensory processing, sensory-based occupational therapy intervention, and issues related to services for children with autism spectrum disorders and emotional and behavioral disorders. Her publications include research and theoretical papers and book chapters.

Watling received her BS and MS in occupational therapy from the School of Medicine at the University of Washington and her doctorate from the College of Education at the University of Washington. Her research focuses on understanding the relationship between sensory processing and behavior, especially among children with autism spectrum disorders. She has volunteered on several AOTA projects and committees, including serving as chair of the Sensory Integration Special Interest Section. She holds faculty appointments at the University of Puget Sound and the University of Washington.

Rondalyn V. Whitney, MOT, OTR/L, has worked in pediatric mental health and school-based practice and has lectured both nationally and internationally on topics related to challenges of parenting, the neurobiology of learning, autism-related disorders, and sensory processing. She most recently authored *Nonverbal Learning Disorder: Understanding and Coping With NLD and Asperger's*. She is a pioneer of innovative social and occupational programs for children and families with disorders of social participation, and her work has served as a model for many programs.

Whitney joined Kennedy Krieger Institute in the spring of 2009 as the research coordinator for a five-site Health Resources and Services Administration study focused on best practices regarding social engagement in school-based practice. She is a doctoral candidate in International Health Sciences at TUI University. Her research focuses on family systems, social participation, and the impact of parenting children with mental health disorders. Whitney is Maryland's Alternate Representative to the Commission on Practice for AOTA and was formerly regional director of the Occupational Therapy Association of California.

Reviewers

Rita P. Fleming-Castaldy, PhD, OT/L, FAOTA
Assistant Professor
Occupational Therapy Department
University of Scranton
Scranton, PA

Penny Kyler, ScD, OTR, FAOTA
Public Health Analyst
Health Resources and Services
Administration
Rockville, MD

Marjorie E. Scaffa, PhD, OTR/L, FAOTA
Professor, Department of Occupational
  Therapy
University of South Alabama
Mobile

List of Boxes, Figures, Tables, and Appendixes

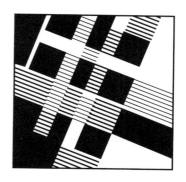

Introduction

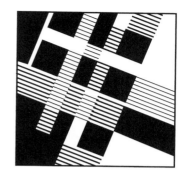

Marian Kavanaugh Scheinholtz, MS, OT/L

Welcome to *Occupational Therapy in Mental Health: Considerations for Advanced Practice,* designed as both an American Occupational Therapy Association (AOTA) Self-Paced Clinical Course (SPCC) and an AOTA Press textbook to address advanced practice in mental health occupational therapy. SPCCs are a means for occupational therapists and occupational therapy assistants to develop skills and knowledge to improve their ability to have a positive impact on the lives of the recipients of their services; readers who successfully complete the SPCC exam can obtain continuing education credit for their efforts (continuing education materials and exam are in a separate packet). As a textbook, the content can be used in the classroom or on its own to provide information and serve as a resource.

Purpose and Objectives

The purpose of this publication is to provide a comprehensive understanding of recent advances and trends in mental health practice, including current theories, standards of practice, literature, and research as they apply to occupational therapy. The learning objectives for readers are as follows:

- To understand the implications of the 2003 President's New Freedom Commission on Mental Health report concerning the transformation of the U.S. mental health system for occupational therapy mental health practice;
- To understand how the Recovery Model promotes the participation of consumers diagnosed with mental illness[1] and how it stands as a framework for occupational therapy practice in mental health, including implications for evaluation and intervention across the lifespan and settings;
- To apply principles of mental health transformation and the Recovery Model to the individual reader's occupational therapy practice;
- To understand current trends in mental health—such as trauma-informed care, consumer-directed care, and the use of evidence-based practices—and recognize their application to occupational therapy; and

---

[1]This volume uses the term *people with mental illness* to describe our patients and clients with mental health issues. The terminology is in no way meant to suggest that mental illness is a singular phenomenon.

- To identify advanced roles for occupational therapists, including advocacy, leadership, private practice, and consultant, and understand ways in which individual readers may evolve their skills and knowledge to assume these roles.

Background

The content was developed on the basis of focus groups and input from occupational therapy advanced practitioners in mental health practice. In addition, this work is informed by leading federal and nongovernmental entities that are shaping current and future mental health systems. These include agencies such as the National Institute of Mental Health, the Substance Abuse and Mental Health Services Administration, the National Empowerment Center, the National Council on Community Behavioral Healthcare, the National Council on Persons With Disabilities, and the National Association of State Mental Health Program Directors.

Occupational therapy began as a mental health profession but has unfortunately lost its recognition as a leading profession that can contribute to the recovery of people diagnosed with mental illness. It is imperative that occupational therapists rise to the challenges of 21st-century mental health care as clinicians, academicians, scientists, and leaders in informing and determining policy and practice parameters. Practitioners with advanced skills and knowledge can develop leadership roles in and outside of occupational therapy realms. Assuming positions of leadership and influence in policy-making, clinical services, and education is vital to the sustainability of occupational therapy practice in mental health.

The President's New Freedom Commission on Mental Health (2003) identified recovery as the guiding principle in a transformed system of mental health care. Occupational therapists are uniquely qualified to assist mental health consumers in the recovery process and to influence general mental health practice to adopt the Recovery Model. However, occupational therapists are little recognized as having these skills and knowledge. The content of this SPCC will assist in bridging that gap by providing a broad range of information on topics determined to be essential to advanced mental health practice in occupational therapy as identified by the competencies for occupational therapists to become AOTA Board Certified in Mental Health. It will also provide an opportunity to develop skills to increase recognition of occupational therapy as a vital service and contributor to a transformed system of mental health care.

The AOTA Board Certification in Mental Health put in place by the AOTA Commission on Continuing Competence and Professional Development provides a process whereby occupational therapists who are members of AOTA may voluntarily apply to be board certified as an advanced practitioner in mental health. The competencies and indicators of the advanced practitioner Board Certification in Mental Health were used to frame the topics in this publication, so it may be used by occupational therapists who are pursuing that certification as an integral part of their professional development.[2] But it is also relevant to practitioners (both therapists and therapy assistants) who are not necessarily interested in advanced certification

---

[2]AOTA Advanced Practitioner Certification in Mental Health (Board Certification) is available only to occupational therapists.

but who wish to maintain their competency and keep current in the field of mental health occupational therapy practice, education, and leadership.

Overview of Chapters

This text has five sections containing 21 chapters. "Section 1. Occupation and Mental Health" describes the relationship between occupational engagement and mental health. Each chapter includes generous use of real-life examples, case examples, and clinical stories from across the lifespan and from a variety of settings to exemplify the concepts and knowledge presented and assist in integrating them as the skills and knowledge of an advanced practitioner. Chapter 1, "Foundation for Advanced Occupational Therapy Practice in Mental Health," provides background information, including definitions of *mental health* and *mental illness* and discussion of the disabling impact of mental illness in the United States and worldwide. It presents the transformation and reform of the U.S. mental health system by presenting an overview of the 2003 report of the President's New Freedom Commission on Mental Health and the development and contents of the *National Consensus Statement on Recovery* (Substance Abuse and Mental Health Services Administration [SAMHSA], 2005). AOTA's efforts to advance mental health practice and the implications of AOTA's (2007) 2017 *Centennial Vision* for mental health conclude the chapter.

Chapter 2, "Defining Occupational Therapy in Mental Health: Vision and Identity," defines the generative influence of occupation on optimizing a person's mental health status and how having a vision and mental health role identity based on an understanding of this influence is vital to advanced practice occupational therapists. This chapter also describes innovative roles for advanced practice occupational therapists, including private practice therapists, and how to brand and market mental health occupational therapy to providers, payers, and the public.

Chapter 3, "Occupation-Focused Community Health and Wellness Programs," is a description of occupation-focused community health programs and models. It includes a discussion of prevention and wellness services and how to promote quality of life and minimize risk from adverse psychosocial circumstances. Consumers and providers of mental health care have considerable concerns about the need to integrate primary care and mental health care, and this chapter considers this issue and provides examples of how this integration can occur and occupational therapy's vital role in this process.

In addition to having a vision and the ability to market oneself in an integrated mental health care arena, one must use evidence-based practice. Chapter 4, "Evidence-Based Practice: Conducting and Understanding Evidence-Based Reviews," provides an understanding of evidence-based practice, defining what it is and how to use evidence-based resources, formulate a focused clinical question, and research the evidence to find direction and support for practice. This chapter also provides an overview of the evidence-based resources available to guide practice and to research focused questions.

"Section 2. Occupational Engagement and Psychiatric Conditions" contains a description of the effect of psychiatric conditions on occupational engagement. The chapters in this section describe the biopsychosocial nature of psychiatric conditions and their impact on functional capacity across children and adolescents, adults, and older adults. Multiple contexts are considered in which functional patterns of occupation occur. Many occupational therapists primarily have knowledge of and experience with adults in hospital settings (inpatient and outpatient). This section presents not only evidence-based information and new perspectives on interventions for adults but also includes information on evaluation and intervention throughout the lifespan with examples and cases to assist readers in integrating current understanding of the functional impact of psychiatric conditions on children, youth, adults, and older adults, evaluating those conditions and providing evidence-based interventions.

Chapter 5, "Occupational Engagement of Children and Youth With Mental Illness"; Chapter 6, "Occupational Engagement of Adults With Mental Illness"; and Chapter 7, "Occupational Engagement of Older Adults With Mental Illness," present evidence, trends, and theories regarding people with psychiatric conditions in each age span and related biomedical and psychosocial interventions. These chapters include how conditions and disorders affect current and potential occupational performance, participation, and quality of life and how contextual influences affect these factors. These chapters also consider the concerns of families and significant others.

Chapter 8, "Evaluation in Mental Health Occupational Therapy Advanced Practice," focuses specifically on evaluation of occupational engagement in various settings, with consideration of constraints posed by length of stay, payment, and so forth. This chapter discusses how to interpret and integrate information gained through evaluation and how to translate findings to consumers, their families, and relevant others (e.g., teachers, employers, residential providers, job coaches, payers).

Chapters 9–11, "Occupational Therapy Intervention for Children and Youth With Mental Illness," "Occupational Therapy Intervention for Adults With Mental Illness," and "Occupational Therapy Intervention for Older Adults With Mental Illness," contain information on how to facilitate environmental and other contextual modifications, how to use naturally occurring or therapeutic groups, and how to monitor effectiveness of services delivered—all to promote consumers' recovery and resilience. Being mindful that many occupational therapists may have limited familiarity with assessments and evaluations for children and youth, Chapter 9 includes a selected listing of those tools and information about their use. Chapter 10 details strategies for evaluation of adults and for forming a partnership with the consumer of services, and Chapter 11 addresses evaluation and intervention strategies for older adults with mental illnesses.

Chapter 12, "Occupational Therapy in High-Risk and Special Situations," describes special situations for evaluation and intervention—specifically, how to provide interventions in difficult situations, such as crisis interventions and consumers with dually diagnosed conditions. This chapter discusses sensory aspects of mental illnesses and how to use sensory modalities to intervene in difficult situations. Chapter 13, "Therapeutic Relationships in Difficult Contexts: Involuntary Commitment, Forensic Settings, and Violence," elaborates further on interventions in difficult situations, considering forensic contexts in which consumers are adjudicated or their mental status is being evaluated pertinent to judicial processes. This chapter focuses on the therapeutic use of self and therapeutic relationships in these types of situations and others in which the consumer is not necessarily receiving intervention by choice. The importance of providing culturally competent services in these situations to gain trust is considered. Chapter 14, "Trauma, Mental Health Care, and Occupational Therapy Practice," focuses on trauma-informed care, another important and emergent area in mental health services. Trauma can be the result of interpersonal violence, crime, disaster, or emotional or physical abuse. This chapter discusses the need to consider the impact of trauma and how to provide trauma-informed services that do not retraumatize the person (e.g., the effect of restraint or seclusion as a treatment modality). Chapters 12, 13, and 14, which discuss difficult situations that are not uncommon occurrences in mental health treatment, use numerous case examples and clinical stories exemplifying the role of occupational therapy. Occupational therapy modalities—including physical, mental, and sensory evaluations and interventions—for these situations and the role of clinical supervision are considered.

The third section of the course, "Consumer-Centered Practice," directly addresses consumer-centered practice and consumer-directed intervention. The chapters in this section consider the engagement of the person diagnosed with a psychiatric condition or illness as a full collaborator and partner in the evaluation and intervention processes. Chapter 15, "Lived Experience: Recovery and Wellness Concepts for Systems Transformation," discusses the role of consumers as providers in consumer-directed programs and self-help groups and the role of occupational therapists in relation to those programs. The chapter discusses how occupational therapists can partner with consumers in promoting self-determination and other avenues of intervention and includes a brief history of the consumer movement and theory and techniques regarding the Recovery Model and process in mental health practice.

Chapter 16, "Client-Centered Principles and Systems," discusses client-centered and relationship-centered models and systems that promote consumer-centered intervention. How to enact consumer-centered principles, including dignity, respect, and unconditional positive regard, to develop therapeutic relationships and promote recovery is described. The chapter also considers advocacy for consumer-centered intervention and establishing systematic changes that promote client-centered processes.

"Section 4. Mental Health Systems and Team Participation" examines mental health systems and the role of occupational therapists as members of the intervention team, as care managers, and as advocates and contributors to mental health policy-making. This section focuses on understanding the complexities of the mental health system and how to have an impact on the system to change it, thereby facilitating coordinated, high-quality services to consumers of mental health services. Chapter 17, "Mental Health Policy and Regulation," provides an overview of federal, state, and local bodies and agencies and how they regulate, direct, and pay for mental health services; gives an overview of the social security system as it is relevant to mental health consumers; and discusses the role of occupational therapists in this process.

Chapter 18, "Collaborative Work With Teams and Policymakers," discusses how to communicate effectively regarding occupational therapy's unique contribution and describes the role occupational therapists can play with key stakeholders in the formulation and transformation of public health policies relevant to mental health. The chapter discusses in particular the issue of occupational therapists being considered as qualified mental health practitioners in state and federal laws and regulations.

Chapter 19, "Community Resources and Care Management," is a discussion of models of care management and the suitability of occupational therapists for these roles. Community resources for care managers are discussed, including how to identify and connect with community resources such as housing, welfare, food stamps, and other entitlements. Chapter 19 also includes a discussion of disability determination for consumers with psychiatric illnesses and an overview of vocational rehabilitation services.

"Section 5. Advocacy" discusses roles for advanced practitioners as leaders and advocates in mental health systems. Chapter 20, "Advocacy for Occupational Therapy and Mental Health Issues," provides information and examples concerning how to advance mental health consumers' access through advocacy for policies and programs that promote engagement in occupations that support participation in multiple contexts. Sociopolitical processes and stakeholders who influence mental health systems are presented, along with consideration of issues such as that many consumers live in significantly impoverished circumstances because of their condition or illness. The effect of deinstitutionalization is explored, as is the ongoing effect of stigma on consumers' health, well-being, and citizenship. In addition to considering these issues, Chapter 20 describes ethical decision-making processes when best intervention options are not available and how social and political advocacy can be used to influence such choices.

Chapter 21, "Leadership in Occupational Therapy and Mental Health," considers leadership skills and assuming the role of a leader in different mental health and health care arenas. This chapter includes a description of organization development, systems analysis, risk management, and change management. The chapter also presents a description of how to conduct program evaluation and continuous quality improvement and how to develop a fieldwork training program for occupational therapy students and other health care practitioners, such as nursing and medical students. The chapter details how to measure outcomes and how to use those data to improve services and outcomes such as consumer satisfaction. Chapter 21 also considers ethical issues relevant to advanced practitioners who are leaders, such as research practices and development of promising innovative, but largely untested, programs.

Use of Term *Occupational Therapist*

Throughout this volume, the term *occupational therapist* is used to indicate both occupational therapists and occupational therapy assistants. This choice does not exclude the occupational therapy assistant's important role in meeting the needs of clients with mental health issues to support their engagement in occupations and their participation in context. The occupational therapist is responsible for all aspects of occupational therapy service delivery and is accountable for the safety and effectiveness of the occupational therapy delivery process. The occupational therapy assistant delivers occupational therapy services under the supervision of and in partnership with the occupational therapist in accordance with the following documents:

- State regulations
- *Standards of Practice for Occupational Therapy* (AOTA, 2005c)

- *Occupational Therapy Code of Ethics (2005)* (AOTA, 2005a)
- *Guidelines for Supervision, Roles, and Responsibilities During the Delivery of Occupational Therapy Services* (AOTA, 2004a)
- *Standards for Continuing Competence* (AOTA, 2005b)
- *Scope of Practice* (AOTA, 2004b).[3]

Summary

The purpose of this SPCC and textbook is to provide current and relevant information on issues and concerns of occupational practice relevant to mental health. This introduction identifies the background and rationale for the development of this text and gives an overview of its contents. Readers are now invited to read and reflect on the material as it applies to their current practice and future pursuits. The field of occupational therapy has a significant potential to contribute to the growing understanding and promotion of resilience and recovery for people with mental illness—to "a life in the community for everyone" (SAMHSA, 2009). It is hoped that occupational therapists who use this text will be leaders in facilitating that goal.

References

American Occupational Therapy Association. (2004a). Guidelines for supervision, roles, and responsibilities during the delivery of occupational therapy services. *American Journal of Occupational Therapy, 58*, 663–667.

American Occupational Therapy Association. (2004b). Scope of practice. *American Journal of Occupational Therapy, 58*, 673–677.

American Occupational Therapy Association. (2005a). Occupational therapy code of ethics (2005). *American Journal of Occupational Therapy, 59*, 639–642.

American Occupational Therapy Association. (2005b). Standards for continuing competence. *American Journal of Occupational Therapy, 59*, 661–662.

American Occupational Therapy Association. (2005c). Standards of practice for occupational therapy. *American Journal of Occupational Therapy, 59*, 663–665.

American Occupational Therapy Association. (2007). AOTA's *Centennial Vision* and executive summary. *American Journal of Occupational Therapy, 61*, 613–614.

President's New Freedom Commission on Mental Health. (2003). *Achieving the promise: Transforming mental health care in America* (Final Report; DHHS Pub. No. SMA–03–3832). Rockville, MD: Author.

Substance Abuse and Mental Health Services Administration. (2005). *National consensus statement on mental health recovery*. Rockville, MD: National Mental Health Information Center. Retrieved January 4, 2009, from http://mentalhealth.samhsa.gov/publications/allpubs/SMA05-4129/

Substance Abuse and Mental Health Services Administration. (2009). *Home page*. Retrieved September 21, 2009, from www.samhsa.gov

---

[3]The only exception is discussions concerning the efforts of AOTA and others to attain Qualified Mental Health Practitioner (QMHP) status in federal and state regulations. This designation would only apply to occupational therapists, not occupational therapy assistants, because of the knowledge and experience requirements in these regulations.

Occupation and Mental Health

CHAPTER 1

Foundation for Advanced Occupational Therapy Practice in Mental Health

Marian Kavanaugh Scheinholtz, MS, OT/L

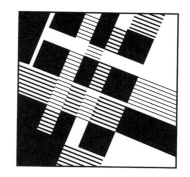

Learning Objectives

After reading this material and completing the examination, readers will be able to

- Identify *mental health* and *mental illness* as they are currently understood,
- Identify the type and extent of disability resulting from mental illness worldwide,
- Recognize the impact of the President's New Freedom Commission on Mental Health (2003) on mental health system transformation in the United States,
- Differentiate the recovery paradigm and its components from traditional mental health service and treatment models, and
- Identify historical aspects of occupational therapy mental health practice and the recent activities of the American Occupational Therapy Association (AOTA) regarding mental health practice and the relation of these efforts to the AOTA *Centennial Vision* (AOTA, 2007b) for occupational therapy.

This chapter provides the framework for this book by describing overarching issues relevant to the prevention and treatment of mental illness. It lays the foundation for advanced occupational therapy practice in mental health as it affects the lives of people diagnosed with mental illness in their journey of recovery.

The treatment of mental illness has advanced considerably in the past 50 years, but significant concerns continue to exist regarding the current diagnosis and treatment of mental illness (Frank & Glied, 2006). Advances include the introduction of medications that have enabled people diagnosed with mental illness to live outside of hospitals and to be spared from ineffective treatments such as frontal lobotomies. Over the years, genetic and biological influences have been recognized as significant determinants of susceptibility to mental illness, and advances have been made in addressing the biological underpinnings of mental illness. Also acknowledged, however, is that the system designed to treat mental illness may in fact be responsible for the continued impairment and disability of the people who live with mental illnesses (Frank & Glied, 2008; President's New Freedom Commission on Mental Health, 2003). Public campaigns to end discrimination against mental illness in insurance, employment, and attitudes of the general public have been mounted; however, noteworthy differences continue to exist in research, treatment, and public acceptance of people diagnosed with these illnesses compared with people living with other physical illnesses and disorders.

Occupational therapists have been effective advocates for people with physical disabilities, enabling children and adults to live, learn, and be full participants in their communities. In turn, occupational therapists, with their knowledge of how to increase and promote occupational performance and function, can be leaders in the transformation of the U.S. mental health system. They can advocate for the growing movement of consumers as providers and the fact that a person with a mental illness can exercise full citizenship in living, working, and learning communities.

Definitions of *Mental Health* and *Mental Illness*

Mental health is reflected in how people think, feel, and act in their daily lives and has been characterized as the way in which people cope with the stress of everyday life. Mental health influences the ways in which people view themselves and their lives and the way in which they interact with others in their lives. It affects people's choices and their reactions to others' choices. Having good mental and physical health is important at every stage of life, from childhood and adolescence through adulthood and older years. Good mental health is possible even in the face of physical illness or disorder or adversity.

In 1999, the U.S. Surgeon General issued the first national report on mental health in the United States (U.S. Department of Health and Human Services [DHHS], 1999). This report defined *mental health* as "a state of successful performance of mental function, resulting in productive activities, fulfilling relationships with other people, and the ability to adapt to change and to cope with adversity" (DHHS, 1999, p. 4). The report defined *mental illness* as "collectively . . . all diagnosable disorders of the brain—health conditions that are characterized by alterations in thinking, mood, or behavior (or some combination thereof) associated with distress and/or impaired functioning" (DHHS, 1999, p. 5). It is noteworthy that the definition of *mental health* emphasizes productivity and adaptability, two of the inherent goals of occupational therapy intervention, and conversely, that the definition of *mental illness* notes impaired functioning, which is the reason for many referrals for occupational therapy.

The World Health Organization (WHO; 2008) defines *mental health* as not just the absence of mental disorder but as "a state of well-being in which every individual realizes his or her own potential, can cope with the normal stresses of life, can work productively and fruitfully, and is able to make a contribution to her or his community" (para. 1). This definition also stresses the relationship of mental health to functional ability and occupational performance.

Mental Illness and Disability

Mental illness affects the person's functioning and thinking processes, greatly diminishing his or her social role and productivity in the community. In addition, because mental illnesses are disabling and last for many years, they take a tremendous toll on the emotional and socioeconomic capabilities of relatives who care for the person, especially when the health system is unable to offer treatment and support at an early stage. In fact, the cost of mental illness must be calculated not only in terms of the cost of treatment but also in the loss of productivity and contribution to family and community life of people disabled by mental illness. The National Council on Disability (NCD; 2008) estimated in 2006 that 24.6 million adults in the United States live with a psychiatric disability, based on the experience of serious psychological distress in people 18 and older—a condition that is highly correlated with serious mental illness. Although the Substance Abuse and Mental Health Services Administration (SAMHSA; 2007) estimated a slight decrease in this number in 2007 (24.3 million adults), it noted that only about two-fifths (44.6%) received mental health services.

Disability resulting from mental illness is not limited to the United States; the *World Health Report on Mental Health* (WHO, 2008) identified the top three leading causes of disability worldwide as behavioral disorders. They are, in order, mental illness, substance abuse, and Alzheimer's disease and dementia (WHO, 2008). Mental disorders are common throughout the world and cost a great deal in economics and human suffering. It is estimated that 877,000 people die worldwide from suicide each year (more than 300,000 in the United States) and that 1 in 4 people who visit a health service have at least one mental, behavioral, or neurological disorder, yet many such disorders are unrecognized and untreated (WHO, 2008). The global disease burden resulting from mental disorders is estimated at 14% (Lancet Global Mental Health Group, 2007), with mental and neuropsychiatric disorders being the leading noncommunicable disease in terms of world morbidity.

Although the worldwide data represent many countries of low- and moderate-income status, these statistics and problems are similar in the United States. The United States has significant problems getting people to seek treatment; for those who do, financial barriers and workforce shortages affect access to services. One of every 2 Americans who needs mental health treatment does not receive it, and for ethnic and racial minorities, the rate is lower and the quality of care is poorer. Of people who commit suicide in the United States, 90% are estimated to have mental disorders (Power, 2007b).

Connection Between Mental and Physical Illness

A research study published by the National Association of State Mental Health Program Directors revealed that people diagnosed with serious mental illness die 25 years earlier than their counterparts (Parks, Svendsen, Singer, & Foti, 2006). The increase in mortality is largely the result of controllable factors such as untreated medical conditions and modifiable risk factors, such as smoking and obesity (Prince et al., 2007). Some have postulated that some of these factors may even be the result of current treatment of mental illness; for example, a side effect of olanzapine, a nontraditional antipsychotic medication used to treat schizophrenia and bipolar disorder, is that it can cause significant weight gain and the resulting problems of obesity (Parks, Radke, & Ruter, 2008). The burden of mental illness is probably underestimated because of a lack of appreciation of the connection between mental illness and other health conditions. Moreover, many health conditions increase the risk of mental illness, and this comorbidity affects help seeking, diagnosis, and treatment. For example, older adults with diabetes, cardiac conditions, arthritis, or other chronic conditions are at higher risk for developing depression, especially when they are isolated or living in substandard conditions.

Effect of Stigma

The NCD (2006) identified six elements for livable inclusive communities for people with disabilities. They are (1) affordable, appropriate, and accessible housing; (2) accessible, affordable, reliable, safe transportation; (3) a physical environment adjusted for inclusiveness and accessibility; (4) work, volunteer, and education opportunities; (5) access to key health and support services; and (6) opportunities for participation in civic, cultural, social, and recreational activities. However, the main barrier faced by people with psychiatric disabilities is that even when physical environmental barriers are eliminated, attitudinal barriers often prevent their full inclusion in the community—the issue is discrimination because of the stigma of mental illness and ingrained negative attitudes and beliefs about people diagnosed with a mental illness (NCD, 2008). In fact, some have suggested that the word *stigma* is itself a source of discrimination and prejudice against people with mental illness. The issue of discrimination and disregard seems to be part of the barrier that affects people's acknowledging that they have symptoms of a mental illness and seeking treatment. This prejudice exists in the belief of many Americans that people with mental illness cannot work or contribute in any way to their community.

Mental Health Reform

In April 2002, U.S. President George W. Bush established the President's New Freedom Commission on Mental Health to address the pressing issues related to disability caused by mental illness. The commission was established to address three obstacles preventing Americans from getting the mental health care they needed: (1) the stigma of mental illness, (2) disparities in mental health benefits in health insurance, and (3) a broken mental health system (referring to fragmentation and lack of coordination of mental health services and benefits in government and nongovernmental systems). Although some controversy regarding the commission existed (related to consideration of universal mental health screening of children and implementation of the Texas Medication Algorithm Project), the final report (President's New Freedom Commission on Mental Health, 2003) generated six recommendations for sweeping change in the mental health system that were positively regarded by consumers, advocates, and mental health providers.

The vision statement of the commission's report stated,

> We envision a future when everyone with a mental illness will recover, a future when mental illnesses can be prevented or cured, a future when mental illnesses are detected early, and a future when everyone with a mental illness

at any stage of life has access to effective treatment and supports—essentials for living, working, learning, and participating fully in the community. (President's New Freedom Commission on Mental Health, 2003, p. 1)

This statement embodies the commission's recommendation that the U.S. mental health system be transformed to one based on the concept of recovery and driven by the wants and needs of consumers, families, and youth (President's New Freedom Commission on Mental Health, 2003). The six specific goals identified by the President's New Freedom Commission on Mental Health (2003) are

1. Americans understand that mental health is essential to overall health.
2. Mental health care is consumer and family driven.
3. Disparities in mental health services are eliminated.
4. Early mental health screening, assessment, and referral to services are common practice.
5. Excellent mental health care is delivered and research is accelerated.
6. Technology is used to access mental health care and information. (p. 5)

Federal and state government agencies have responded to the New Freedom Commission's report by developing plans and initiating activities to address these six goals and transform their state's system of mental health care. One agency that has taken a leading role in the implementation of the New Freedom Commission report is SAMHSA.

Substance Abuse and Mental Health Services Administration

SAMHSA is a federal agency in the DHHS. It was created in 1992 and is shepherding federal efforts to respond to the President's New Freedom Commission on Mental Health (2003). With its vision of a "life in the community for everyone" (SAMHSA, 2009), the agency informs, directs, and contributes to national mental health and substance abuse policy; makes grants to develop service capacity; develops, sponsors, and disseminates evidence-based practices; and facilitates collection of data on prevalence of mental illness and service use by people with mental illness. SAMHSA has three centers and supporting offices to carry out its mission: the Center for Mental Health Services, the Center for Substance Abuse Prevention, and the Center for Substance Abuse Treatment. In 2007, SAMHSA had a budget of approximately $3.3 billion, which it used in part to administer block grants to the states, discretionary grants, and contracts. These funds support efforts of the states and local communities to engage in prevention, early intervention, and a range of substance abuse treatment and mental health and recovery support services.

One of SAMHSA's priorities has been the transformation of the mental health system. In the words of Kathryn Power (2007a), director of the Center for Mental Health Services, "CMHS is leading the Federal Government in a collaborative effort to transform our national mental health system into one that holds the promise of hope for recovery for the millions of Americans we serve" (slide 16). *Transformation* is envisioned as the broad-based approach SAMHSA has adopted to introduce fundamental change in the way in which mental health services are perceived, accessed, delivered, and financed:

In a transformed system of care:

- Recovery is the guiding principle.
- Consumers—working in partnership with their care providers—direct their own care.
- Prevention is as important as treatment.
- Everyone shares equally in the hope of recovery from mental illnesses, regardless of race, gender, ethnicity, or geographic location.
- The use of evidence-based, state-of-the-art treatments and supports is standard practice.
- Services and supports are readily available and accessible and coordinated across multiple systems. (Power, 2007b, p. 2)

Recovery is a critical concept to transformation because it represents a journey of hope to consumers and has a variety of other implications. Recovery is the process that enables people to participate fully in their daily occupations as citizens of their communities despite being diagnosed with or having a history of mental illness. It can also mean a reduction or complete remission of symptoms of mental illness. Recovery is also regarded as the process of striving for these goals.

This course has recovery and mental health system reform as its basis. Occupational therapy has a clear role in a system that focuses on recovery because the basic tenets of occupational therapy are consistent with the components of recovery. With its emphasis on full community participation for all people through direct enhancement of functional performance, occupational therapy could be a driving force in the transformation of mental health services.

Definition and Components of Recovery

The National Consensus Statement on Recovery (SAMHSA, 2005) was developed by 110 expert panelists, including mental health consumers, family members, providers, advocates, researchers, academicians, managed care representatives, accreditation organization representatives, and state and local public officials. On the basis of their findings, the following consensus statement was derived:

Mental health recovery is a journey of healing and transformation enabling a person with a mental health problem to live a meaningful life in a community of his or her choice while striving to achieve his or her full potential. (SAMHSA, 2005, para. 3)

The National Consensus group identified 10 fundamental components of recovery, each of which is important to the recovery of a person with mental illness:

1. *Self-direction* refers to consumers being the drivers of their own recovery process by defining their life goals and how to achieve them. It emphasizes autonomy, independence, and control over resources as underlying components of a self-directed life.
2. Recovery is *individualized and person centered* because it is based on the person's strengths and resilience, needs, preferences, and experiences. Recovery is an end process, but it also is a journey to achieve wellness and optimal health.

3. *Empowerment* refers to consumers having choices over various options and the opportunity to participate in all decisions that affect their lives. Moreover, they are educated and supported to do this and have the opportunity to participate collectively with other consumers to speak about their wants and aspirations. Empowerment enables consumers to express the control they have over everyday decisions and their life path.

4. Recovery is *holistic* because it encompasses the person's mind, body, and spirit and views him or her in relation to peers, family, and community. It is concerned with housing, employment, education, mental and physical health care, spirituality, and creativity.

5. The *nonlinear* aspect of recovery is the understanding that recovery is not unidirectional; rather, it is a process of growth, setbacks, and learning from these experiences. Recovery begins with the awareness that positive change can occur, and this awareness is the first step in engaging in the recovery process.

6. Recovery is *strengths based* in that it focuses on the person's inherent worth. The person is viewed as having strengths, capacities, and talents that can be built on as he or she engages in productive life roles and leaves behind the role of patient with its implication of incompetence and need for care giving.

7. *Peer support* is invaluable in recovery because the person shares his or her experiences to encourage and engage other consumers in the recovery process. It provides a sense of belonging, a valuable role, and a community of mutual support.

8. *Respect* from other members of the community is vital to recovery. This aspect directly addresses the elimination of the stigma of mental illness and the discrimination people experience because of their history of mental illness.

9. Consumers have *responsibility* for their own journey of recovery and for taking care of themselves throughout the journey. This level of responsibility can require courage and fortitude as challenges arise and growth ensues.

10. *Hope* is an essential component of recovery because it motivates the person toward the future and the promise of a better life. The knowledge that people can and do overcome barriers underpins the ability to surmount everyday challenges and overcome periodic setbacks. Hope is "the catalyst of the recovery process" (SAMHSA, 2005, para. 14).

Promoting Mental Health Recovery

Onken, Dumont, Ridgway, Dornan, and Ralph (2002) reported on a research project that used a diverse cross-section of consumer–survivors to identify what hinders and what helps mental health recovery. Their definition of *recovery* envisions a dynamic interaction between the person (self–whole person, hope–sense of meaning and purpose) and the environment (basic material resources, social relationships, meaningful activities, peer support, formal mental health service staff) as well as the characteristics of the exchange between the person and the environment. This definition closely parallels occupational therapy's understanding of people and their environment as they engage in occupation.

Having basic material resources moves people toward recovery, that is, a livable income, a safe and decent place to live, affordable and accessible health care and transportation, and a means of communication. In addition to basic resources, people need opportunities and supports to engage as citizen members of a community. Recovery involves having mutually supportive and satisfying social relationships with family, friends, coworkers, and neighbors. Conversely, recovery is impeded by isolation, poverty, controlling relationships, poor social skills, disabling health conditions, immigrant status, past trauma, and social stigma. Being connected to the community by a job or career can provide a sense of identify and mastery that is important to recovery. Involvement in advancing one's education and volunteering or participating in group advocacy efforts can also provide this sense of full citizenship and move a person toward recovery. In Onken et al.'s (2002) research study, many participants reported high rates of unemployment, underemployment, and exploitation. Moreover, they reported that few educational and training opportunities, loss of entitlements and benefits and other employment disincentives, and prejudice and discrimination also hampered participants' efforts to lead a productive and meaningful life (Onken et al., 2002).

Occupational Therapy and Mental Health

Occupational therapy has its roots in the treatment of mental illness, but concerns about practice and education in this area have existed for many years. The profession of occupational therapy began in the United States as part of the 20th century's mental hygiene movement. Moral treatment philosophy was used to address institutionalization and urbanization by developing a humanistic and holistic approach to health care using a biopsychosocial model. In the 1930s and 1940s, occupational therapists became aides to psychiatrists in the treatment of people with mental illness in hospitals, using music, drama, work, recreation, and crafts for diversion and relaxation and for symptom reduction secondary to medical treatments. In the 1950s and 1960s, psychoanalytic theory advanced occupational therapy as a psychodynamic modality that emphasized the dynamic relationship between the therapist and the patient and the use of self as a therapeutic tool. In the 1960s and 1970s, widespread use of tranquilizers, the passage of the Community Mental Health Centers Act, and the enactment of Medicare and Medicaid legislation led to deinstitutionalization of state hospitals and the rise of community care in hospitals and community agencies. At this time, occupational therapists were working in private and state psychiatric hospitals, community and university hospitals, community mental health centers, partial hospitalization programs, and day treatment programs (Scheinholtz, 2003).

The psychosocial rehabilitation movement grew during the 1980s and beyond with the support of federal groups such as the Community Support Program of the Alcohol, Drug, and Mental Health Administration (McDonel Herr, English, & Brown, 2003), which eventually became a part of SAMHSA's Center for Mental Health Services. The Fountainhouse Model (McDonel Herr et al., 2003) advanced consumer empowerment and principles such as the importance of belonging (membership), social networking (drop-in centers), and productive activity (clubhouse work units and transitional employment programs).

Some occupational therapists began working in these types of programs, which put the consumer at the center of the intervention model and focused on making mental health services consumer and family driven. However, many therapists continued to work in hospital settings because of salary differentials, lack of acceptance of occupational therapy as a mental health profession, and lack of role induction by occupational therapy educational programs for mental health practice outside hospitals. As managed care became a reality in health care in the late 20th century, many psychiatric hospitals closed or were significantly downsized, which, along with other factors, led to a diminished number of occupational therapists working in mental health over the past 40 years.

A strong belief in occupational therapy's efficacy and skill in aiding the recovery of people with mental illness has persisted, as has the inherent value of understanding and treating the mental health or psychosocial aspects of the person. The American Occupational Therapy Association (AOTA) has engaged in various activities in recent years to understand the trends in mental health practice and promote occupational therapists as providers of mental health care. On the basis of the work of leaders in the field of occupational therapy mental health practice, the AOTA Mental Health Partnership Project was initiated in 1998. The project (Scheinholtz, 1998) focused on promoting high-quality service to consumers with mental illness and their families but also incubated occupational therapists who would become leaders in the profession in the area of education, practice, and governance of the association.

In the intervening years, AOTA has invested in developing guidelines for evidence-based practice in mental health, initially addressing evidence-based practices for substance misuse (Stoffel & Moyers, 2004) and mental health disorders of children and youth. AOTA also has pursued an emphasis on the mental health problems of and interventions for children and youth, resulting in increased attention to and interest in this area among many pediatric occupational therapists. Most recently, the AOTA Board of Directors successively appointed two ad hoc groups to identify issues, opportunities, and barriers to occupational therapy practice in mental health (Brown et al., 2006; Pitts et al., 2005).

The AOTA Representative Assembly and the AOTA Board considered these reports and the concerns of AOTA members about the importance of mental health practice in occupational therapy. The Representative Assembly recommended that AOTA initiate short- and long-term activities to address the areas of concern, initially targeting the regulatory and legislative barriers to the identification of occupational therapists as qualified mental health practitioners in state and federal law (AOTA, 2007a). In 2007, AOTA established a long-term plan to advance occupational therapy in mental health practice. This work will support AOTA's work as it pursues its *Centennial Vision* of occupational therapy as "a powerful, widely recognized, science-driven, and evidence-based profession with a globally connected and diverse workforce meeting society's occupational needs" (AOTA, 2007b, p. 613). Addressing the promotion of good mental health and the alleviation of disability resulting from mental illness has been identified as an integral part of the *Centennial Vision*. Along with five other broad areas of practice, AOTA has identified mental health as vitally important to achieving the 2017 *Centennial Vision* and to education, practice, and research in occupational therapy in the 21st century (AOTA, 2009).

The choice to make mental health one of the priority areas for strategic planning coincides with an exciting era for mental health in the United States. This era was launched by the passage in 2008 of the Paul Wellstone and Pete Domenici Mental Health Parity and Addiction Equity Act, the considerable emphasis by federal and state agencies on transforming the mental health system, the recognition of the significant mental health needs of veterans returning from foreign conflict, and the direction that mental health be viewed as a public health issue. It is indeed appropriate for occupational therapy to educate its practitioners and the public in occupation's powerful role in enhancing the participation of all citizens, including people who have been diagnosed with or treated for a mental illness or disorder.

References

American Occupational Therapy Association. (2007a). *Advancing occupational therapy in mental health practice: Long-term plan.* Unpublished document.

American Occupational Therapy Association. (2007b). AOTA's *Centennial Vision* and executive summary. *American Journal of Occupational Therapy, 61,* 613–614.

American Occupational Therapy Association. (2009). *Practice areas: Occupational therapy practice areas for the 21st century.* Retrieved January 13, 2009, from www.aota.org/practitioners/practiceareas.aspx

Brown, C., Moyers, P., Haertlein Sells, C., Learnard, L., Mahaffey, L.M., Pitts, D.B., et al. (2006). *Report of the Ad Hoc Committee on Mental Health Practice in Occupational Therapy.* Unpublished report to the AOTA Board of Directors.

Community Mental Health Centers Act, Pub. L. 88–164, 42 U.S.C. 2689 *et seq.*

Frank, R. G., & Glied, S. A. (2006). *Better but not well: Mental health policy in the United States since 1950.* Baltimore: Johns Hopkins University Press.

Lancet Global Mental Health Group. (2007). Scale up services for mental disorders: A call for action. *Lancet, 370,* 1241–1252.

McDonel Herr, E. C., English, M. J., & Brown, N. B. (2003). Translating mental health services research into practice: A perspective from staff at the US Substance Abuse and Mental Health Services Administration. *Alzheimer's Care Quarterly, 4,* 241–253.

National Council on Disability. (2006). *Creating livable communities, 2006.* Retrieved January 4, 2009, from www.ncd.gov/newsroom/publications/2006/livable_communities.htm

National Council on Disability. (2008). *Inclusive livable communities for people with psychiatric disabilities.* Retrieved January 4, 2009, from www.ncd.gov/newsroom/publications/2008/LivableCommunities.html

Onken, S., Dumont, J. M., Ridgway, P., Dornan, D. H., & Ralph, R. O. (2002). *Mental health recovery: What helps and what hinders? A national research project for the development of recovery facilitating system performance indicators.* Alexandria, VA: National Technical Assistance Center for State Mental Health Planning, National Association of State Mental Health Program Directors.

Parks, J., Radke, A. Q., & Ruter, T. J. (2008). *Obesity reduction and prevention strategies for individuals with serious mental illness* (Medical Directors Council Technical Report). Alexandria, VA: National Association of State Mental Health Program Directors.

Parks, J., Svendsen, D., Singer, P., & Foti, M. E. (2006). *Morbidity and mortality in people with serious mental illness* (Medical Directors Council Technical Report). Alexandria, VA: National Association of State Mental Health Program Directors.

Paul Wellstone and Pete Domenici Mental Health Parity and Addiction Equity Act of 2008, Pub. L. 110–343.

Pitts, D. B., Lamb, A., Ramsay, D., Learnard, L., Clark, F., Scheinholtz, M., et al. (2005). *Promotion of occupational therapy in mental health systems: Report of Ad Hoc Workgroup to AOTA Board of Directors.* Unpublished report.

Power, A. K. (2007a). *Center for Mental Health Services* [Slide presentation]. Rockville, MD: Center for Mental Health Services National Advisory Council.

Power, A. K. (2007b). *Putting consumers at the center of care: Remarks.* Rockville, MD: Center for Mental Health Services National Advisory Council Subcommittee on Consumer Survivor Issues.

President's New Freedom Commission on Mental Health. (2003). *Achieving the promise: Transforming mental health care in America* (Final Report, DHHS Pub. No. SMA–03–3832). Rockville, MD: Author.

Prince, M., Patel, V., Saxena, S., Mah, M., Maselko, H., Phillips, M. R., et al. (2007). No health without mental health. *Lancet, 370,* 859–877.

Scheinholtz, M. (1998, October). *Mental Health Partnership Project.* AOTA Mental Health Special Interest Section Practice Conference Presentation, Boston.

Scheinholtz, M. K. (2003, January). *Occupational therapy in mental health: Past, present, and future.* Presented to the American Occupational Therapy Association Board of Directors, Bethesda, MD.

Stoffel, V. C., & Moyers, P. A. (2004) An evidence-based and occupational perspective of interventions for persons with substance-use disorders. *American Journal of Occupational Therapy, 58,* 570–586.

Substance Abuse and Mental Health Services Administration. (2005). *National consensus statement on mental health recovery.* Rockville, MD: National Mental Health Information Center. Retrieved January 4, 2009, from http://mentalhealth.samhsa.gov/publications/allpubs/SMA05-4129/

Substance Abuse and Mental Health Services Administration. (2007). *Results from the 2006 National Survey on Drug Use and Health: National findings* (NSDUH Series H–32, SMA 07–4293). Rockville, MD: Author.

Substance Abuse and Mental Health Services Administration. (2009). *Home page.* Retrieved September 21, 2009, from www.samhsa.gov

U.S. Department of Health and Human Services. (1999). *Mental health: A report of the Surgeon General.* Rockville, MD: U.S. Department of Health and Human Services, Substance Abuse and Mental Health Services Administration, Center for Mental Health Services & National Institute of Mental Health. Retrieved November 17, 2009, from www.surgeongeneral.gov/library/mentalhealth/home.html

World Health Organization. (2008). *WHO urges more investments, services for mental health.* Retrieved March 24, 2008, from www.who.int/mental_health/en/

CHAPTER 2

Defining Occupational Therapy in Mental Health: Vision and Identity

Susan Haiman, MPS, CPRP, OTR/L, FAOTA, and Linda T. Learnard, OTR/L

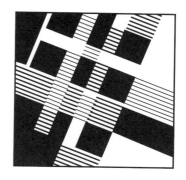

Learning Objectives

After reading this material and completing the examination, readers will be able to

- Identify the role of vision in advanced practice,
- Recognize the importance of branding and its relevance for occupational therapy practice,
- Identify the elements of branding, and
- Identify how brands are sustained as examples of excellence.

In this chapter, readers are encouraged to have or develop a vision, to define his or her product, to be an agent of change, and to focus a new lens on the mental health arena. The chapter explores the importance of establishing clarity about current roles and introduces future roles for "therapists of vision." Finally, it addresses the issue of selling occupational therapy's "products" in new ways, in new venues, and with an eye toward marketing and the methodology of branding.

Being Visionary

Being a visionary requires one to say "if" rather than "but" and not to be impeded by people who say "but." *Merriam-Webster's Collegiate Dictionary* (2001) defined *visionary* as "having or marked by foresight and imagination" (p. 1316). Having vision requires one to make a firm commitment to the pursuit of innovation while continually nurturing one's political awareness and social values and sustaining a sense of the global community. The profession of occupational therapy requires practitioners engaged in quality practice to have a vision of what they are doing and how their practice contributes to and weaves into the fabric of society in a global community.

Being a therapist of vision is about hope. It's about giving hope—to consumers who have almost given up; to service providers who feel used up; and to payers who are looking for the results of the monies expended. "Call in the Hope Lady!" the psychiatrist bellows, "the lady who comes up with new and different ways to help my patients and treatment team get *real* outcomes or results." Just meeting daily quotas and reimbursement guidelines is not enough. Having vision is about providing quality service and generating results that help set guidelines that enhance one's practice and guide the reimbursement system.

"Viewing health in the context of life performance has been a distinguishing characteristic of occupational therapy since its inception early in the twentieth century" (Christiansen & Baum, 1991, p. 4). The founders of occupational therapy created this vision and designed a model of practice to support it. To survive in the current health care environment, a clear vision of practice is even more critical.

One the profession's greatest visionaries, Mary Reilly (1962) stated, "If we wish to exist as a profession, we must identify the vital need of man which we serve and the manner in which we serve it." (p. 9). Identifying the needs of humankind can seem like an ever-moving target. A therapist of vision is not afraid to keep reaching beyond the horizon. Occupational therapists, especially those who practice in the mental health arena, must do more than survive. Without a vision to guide an advanced professional practice, one becomes just a technician, mimicking and carrying out the practices of others. Occupational therapy professionals use a wide range of knowledge and concepts, including client centeredness, clinical reasoning, evidence-based practice, theoretical perspectives, and the wisdom of the past, to develop a vision that infuses their work. From there, it is a short leap to infusing consumers with the hope of achieving the greatest engagement in occupations that supports mastery over their lives and participation in society (American Occupational Therapy Association [AOTA], 2007).

Developing a Vision

Therapists of vision must hold principles and beliefs developed through lifelong learning, mentoring, sound clinical reasoning, use of evidence or contributions to evidence-based practice, and a long and complex visioning process. AOTA (2007) has developed a *Centennial Vision* of the profession by its 100th anniversary:

> By the year 2017, we envision that occupational therapy [will be] a powerful, widely recognized, science-driven, and evidence-based profession with a globally connected and diverse workforce meeting society's occupational needs. (p. 613)

This *Centennial Vision* serves as a roadmap for the profession as a whole, but it is *not* a prescription for the individual therapist's practice. Being a visionary requires one to look to the future, asking "What if my practice knew no bounds?" "What if my only limit was beyond the horizon?" and "What if those in need of service could share this vision with me?"

Some occupational therapists ask, "How can we survive in the current care delivery system?" They should instead be asking, "How can I envision and lead the future of our care delivery?" Therapists of vision, like the mouse in *Who Moved My Cheese?* (Johnson, 1998), have their eyes on the horizon; they are not just anxious about change but also are leading it. The authors of this chapter, for example, asked themselves, "How can I mold my future to encompass the values and philosophy embedded in occupational therapy while being an agent of change throughout systems and society?" Therapists of vision have to be comfortable in their own skin and willing to articulate potentially unpopular thoughts. Above all, they must be willing to take risks. "Dream. Talk out loud. Think outside the box. Imagine what your organization's future could be without fear of laughter or ridicule" (Wilbanks, 2007, p 63). Yes, this process may be difficult or feel uncomfortable, but it is essential to continuing to provide occupational therapy services in the mental health arena.

In working with clients, therapists of vision need to look at the potential of products and services to aid their clients' recovery and their role in that recovery. Most of all, visionaries must consider the clients' environments. Without this vision, those environments cannot be shaped to support the recovery process.

Therapists of vision must see the community as the clinic without walls. Working with clients in their natural environments reveals issues in performance that may be hidden by the formality of the clinic. In the supermarket, coffee shop, or clothing store, for example, practitioners can be observers of how clients operate in "real life." *Mental Health: A Report of the Surgeon General* (U.S. Department of Health and Human Services, 1999) cited the 1990 Harvard Public Health Study (Murray & Lopez, 1996) revealing that mental illnesses encompass three of the top seven leading causes of disability in worldwide market economies. Turning the community into a clinic may help clients to feel destigmatized and promote seeking help on an individual basis, while addressing this global reality without the cost of maintaining treatment facilities.

Visionaries are the leaders who can guide our institutions, agencies, and communities to seek roles for themselves in enabling the recovery of people with mental illness. Envisioning the attitudes and values of society and the global community can enhance its citizens' occupations. The domain of occupational therapy and the mastery of activity analysis skills provide excellent tools for learning and understanding clients' needs, their environments and systems, and the global village in which we all live.

Envision occupational therapy as part of health and preventive medicine. For example, designing community systems and structures to be supportive of people's lifestyles as community citizens will help them as they age and live longer. Why not design houses and systems to prevent injuries and accidents? Why not plan for wellness in later years rather than disease and decay?

Examine the perceived needs of stakeholders in the mental health service delivery system: clients, families, payers, communities that receive services, government systems, and institutions. Then find ways to provide results that truly have meaning for the stakeholders. The skill learned must be one that will truly meet a need. Writing one's name legibly is a good skill, but knowing how to dial the phone for help may be more important.

The skills needed for visionary thinking are well within the grasp of every occupational therapist. They are available through training and from mentors and supervisors, but they can also come from numerous opportunities for creativity in practice with clients engaged in recovery from mental illness. A mission statement and vision are helpful in both academic and clinical training programs and throughout life. Such skills support the process used by many occupational therapists as they evaluate the person–environment–occupation fit, envision the best possible outcome, and design steps to reach that outcome. Mary Reilly (1962) envisioned that such a process would enable "OT to be one of the great ideas of the 20th century" (p. 9). Reilly listed the necessary skills as critical thinking, thoughtful judgment, analysis, interpretation of data, and synthesis.

Strategic Thinking at the Individual Level

Another skill that helps develop a vision is *strategic thinking*, which "strives to uncover opportunities that will create new, professional value. During this process we must consciously challenge old assumptions about the [profession's] value proposition" (Wilbanks, 2007, p. 62).

Strategic thinking at the individual level encompasses a holistic understanding of the profession, an understanding of its environment, and an understanding of its vision. A prerequisite for this thinking is creativity, in particular the ability to question prevalent concepts and perceptions (de Bono, 1999) and to recombine or make connections between issues that may seem unconnected (Robinson & Stern, 1997). This ability requires strategic thinkers to understand their own behavioral patterns and existing concepts and perceptions within the care delivery system. Strategists should enjoy the challenge of thinking "outside the box" and of using imagination and creativity to explore whether there are alternative ways of doing things (Wilbanks, 2007). For Senge (1990), having a vision is more like having a calling than having a good idea. In his view, visions are "pictures or images people carry in their heads and hearts" (p. 206). Visions represent what one truly wants, based on fundamental intrinsic values and a sense of purpose that matters deeply to the people in the profession (and to the consumers they are seeing).

Strategic thinking never stops; its task is to get buy-in and lead others who can implement and manage. One of the great managers and business visionaries of our time was Jack Welch of General Electric. Welch defined the following "rules" for vision (Tichy & Sherman, 1993, pp. 26–36):

- Rule your destiny, or someone else will.
- See reality as it is, not as it was or as you wish it were.
- Be candid with everyone.
- Manage; lead before you have to.
- You don't have a competitive advantage if you don't compete.

Hickman (1992) analyzed the relationship between the vision and its practical implementation as the two opposite ends of a spectrum. He concluded that an objective should be to blend strong visionary leadership and effective management into one integrated whole in which the strengths of both combine synergistically to the advantage of the enterprise. Advanced practice means having a vision before one offers services to clients, be they individuals, agencies, or systems.

Visions Realized

To create a vision for mental health recovery and transformation of the mental health care delivery system, a panel of experts at the National Consensus Conference on Mental Health Recovery and Mental Health Systems Transformation developed the following vision statement:

> Mental health recovery is a journey of healing and transformation enabling a person with a mental health problem to live a meaningful life in a community of his or her choice while striving to achieve his or her full potential. (Substance Abuse and Mental Health Services Administration [SAMHSA], 2005, pp. 1–2)

As occupational therapists practicing in mental health, advanced practitioners need visions that mirror those of SAMHSA and AOTA, putting words into action and bringing interventions to life in new paradigms. What follows are brief examples of how experienced and visionary occupational therapists brought vision into practice. What these visionaries share is the intent to bring services to clients and consumers where they live. They moved practice from inpatient settings and partial hospitalization programs into the real community, providing psychosocial rehabilitation in clinics without walls.

Example 1

This example involves envisioning the provision of service to the community at large rather than to one person at a time. Occupational Therapy Consultation and Rehabilitation Services, Inc., in Lincolnville, Maine, is a private practice that has been in operation for more than 25 years. This practice contracts with a variety of state departments, private for-profit and nonprofit agencies, schools, and families or individuals. Through its connections to this wide variety of entities, the practice is able to provide services in any environment in which they are needed rather than in the narrow range delineated by traditional practices linked to single institutions and rigidly defined reimbursement formulas. Defining the products and services the practice offers to this community is critical to its marketing (Learnard, 1996; Learnard & Devereaux, 1992).

Example 2

This example centers on the role an occupational therapist played in a faith-based organization providing social rehabilitation for Jewish adults living in Philadelphia's large metropolitan area and suburbs.

Tikvah was founded 17 years ago by parents to serve their adult children with mental illness, behavioral health issues, or complex brain disorders. The founders believed that their faith-based community was not offering the resources or support to enable their loved ones to fully participate in the social and spiritual contexts so important to their self-esteem and self-image. The occupational therapist envisioned a faith-based community social club that would provide a meaningful theoretical framework within which to offer environmental intervention in a variety of programs that facilitate but are not limited to spiritual participation, empowerment, social participation, work, and home maintenance. In some instances, consultation about activities of daily living and instrumental activities of daily living is included (Haiman, 1995, 2004).

Example 3

Another example of using vision to guide practice can be found in the work of Margaret Swarbrick (2007). Following her passion, Dr. Swarbrick spearheaded the development of consumer-operated services through the creation of a consumer-operated self-help center model that has evolved in New Jersey. This model is a viable alternative to overburdened traditional mental health centers and has the recovery model and a wellness focus at its core.

Example 4

Twelve years ago, the Mental Health Task Force of the Metropolitan New York District of the New York State Occupational Therapy Association began to align itself with critical stakeholders in the community, beyond institutions, to include families and consumers who were members of local chapters of the National Alliance on Mental Illness (NAMI). This alliance, nurtured over the years, resulted in fertile ground into which the seeds of an idea were planted. Task force members, including Suzanne White and Eileen LaMourie of the State University of New York Downstate Occupational Therapy Program, envisioned an innovative program that would empower mental health consumers to alter their lifestyles to incorporate new routines and community inclusion. The program worked to prepare members to participate with occupational therapists in the first springtime regional NAMIWalks awareness activity, a grassroots advocacy effort to raise awareness and funds. The program included 12 sessions of an ongoing walking program that enabled consumers to participate in the NYC–METRO Walkathon (a video on YouTube describes the experience; lamoureaux1968, 2008). Their efforts show the trajectory from the visions generated through the AOTA Mental Health Partnership Program in 1999 to realization on the ground in 2008.

These four examples differ in the type and nature of occupational therapy service delivered, the receiver of service, and the outcome. However, each example demonstrates that realizing a vision is an ongoing effort that takes time, commitment, and the capacity to be resilient in the face of challenges. A vision is effectively implemented through bold action and forceful articulation.

Branding Your Practice, Defining Your Product

Many businesses and nonprofit organizations have realized the need to establish a brand. This approach includes not only corporate or industrial markets but also branding of services such as occupational therapy (Rooney, 1995). Nontraditional branding environments are the future, as are new branding techniques. But these new strategies, techniques, and arenas for branding must be managed. In an advanced practice, the occupational therapist's organization must support and identify with a particular branding strategy. The goals, objectives, and mission of any organization should be in line with the strategy used (Rooney, 1995).

A brand is a product or service, but not every product or service is a brand. Rather, a *brand* is the established relationship between the product or service and the user. For instance, the United of Way of America undertook the process of looking at its brand. It could say with conviction that the United Way collected donations and allocated funds to agencies—but what was its actual product? The United Way's intention was to serve communities in need. However, the public is not interested in intentions; they care about what is done. Rather than just doling out money to various groups, the United Way invites groups to submit grant applications for specific projects in their communities. The most beneficial projects are given seed money to make a real difference in their communities. Thus, the United Way is valued for helping solve community problems—its brand.

Typically, occupational therapists have good intentions, but what is it that they really do? What is the service or product of advanced practice occupational therapists in the mental health system? What are the outcomes that are meaningful to others? Are skills taught or supports built that are meaningful and valuable to the person? Do occupational therapists enable people to access opportunities for skills acquisition, role acquisition, or both and to support themselves as integrated members of the community?

Brand is the occupational therapist's greatest equity. It needs to be protected, cultivated, and nurtured to strengthen, grow, and thrive over the course of time. The user needs to feel a powerful emotional bond with the product or service, a bond that determines not just how consumers feel about the product but also how the product makes them feel about themselves. For example, McDonald's Golden Arches evoke myriad experiences—hunger, emotions, visual images, tastes, convenience, fast food, and so forth (United Way of America, 2000b). This brand is so consistent that many children can recognize it before they can read.

What is the product of an occupational therapy advanced practice? What is its brand? Is it recognizable? Product image must communicate quality backed up by consistent performance. Measuring the success or failure of one's product is purely a function of its recognizable results.

Developing a new assessment tool, creating or changing a philosophy of practice, or coming up with a brand should not be done in a random fashion but rather should be based on supporting and cultivating the occupational therapy brand. All advanced occupational therapy practitioners need to ask themselves the following questions:

- Do clients feel more enabled after services are provided for, to, or with them?
- Do clients feel smarter or have a better sense of accomplishment or self-importance when they are enabled to learn skills and to seek supports?
- Do the services make clients feel more able or more disabled?
- Which is more valuable—fixing things for clients or empowering them to create their own solutions and become contributing citizens of the community?
- What is being fixed—what the occupational therapist thinks needs to be fixed or what the client views as necessary? What questions are being answered—the therapist's or the client's?

Four Measures of the Effectiveness of a Good Brand

Knowledge

Knowledge is related to consumer experience or interaction with a brand. Occupational therapists practicing in mental health hold a strong and unique knowledge base of both the art and the science of activity analysis—skill in observation, knowledge of creative problem solving, understanding of the sciences of human functioning, knowledge of building relationships and interacting with people, and experience in the skills and requirements of life's roles and occupations. Occupational therapy is one of the few professions in which therapists are trained to have a holistic view of people, to work across people's lifespan, and to perceive both the physical and the mental aspects of functioning. Knowledge must be the core of the product that is defined. Do consumers know what therapists do or know?

In Example 1, the Lincolnville group works to maintain the highest level of knowledge and information on the latest practices because part of their brand is that they are the best at delivering high-quality, cost-effective, community-based mental health services to individuals, businesses, and group homes. Much of their work is funded through contracts with Medicaid and Medicare at the state level. Thus, the group maintains a high quality of competency by budgeting well for continuing education in their business plan. They attend both workshops and conferences and purchase new books and assessment tools each year.

Esteem

What word recognition occurs when one sees the terms *occupational therapist* or *OT*? Is the term *occupational therapy* held in high regard? What is the response when one sees the business name of an occupational therapist or results of that practice? A consistently high-quality product is necessary for strong recognition to occur. Occupational therapists often hear that their product is of high quality and useful, then they are asked why the reports and services received before provide the same level of information and service. As resources shrink and other disciplines continue to encroach, occupational therapy's ability to be considered unique and generally helpful versus highly regarded in just a few practices will be narrowed significantly. In many cases, an occupational therapy intervention may not be requested until considerable loss of function occurs.

For a product to be recognized, its quality must be consistent. In a branded practice with a defined product, all staff must work at the same high level of performance and with a comprehensive approach to service delivery that is meaningful for clients receiving or paying for services, thus making the product highly recognizable as a pathway to problem solving and environmental design that enables occupational performance. Standards need to include a high level of expectation for future practice, which must be based on vision and values and supported by evidence. Practice must imagine what it will be tomorrow rather than just reflect what it is today. Outcomes and services need to be easily recognized as the product (United Way of America, 2000a, 2000b).

In the Lincolnville private practice, time is spent listening to the clients' issues, concerns, and needs; referral source; and payment source. Follow-up meetings are held to discuss how providers can use and learn from the information provided in the functional assessments. A result of this process is that at a time when agencies and service providers are experiencing difficulties, the Lincolnville private practice is the first to be called. Their services are well worth their cost to the payer.

Relevance

What is the ultimate nature of the product, its special qualities? Apple Computers (Apple, Inc., 2008) established its essence as the educator of the future, promoting a unique understanding of the future and a focus on being the first to develop new educational tools, a result of which is that for many years the Apple symbol dominated our schools. In another example, the Disney name and symbols have come to represent fantasy, magic, and fun to the people interacting with them. At its essence, Disney represents wholesome family values.

To have a strong product, core values and beliefs must illustrate one's professional values and philosophies, distilling the essentials of practice. Although the tools used may change, the values, vision, and purpose must remain constant. The product's essence needs to be conveyed through the product and its performance. It must be known and sensed by the people who acquire it. The occupational therapist's essence enables consumers to embrace and develop their own unique spirit in their everyday lives. Leadership requires having a sense of one's direction, being able to lead with conviction, and taking the risk to proceed.

Does the product solve a problem for the purchaser? For a product to be relevant, one needs to feel a personal connection, a personal sense of gain or usefulness, before value is perceived. Products that make people feel smarter, more attractive, or unique tend to sell well. Kodak promises a way to preserve memories, a very personal touch. The United Way is valued for solving community problems.

In Example 1, clients and support providers feel enabled to start the process of actually doing something. Their occupational therapists are often called on to bring some hopefulness into the case or situation. They work hard to point out what providers have done well and specifically point out the next step. Thus, when support providers and clients leave the situation, they know what to do next and feel more hopeful. The occupational therapists' work is relevant to the clients' needs.

Differentiate

Occupational therapists should ask several questions regarding their practice:

- Is the service or product unique?
- Is it the quality or the cost of the product the draw?
- Is the service particularly unique to the provider?
- What information or product is brought to the treatment team?
- Is the product a problem solver, using the knowledge of function and occupation?

Delivering the highest quality of services; specializing in assessment of functional performance; and providing recommendations for shaping the environment to enable function, specific problem solving, or both are the products in the earlier practice examples. The Lincolnville group differentiates itself by being the group that provides results in difficult situations. This consistency of high-quality practice with a focus on function and the environment helps it stand out as unique. Thus, when the warden at the state prison has ongoing problems with an inmate on the mental health unit, he has his assistant call the person who "solves these messes for him" and is willing to pay a healthy fee for the service out of his own administrative budget.

Service Provision Arenas

It is important not only to consider current practice arenas but also to imagine other possible arenas in which the product can be useful and valued and one's brand can shine. Occupational therapists practice direct service and consultation in community and private hospitals and in rehabilitation, general, and psychiatric-specialty hospitals, both state and private. Practice also occurs in partial hospital or intensive outpatient environments and in geriatric psychiatry and dementia care. Community practice environments include working on assertive community treatment teams and in community mental health centers, schools, private practices, clubhouses, psychosocial rehabilitation programs, supportive housing, and home care. Occupational therapists must establish their brand in those arenas.

Product determination and service delivery should support and enhance the brand. Are services provided directly to the client, to a group, or to care providers? Are care providers taught how to provide services or give educational information? Is service provision managed or created? Is service provision merely envisioned, or is a policy developed to carry out visionary service delivery?

Although the AOTA Mental Health Partnership Project (Scheinholtz, 1998) occurred more than 10 years ago, it is significant to the development of current occupational therapy mental health practice. As part of the project, 10 characteristics for excellence in practice were delineated. We list them here with descriptions that identify appropriate attitudes and avenues for advanced occupational therapy practitioners:

1. *Recognize opportunities and take advantage of them.* It is important to view change or challenge as an opportunity. Fighting change is not likely to gain much for one's practice, but helping with change is an opportunity to blend vision into the change.
2. *Be resourceful (know how to access resources).* Always be aware of your resources. Keep track of contacts and connections. Know what others need and value. Know others' strengths and weaknesses. Know who has which resources to offer. Nurture and develop all contacts and resources. Start the process by having lunch with different groups of people rather than with your usual group of friends.
3. *Be creative.* Avoid doing things the same way. Make an effort to do them differently. Change a little each day. There's more than one right way to do things.
4. *Be an independent thinker (stand up with conviction).* Don't be afraid to say what you think. Share your accomplishments. Have something valuable to contribute to each team meeting, even if it is to question the status quo.
5. *Be a hard worker.* Being a professional is not a 9-to-5 job. Always develop, practice, and think of improving yourself as a therapeutic agent.
6. *Be optimistic.* Have a "can-do" attitude. See the one thing you can do in each situation, no matter how bleak. Always contribute hopefulness to each situation.

7. *Be an innovator.* Think outside the box. Value being a change agent.
8. *Be a risk taker.* Don't be afraid to take a risk. Throw that idea on the table. Don't be afraid someone will criticize your idea. If they do, it doesn't necessarily mean they don't like you.
9. *Be a visionary.* See yourself as part of the health care delivery system, not just a cog in the wheel.
10. *Be a leader.* Take the initiative and lead the pack. Don't be afraid to take charge.

Only when occupational therapists develop these 10 characteristics, define their vision, establish their brand, and determine their product can they call themselves *advanced.* It is good to measure one's work against the models of practice that have been explored. As mental health parity becomes a reality in 2010, the occupational therapy brand has the opportunity to become a recognizable lower-cost, highly effective product that will sell. Rather than miss the opportunity, meet it with vision! It really is about giving hope.

References

American Occupational Therapy Association. (2007). AOTA's *Centennial Vision* and executive summary. *American Journal of Occupational Therapy, 61,* 613–614.

Apple, Inc. (2008). *Learning interchange: Apple Distinguished Schools.* Retrieved September 22, 2008, from http://edcommunity.apple.com/ali/collection.php?collection=2542

Christiansen, C., & Baum, C. (Eds.). (1991). *Occupational therapy: Overcoming human performance deficits.* Thorofare, NJ: Slack.

De Bono, E. (1999). *Six thinking hats.* Toronto, ON: Knightsbride/MICA.

Haiman, S. (1995). Occupational therapy update: Dilemmas in professional collaboration with consumers. *Psychiatric Services, 46,* 443–445.

Haiman, S. (2004, September). A parent/consumer–driven community program: Authentic occupational therapy. *Home and Community Health Special Interest Section Quarterly, 11,* 1–4.

Hickman, C. R. (1992). *Mind of a manager, soul of a leader.* New York: Wiley.

Johnson, S. (1998). *Who moved my cheese? An amazing way to deal with change in your work and in your life.* New York: Penguin.

lamoureaux1968. (2008). *OTs walk with NAMI* [Video file]. Video posted to www.youtube.com/watch?gl=GB&hl=en-GB&v=D076_98OhKw

Learnard, L. T. (1996). A community-based future. *OT Practice, 1*(7), 14–17.

Learnard, L. T., & Devereaux, E. (1992). A model for community practice. *Hospital and Community Psychiatry, 43,* 869–871.

Merriam-Webster's Collegiate Dictionary. (2001). Springfield, MA: Merriam-Webster.

Murray, C. J. L., & Lopez, A. D. (Eds.). (1996). *The global burden of disease: A comprehensive assessment of mortality and disability from diseases, injuries, and risk factors in 1990 and projected to 2020.* Cambridge, MA: Harvard School of Public Health.

Reilly, M. (1962). Occupational therapy can be one of the great ideas of 20th century medicine (Eleanor Clarke Slagle Lecture). *American Journal of Occupational Therapy, 16*(1), 1–9.

Robinson, A. G., & Stern, S. (1997). *Corporate creativity: How innovation and improvement actually happen.* San Francisco: Berrett-Koehler.

Rooney, J. A. (1995). Branding: A trend for today and tomorrow. *Journal of Product and Brand Management, 4,* 48–55.

Scheinholtz, M. (1998, November). *Mental Health Partnership Project.* Presentation at the American Occupational Therapy Association Special Interest Section Practice Conference, Boston.

Scheinholtz, M. (2007, November). *Mental health occupational therapy for today and tomorrow.* Presentation at the American Occupational Therapy Association Student Conclave, Pittsburgh.

Senge, P. M. (1990). *The fifth discipline.* Sydney, New South Wales, Australia: Random House.

Substance Abuse and Mental Health Services Administration. (2005). *National consensus statement on mental health recovery.* Rockville, MD: National Mental Health Information

Center. Retrieved November 17, 2009, from http://mentalhealth.samhsa.gov/ publications/allpubs/SMA05-4129/

Swarbrick, M. (2007). Consumer-operated self-help centers. *Psychiatric Rehabilitation Journal, 31*(1), 76–79.

Tichy, N., & Sherman, S. (1993). Walking the talk at GE. *Training & Development, 47*(6), 26–36.

United Way of America (2000a). *The BRAND new United Way. Living the brand: A guide.* Alexandria, VA: Author.

United Way of America. (2000b). *News you can use* (Research Pub.). Alexandria, VA: Author.

U.S. Department of Health and Human Services. (1999). *Mental health: A report of the Surgeon General.* Rockville, MD: U.S. Department of Health and Human Services, Substance Abuse and Mental Health Services Administration, Center for Mental Health Services & National Institute of Mental Health. Retrieved January 17, 2009, from www. surgeongeneral.gov/library/mentalhealth/home.html

Wilbanks, L. (2007, September/October). Strategic thinking, practical dreaming. *IT Professional, 9*(5), 62–63.

CHAPTER 3

Occupation-Focused Community Health and Wellness Programs

Margaret Swarbrick, PhD, OTR, CPRP

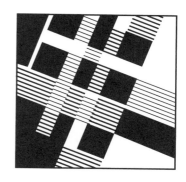

Learning Objectives

After reading this material and completing the examination, readers will be able to

- Identify how social determinants of health may contribute to medical and mental health conditions that affect occupational performance,

- Identify the federal initiatives—including *Healthy People 2010* (U.S. Department of Health and Human Services, 2000) and the Center for Mental Health Services National Wellness Summit for People With Mental Illness—that are focused on disease prevention and management and health and wellness promotion,

- Identify roles and opportunities for occupational therapy practice in health and wellness practice models and arenas, and

- Identify how to apply health promotion and wellness principles to people living with mental illness and others living with chronic medical conditions.

The occupational therapy profession can play an important role in and make a positive impact on the nation's health by understanding health promotion and wellness models that are adaptive, holistic, and congruent with the profession's philosophy. The profession faces challenges in meeting the total heath needs of people and their communities. Occupational therapy is in an ideal position to assume a leadership role in the arena of health promotion and wellness because the profession is client centered and occupation based and recognizes how context affects performance.

This chapter explores a variety of health and wellness topics relevant to occupational therapy practice, including social determinants of health, health promotion, public health initiatives, mental health disparities, integrated models, peer-delivered self-management programs, and the emerging role of mind–body medicine. It discusses health concerns facing the nation and particularly people living with serious forms of mental illness, outlines health promotion practices and a wellness model, and suggests implications for occupational therapy practice.

Health

As our society continues to progress in terms of scientific and technological advancements, the right of all citizens to good health and quality health care is not guaranteed. Although the general population is now living longer, people who are disadvantaged and disenfranchised often experience a shorter lifespan and live with chronic, disabling medical conditions. The Public Health Model reveals determinants of health across populations, recognizing that health is affected by many factors including where people live and their income, educational status, and social relationships, known as *social determinants of health.* Social determinants of health are the economic and social conditions under which people live that determine their health. Some conditions are a result of social, economic, and political forces (Wilkinson & Marmot, 2003). Social determinants of health have been recognized by the World Health Organization and include income and social status, social support networks, education and literacy (i.e., health literacy), employment and working conditions, social and physical environments, personal health practices and coping skills, child development, genetic factors, access to health services, gender, and culture (Wilkinson & Marmot, 2003). Researchers have pinpointed social determinants—the specific exposures through which members of different socioeconomic groups come to experience varying degrees of health and illness. A social gradient in health runs through society, with the people who are poorest generally suffering the worst health. Although it has been well documented that people in different socioeconomic groups experience differing health outcomes, the specific factors and means by which those factors lead to illness are unclear. Many major diseases are determined by a network of interacting exposures that increase or decrease the risk for the disease. Later in this chapter, I examine how people living with serious forms of mental illness are at increased risk for serious disabling medical conditions and a shortened lifespan.

Public Health Initiatives

Given the inequities of health and a desire to promote good health for all citizens, a public health agenda has been set for the nation. *Public health* is the science and art of preventing disease, prolonging life, and promoting health through the organized efforts and informed choices of society, organizations (public and private), communities, and people. In the United States, the Centers for Disease Control and Prevention's National Center for Chronic Disease Prevention and Health Promotion (www. cdc.gov/nccdphp/) is a federal agency at the forefront of the nation's efforts to understand, prevent, and control chronic diseases. The center conducts studies to better understand the causes of diseases, supports programs to promote healthy behaviors, and monitors the health of the nation through national surveys.

The *Healthy People 2010* (U.S. Department of Health and Human Services [DHHS], 2000) initiative was formed with the goal of improving the health of Americans in terms of health problems, health status, and access to available health services. The initiative is designed to increase people's lifespan and health status;

reduce disparities; and secure access to health services, particularly preventive services, for all Americans. The leading health indicators include mental health, physical activity, tobacco use, responsible sexual behavior, injury and violence, environmental quality, immunization, and access to health care (DHHS, 2000).

Healthy People 2010 focuses on health promotion and prevention. *Health promotion* is a process of enhancing health through education, guidance, and support and is believed to contribute to positive behavioral change. *Health promotion* is a planned approach that is considered educational, political, and organizational. Educational strategies are used to empower people to assume responsibility for their own lifestyles. Health promotion models are based on the belief that people should be supported in their effort to exert control over social determinants of health. Health promotion strategies include creating supportive organizational environments and strengthening social empowerment through community action.

Prevention is a process using actions designed to prevent health problems before they start. *Secondary prevention* is the recognition of problems early in development. The goal is to identify underlying causes and change contributing behaviors in an effort to halt disease development or progression. Many untimely deaths and hospitalizations in the United States are linked to largely preventable behaviors, such as tobacco use, alcohol abuse, sedentary lifestyle, and overeating (DHHS, 2000). Healthy lifestyle habits and behaviors such as eating nutritious foods, being physically active, and avoiding tobacco use can prevent or control the devastating effects of many diseases. Public health models address the impact on health of individual behaviors and risk factors to population-level issues such as inequality, poverty, and education.

Health promotion and prevention campaigns target many of these lifestyle habits; the goal is to prevent disease and associated disabilities. Another example of this concept is the focus on establishing habits and strategies to prevent recurrence rather than waiting until the point at which the problem needs fixing. Smoking has been identified as hazardous to physical health by shortening the lifespan and reducing the quality of life lived, and public health efforts have focused significant attention on smoking cessation efforts for the general population, with great success. Smoking rates in the United States have diminished significantly except for people living with serious forms of mental illness, who smoke half of all cigarettes produced. Many more people living with mental illness are smokers compared with the larger society. I review smoking cessation initiatives for this population later.

Mental Health

Mental health is one of the *Healthy People 2010* leading target health indicators (DHHS, 2000). Mental health problems are more common than heart disease, lung disease, and cancer combined (Kessler, Berglund, Demler, Jin, & Walters, 2005; Kessler, Chiu, Demler, & Walters, 2005). According to the National Institute of Mental Health (NIMH; 2008), an estimated 26.2% of Americans ages 18 and older—about 1 in 4 adults—suffer from a diagnosable mental disorder in a given year. When applied to the 2004 U.S. Census residential population estimate for ages 18 and older, this figure translates to 57.7 million people. Even though mental disorders are widespread in the population, the main burden of illness is concentrated in a much smaller proportion—about 6%, or 1 in 17 adults—who suffer from a serious mental illness. In addition, mental disorders are the leading cause of disability in the United States and Canada for people ages 15 to 44. Many people suffer from more than one mental disorder at a given time: Nearly half (45%) of those with any mental disorder meet criteria for two or more disorders, and severity is strongly related to comorbidity (NIMH, 2008). People assume that mental illness is something that affects other people and is unlikely to have an impact on their own lives. In fact, mental illness affects everyone in today's society—families, workplaces, educational settings, places of worship, and the community in general.

Mental disorders were once thought to affect few people, but today the opposite is known to be true. Not too long ago, people commonly believed that those with mental illness should be confined in institutional settings for the rest of their lives. It is now known that a significant number of people in today's society live with an identified mental illness and lead full, productive, and satisfying lives. Many people living with a diagnosis of a mental disorder (anxiety disorder, posttraumatic stress disorder, obsessive–compulsive disorder, substance use, eating disorder, depression, bipolar disorder, schizophrenia) work, vote, and own homes and businesses. They successfully contribute to their communities and the economy. There is hope and a renewed optimism regarding the outcomes of living with a mental illness.

Mental health and mental illness are points on a continuum. Mental health is often judged through one's ability to engage in productive activities, fulfill relationships with others, adapt to change, and cope with adversity. It is something we aspire to and work toward every day. *Mental health* includes having a sense of balance and the capacity to be flexible in dealing with inevitable stress and crisis. Having good mental health affects personal well-being, families, relationships, and the ability to participate productively in society. *Mental illness* refers collectively to all diagnosable mental disorders. *Mental disorders* are health conditions characterized by alterations in thinking, mood, or behavior (or some combination thereof) and are associated with distress that possibly affects the ability to function in daily life activities. The line between health and illness can be quite thin.

Many people who may need treatment for a mental health problem or condition may not seek such help because of mental health stigma. Stigmatizing attitudes and beliefs about mental illness are widespread, and the ramifications are serious. *Stigma* refers to a cluster of negative attitudes and beliefs that motivate the general public to fear, reject, avoid, and discriminate against people with mental illness (President's New Freedom Commission on Mental Health, 2003). Many people would rather suffer in silence from the mental health condition than suffer the effects of the stigma and discrimination if they seek help. Stigma assumes many forms, both subtle and overt, and can negatively affect all areas of life—housing, employment, and relationships. Stigma can appear as prejudice, discrimination, fear, distrust, and stereotyping. Stigma may not only prevent people from seeking help, it may even prevent them from acknowledging that they may need help. Stigma may have an impact on their access to care and the quality of care they receive; perhaps worst of all, it can result in the person internalizing the stigmatizing attitudes, referred to as *self-stigma*.

Many people living with mental illness have reported that fighting the stigma associated with the illness is often more difficult than battling the illness itself. As occupational therapists and members of communities, it is important that we not label the person who may be living with a mental illness or problem. People with mental health conditions or problems, regardless of severity, are, first, people. They should not be defined by their condition (e.g., by terms such as *depressives* or *schizophrenics,* which are derogatory); those terms are considered disrespectful and a formidable barrier to recovery. Stigma is considered a significant barrier to recovery. Occupational therapists should educate other professionals who may use derogatory terms regarding patients. Stigma among health care professionals and even among mental health professionals is a reality and can affect good patient care.

Occupational therapists can play an important role in addressing stigma. The Substance Abuse and Mental Health Services Administration's Resource Center to Promote Acceptance, Dignity and Social Inclusion Associated With Mental Health (http://stopstigma.samhsa.gov/) is an excellent resource for occupational therapists to counter discrimination and prejudice through information, technical assistance, and access to research.

Health Disparities

Premature mortality resulting from comorbidity of many serious medical conditions with serious mental illness is a challenge for society and the health care system. Recent findings have suggested that people living with serious mental illness develop serious medical comorbidities that result in a lifespan shorter by 25 years than that of the general population (Parks, Svendsen, Singer, Foti, & Mauer, 2006). Many people receiving psychiatric care are at increased risk for developing chronic disabling medical conditions and may possibly have a shortened lifespan. The National Association of State Mental Health Program Directors' *Morbidity and Mortality in People Living With Serious Mental Illness* (Parks et al., 2006) highlighted this health disparity and identified factors contributing to the incidence of chronic health conditions and early death.

Comorbid Medical Conditions

The medications prescribed to ameliorate the symptoms of mental illness seem to have some negative impacts on physical health. The newer class of antipsychotic medications, such as quetiapine (Seroquel), may induce several serious adverse health issues, including the metabolic syndrome, diabetes, dyslipidemia, obesity, hypertension, osteoporosis, periodontal disease, and sexual dysfunction (Enger, Weatherby, Reynolds, Glasser, & Walker, 2004; Joukamaa et al., 2006; Meltzer, 2005). People taking newer generation antipsychotics are at increased risk for abnormal glucose and lipid metabolism (Lieberman et al., 2005; Nasrallah et al., 2006), and those who develop complications are frequently not treated for them or are treated inadequately. The strong association of both conventional and second-generation antipsychotic medications with obesity and related conditions has become central to the consciousness of clinicians prescribing antipsychotic medication, just as motor side effects and tardive dyskinesia have previously been central considerations. At the onset of prescribing this medication, weight, glucose, and lipid monitoring should commence, as should preventive measures in diet and exercise that will reduce the risk of obesity. This monitoring is not yet standard practice, and occupational therapists can play a role by informing consumers with whom they work. A clear need to monitor and treat cardiovascular risk factors also exists in this population.

Poor health habits are also a powerful contributor to the disability experience and recovery efforts (Hutchinson et al., 2006). Adults living with serious forms of mental illness are likely to be overweight, be smokers, and live a sedentary lifestyle. Mental illness often co-occurs with diabetes, increased risk of infectious disease, and increased incidence of alcohol and substance abuse. Lack of knowledge of correct dietary principles, lower self-efficacy, limited social support, and psychiatric symptoms often influence health-related behavior (Leas & McCabe, 2007). Occupational therapists can help people seeking to make health-related behavior changes by incorporating health promotion principles and guidelines.

Health Promotion and Occupational Therapy Approaches to Addressing Health Issues

The excess comorbidity in people with serious mental illness and others who are disadvantaged consists of largely preventable health conditions that can be addressed. A growing evidence base of effective heath promotion and education practices addresses physical activity, nutrition education, diet and glucose monitoring, dental health practices, smoking cessation, and prevention of transmission of HIV/AIDS.

The benefits of physical activity on health outcomes of people living with mental illness are similar to the positive response found among the general population. Not only does physical activity have known health benefits regardless of illness type, but research has also documented that it can alleviate secondary symptoms such as low self-esteem and social withdrawal (Biddle, Fox, & Boutcher, 2000; Faulkner & Carless, 2006). Guidelines are available to assist in the provision of evidence-based physical activity interventions that educate consumers and promote improved health (Richardson et al., 2005). Physical activity programs that integrate education about the importance of activity and incorporate the supported activity are recommended. Education strengthens self-efficacy, which is one of the most important predictors of adherence to an active lifestyle (Richardson et al., 2005). Physical activity and educational interventions are feasible and can result in significant behavior change, which improves physical health outcomes.

Occupational therapists can play an important role in helping people to engage in meaningful activities and daily routines that promote physical well-being by taking part in programs such as OTs Walk With NAMI. Members of the Mental Health Task Force of the Metropolitan New York District of the New York State Occupational Therapy Association collaborated with the National Alliance on Mental Illness (NAMI). Occupational therapy faculty and students were encouraged to form partnerships with mental health facilities throughout New York City to support and encourage consumers to actively engage in the NAMI NYC–METRO Walkathon, crossing the Brooklyn Bridge.

Metropolitan New York District Mental Health Task Force leaders envision that occupational therapy students, supported by faculty and clinicians, will introduce this walking protocol to consumers during their fieldwork and will start walking groups throughout New York City. Supported by evidence that weight control and physical exercise are effective physical and mental health interventions for this population, this protocol includes detailed goals, session plans, and outcome measurements. Possibilities for research are embedded in the protocol as well. To share the program protocol, materials, and inspiration with participants, the project coordinators have created a group page on Facebook (http://downstate.facebook.com/group.php?gid=5876819365).

Another health concern for people living with mental illness is tobacco use. Whereas tobacco use has decreased in the general population largely as the result of aggressive health promotion campaigns, people living with serious mental illness continue to smoke at alarming rates. According to the Robert Wood Johnson Foundation Smoking Cessation Leadership Center (2008, para. 1), "Persons with mental illness smoke half of all cigarettes produced and are only half as likely to quit as smokers" without mental illness. It is not a surprise that tobacco use is a significant issue contributing to the poor health of people living with mental illness. Smoking cessation interventions and strategies have been shown to be effective for both the general population and people living with serious mental illness. Various effective methods are available to facilitate smoking cessation. A manual for successful smoking cessation among people with serious mental illness, *Tobacco-Free Living in Psychiatric Settings,* has been developed by physician Jill Williams and her colleagues (National Association of State Mental Health Program Directors, 2007) and is available on the National Association of State Mental Health Program Directors Web site (www.nasmhpd.org). Williams has also worked with colleagues to develop *Learning About Healthy Living* (Williams et al., 2005).

Behavioral approaches are effective in achieving modest weight loss for people with psychiatric disabilities, which is associated with important health-protective outcomes (Ussher, Stanbury, Cheeseman, & Faulkner, 2007). An occupational therapist working collaboratively with a nurse has developed dietary and exercise interventions to address weight loss and control of glucose levels (Brown, 2006; Brown & Chan, 2006). An evidence-based food education program assists people to more effectively manage their weight and counteract the ill effects of weight gain associated with lifestyle and medications (Brown, Goetz, Van Sciver, Sullivan, & Hamera, 2006). This manualized rehabilitation intervention includes goal setting, skills training, skills practice, and the provision of social support around nutrition that supports the recovery process.

NAMI (n.d.) has also developed the Hearts & Minds program to address physical health needs. The program is designed to raise awareness and provide information on diabetes, diet, exercise, and smoking. Along with information on diabetes and sleep apnea, Hearts & Minds contains tips on exercise and diet and includes a shopping list template, recipes, and a food diary. This program includes a 13-minute inspirational video and a 26-page booklet, available online.

In response to the alarming rates of mortality and morbidity among people living with mental illness, the Center for Mental Health Services (CMHS) sponsored a National Wellness Summit for People With Mental Illness in Rockville, Maryland, in September 2007. As a result of the summit, a target was set that "within 10 years we will eliminate 10 years of the 25-year disparity in lifespan of public mental health consumers" (Manderscheid & del Vecchio, 2008).

Integrated Models of Care

A clear message exists that the mental health system needs to be holistic and emphasize health promotion and improved access to and interface of physical and mental health (CMHS, 2005; DHHS, 2005; Mental Health America, 2007; President's New Freedom Commission on Mental Health, 2003).

The Bazelon Center for Mental Health Law published *Get It Together: How to Integrate Physical and Mental Healthcare for People With Serious Mental Disorders,* which focuses on integration and problems stemming from a fragmented health care system (Koyanagi, 2004). Both Mental Health America and NAMI have also issued statements calling for increased action to promote access to quality health care for people with mental illness.

Cherokee Health Systems is a model organization with 23 sites in 13 Tennessee counties that is both a primary care provider and a specialty behavioral health provider (www.cherokeehealth.com). Cherokee Health Systems is integrated both structurally and financially, which supports its focus on clinical integration. Integrated care is embedded in the organization's vision and mission and practiced across an array of comprehensive primary care, behavioral health, and prevention programs and services (Koyanagi, 2004). A behavioral health consultant is an embedded, full-time member of the primary care team, with a psychiatrist available, generally by telephone, for medication consults. The behavioral health consultant provides brief, targeted, real-time interventions to address the psychosocial aspects of primary care.

For people who need specialty behavioral health services, a primary care provider is embedded in the specialty behavioral health team. According to the Bazelon report (Koyanagi, 2004), Cherokee hires primary care providers who are comfortable with mental health issues and believes that all front-line, administrative, and support staff must be essential players, committed to the holistic approach (Koyanagi, 2004). The local community is aware that Cherokee treats people for all types of illnesses. Collaborative care is built into Cherokee's unified program model because the organization focuses on clinical integration as its mission. However, placing both the behavioral health and the primary care functions under the same organizational structure or within the same physical facility can still be only a co-location, not collaborative care. The focus on the clinical process is what creates collaborative care. Other models are being developed across the country (Mauer, 2003; Unutzer, Schoenbaum, Druss, & Katon, 2006). A good resource is a publication produced by the National Institute for Mental Health in England (2005) titled *Mental Health Promotion in Primary Healthcare.*

Peer-Delivered Self-Management Programs

Disease and illness self-management programs have become more widely available to help people with chronic medical conditions. In this section, I discuss how peer-delivered self-management models for chronic physical health conditions are being applied to the management of medical conditions encountered by people with psychiatric disabilities. The most widely studied of the self-management programs is the Chronic Disease Self-Management Program developed by Stanford University's Patient Education Research Center. The Chronic Disease Self-Management Program is a community-based program with prescribed curricula for people managing several different chronic physical illnesses (Lorig, Hurwicz, Sobel, Hobbs, & Ritter, 2004). Typically, it includes education, skills training, and peer support, and it has been applied in populations with asthma, diabetes, HIV, and back pain (Bruce, Lorig, & Laurent, 2007; Lorig et al., 2004).

Another key factor in disease self-management programs is the use of peer-led interventions. Trained peers with similar health issues have been shown to be positive role models and to increase a person's sense of self-efficacy (Lorig et al., 2004). Short-term action plans or goals are central to self-management (Bodenheimer, Lorig, Holman, & Grumbach, 2002). The proposed intervention uses peer wellness coaches to assist people in developing a personalized goal in the area that they feel is of most concern. The coaches will then provide support and follow-up for attainment of personal goals.

Although no published studies address disease self-management of physical health issues for people with psychiatric disabilities, at least two such studies are under way. The Health and Recovery Peer Project is being conducted by Benjamin Druss in Atlanta, Georgia (Druss, 2007). Other techniques to self-manage symptoms of psychiatric disorders have been addressed, including the evidence-based practice Illness Management and Recovery and Wellness Recovery Action Plan (WRAP) developed by Mary Ellen Copeland. WRAP is an excellent example of a peer-delivered self-management model designed to teach people with mental illness to identify self-care strategies to maximize health (Copeland, 1997, 2001). WRAP provides a structure to increase support and develop an action plan for creating good health through management of distressing mental and physical symptoms. This model prepares people to assume personal responsibility for their health as a fundamental process of their personal recovery and wellness. WRAP is an excellent strategy to help people develop daily plans and other self-awareness processes to help restore and maintain personal wellness (Swarbrick, 2006). WRAP offers a "train the trainer" approach to provide facilitation skills and strategies that promote the dissemination of these curricula and train both providers and peer providers in the competencies needed to teach self-management skills. Occupational therapists can assume an important role by offering people in recovery training on how to conduct WRAP sessions individually or in a group context.

Using peer-to-peer education to improve health emphasizes the centrality of personal medicine (Deegan, 2005) and shared decision making (Deegan, 2006). Peers help one another to articulate the personal medicine that supports their recovery, to identify their health concerns, and to prepare to work with medical providers to ensure their needs are met. A provider component helps providers assist people in their medication decisions and dilemmas, and a software program prepares people to engage as proactive participants in their health encounters (Deegan, 2006).

Shared decision making is an interactive and collaborative process between people and their health care practitioners about decisions pertinent to their treatment; services; and, ultimately, their personal recovery. An *optimal decision* is one that is informed, consistent with personal values, and acted on (del Vecchio, 2008). Shared decision making is particularly relevant when uncertainty about a particular decision exists. Uncertainty may stem from multiple or competing options, each with advantages and disadvantages; incomplete or inconclusive scientific outcome evidence; or individual factors such as personal values and beliefs, a limited knowledge about the options, or lack of support to make a clear choice.

The Ottawa Health Research Institute maintains the Ottawa Health Decision Centre (http://decisionaid.ohri.ca), which has an inventory of decision aids for physical health care that can be used or adapted by occupational therapists to promote the consumers' role in shared decision making. The Dartmouth–Hitchcock Medical Center Decision Support Center, with funding from the Foundation for Informed Medical Decision Making and Health Dialog, Inc., has established an onsite decision-support center for patients and also provides limited online resources (www.dhmc. org/webpage.cfm?site_id=2&org_id=108&gsec_id=0&sec_id=0&item_id=2486).

Professional Training and Education

Professional academic training and education that incorporates health promotion principles, health knowledge, skills, and strategies is necessary in transforming the mental health system into one that supports recovery (Hutchinson et al., 2006). Health promotion efforts require that professionals shift from an orientation focused on illness to one focused on health and wellness. This shift will require some changes in terms of education and training for occupational therapists. Health promotion should be included in the training curriculum and training experiences of all providers, including occupational therapists (see Figure 3.1 for health promotion principles).

Educational, behavioral, and cultural approaches that promote health are essential components of education. Specific skills and knowledge that are essential for all professionals who work on health issues with people living with mental illness include active teaching skills; consultation skills; communication skills, including shared decision making, information sharing, and partnering; cultural competency skills; trauma-informed health knowledge; and basic health literacy skills (Bussema & Nemec, 2006; Koyanagi, 2004).

The lack of relevant training and education about health issues and health promotion is an identified barrier that impedes the achievement of optimal health for people in recovery (CMHS, 2005). The inability to transfer education and training into daily practices and lifestyles underlies this barrier and has long been recognized as the most difficult aspect of creating change and achieving desired outcomes (Swarbrick, Hutchinson, & Gill, 2008). That people living with mental illness need functional health as a foundation for their recovery is clear (Hutchinson et al., 2006). Health promotion is a process of enhancing wellness through education, guidance, and support and contributes to positive behavioral change (Swarbrick et al., 2008). Occupational therapists need to have a better understanding of health education and create health promotion guidelines for practice.

Health literacy is an important concept, and the availability of health information and access to health education and promotion services is important to create opportunities to obtain health resources. The Institute of Medicine (2004) defined *health literacy* as the ability to find, understand, and use health information and services to make appropriate health decisions and act on health information. Improving health literacy is a *Healthy People 2010* objective (DHHS, 2000). Many of the skills people use to manage their lives are contingent on health literacy— the ability to read and understand a prescription label, understand a physician's order, read educational brochures provided by health care providers, comprehend a written consent form before a medical procedure, figure out health benefits available from third-party payers, and negotiate our complex health care delivery system (Costa, 2008). As occupational therapists, it is important that we understand the complex skills involved in health literacy: Reading, listening, comprehending,

1. Health and access to health care are universal rights of all people.

2. Health promotion recognizes the potential for health and wellness of mental health consumers.

3. Active participation of mental health consumers in health promotion activities is ideal.

4. Health education is the cornerstone of health promotion for mental health consumers.

5. Health promotion for consumers addresses the characteristics of environments in which people live, learn, and work.

6. Health promotion is holistic and eclectic in its use of many strategies and pathways.

7. Health promotion addresses each person's resource needs.

8. Health promotion interventions must address differences in people's readiness for change.

Figure 3.1. Eight principles of health promotion.
Source. Hutchinson et al. (2006).

problem solving, and analyzing are among the skills required to understand and apply health information (Costa, 2008). An occupational therapist has developed a Web site (www.healthliteracy.com) and written a book on this topic for health care practitioners: *Health Literacy A to Z: Practical Ways to Communicate Your Health Message* (Osborne, 2005).

With the National Ad Council, the Agency for Healthcare Research and Quality has launched a public education campaign, "Questions Are the Answer," to encourage health literacy by getting people involved in their health care. It includes public service announcements and online tools to prepare consumers for doctors' visits (see www.ahrq.gov/questionsaretheanswer).

Wellness

Health promotion focuses on wellness. Wellness is a conscious, deliberate process that requires a person to become aware of and make choices for a more satisfying lifestyle (Swarbrick, 1997, 2006). A wellness lifestyle includes a "self-defined balance" of health habits, including adequate sleep, rest, and good nutrition; productivity and exercise; participation in meaningful activity; and connections with supportive relationships (Swarbrick, 1997, 2006). Wellness is holistic and includes the following dimensions: physical, emotional, social, financial, occupational, spiritual, and intellectual. The Wellness Model expects the person to assume personal responsibility and be proactive in the preservation of his or her own health. The person served should be encouraged to assume an active role in self-monitoring his or her own health behaviors and increasing activity on the dimensions on which he or she perceives an imbalance. This model is different from the traditional one, in which the health care provider defines the problem and prescribes the methods to be used for change. In the Wellness Model, the occupational therapist should collaborate and act as a coach, helping to guide the person toward successful behavioral change. Traditionally, people tend to have problems achieving compliance with health initiatives because they perceive the recommendation as punitive rather than collaborative and supportive, causing rebellion and lack of follow through.

The Wellness Model views motivation for compliance and commitment to change through personal control and good health (whereas in the traditional model, fear is used to drive change and instill compliance). People's strengths and their capacity to achieve their goals are supported. Focusing on limitations and weaknesses can create barriers to progress and self-fulfillment rather than support positive change. If one has impairment on one dimension, the unimpaired dimension can be emphasized in a program of change. For many people, regular exercise and routine are important strategies to manage symptoms of depression and anxiety and deal with stress. More than 30 years ago, when I was quite disabled by signs and symptoms of mental illness, I found swimming to be an effective tool to help me manage severe symptoms (Swarbrick, 2006). In addition to using swimming as a key aspect of my daily maintenance plan, I also adhere to a regular sleep–wake routine (fall asleep and wake up at the same time 7 days a week), do not work on the computer after 8:00 p.m., and schedule a productive activity every day. My mental and social well-being are strongly influenced by those activities and routines. Helping people to create a self-defined balance of health habits and routines that support personal wellness is a core tool of occupational therapy practice.

The Wellness Model recognizes protective factors and the valuable role of social support in helping people to strengthen their ability to cope with stress and adversity in many of life's crises. Social support, in addition to other protective factors (coping skills, self-care, and self-esteem), has a powerful impact on lessening the incidence of illness (mental disorders and stress-related illness). A person may encounter risk factors such as organic factors, exposure to stress, exploitation, and trauma. Incidence of illness or disorder can be reduced by strengthening protective factors such as coping skills, self-esteem, self-care skills, and social support systems. As occupational therapists design, deliver, and evaluate occupational therapy services, they must keep all of those wellness factors in mind.

The National Center for Complementary and Alternative Medicine is 1 of the 27 institutes and centers that make up the National Institutes of Health of DHHS. Its mission is to explore complementary and alternative healing practices in the context of rigorous science; to train complementary and alternative medicine researchers; and to disseminate authoritative information to the public and professionals.

Alternative and complementary medicine are often referred to as *mind–body medicine*. Practices range from deep breathing and progressive muscle relaxation to meditation, hypnosis, and guided imagery. A large percentage of physician visits are believed to be for stress-related complaints. Herbert Benson and his colleagues have researched the effectiveness of mind–body medicine in helping people reduce stress that can cause or exacerbate conditions such as heart disease, infertility, gastrointestinal disorders, and chronic pain. The Benson–Henry Institute's work is based on the inseparable connection between the mind and the body and the complicated interactions that take place among thoughts, the body, and the outside world. (More information is available at www.massgeneral.org/bhi.)

Mind–body medicine integrates modern scientific medicine, psychology, nutrition, exercise physiology, and the power of belief (intention) to enhance the natural healing capacities of body and mind. The outcome is self-care and self-management, which complement the conventional medical paths of surgery and pharmaceuticals. The mind–body approach has important implications for the way in which therapists view illness and treat disease. The model takes into account that physical health is influenced by thoughts, feelings, and behaviors and, conversely, that thoughts, feelings, and behaviors can be influenced by physical symptoms. Mind–body medicine incorporates the relaxation response, cognitive–behavioral approaches, and the role of physical activity and nutrition. It is an educational approach that helps people take control of their lives and learn to use their own healing power to reduce stress and other negative thoughts and behaviors to maintain and regain health. Mind–body approaches play an important role in promoting wellness and recovery for people living with mental illness and other chronic health conditions and could possibly play a role in preventing development or exacerbation of other chronic health conditions.

Many Americans are using mind–body interventions. Practices range from deep breathing and progressive muscle relaxation to meditation, hypnosis, and guided imagery. Between 60% and 90% of all physician visits are believed to be for stress-related complaints. Mind–body approaches have the potential to assume an important role in promoting wellness and recovery for people living with mental illness (and could possibly play a role in preventing relapse and the development of other chronic health conditions).

Russinova, Wewiorski, and Cash (2002) explored the perceived benefits of alternative health care practices by people with serious mental illness They found that people in recovery access a variety of integrative and complementary health practices and treatments to improve well-being. Although their sample size was small and their cohort was a nonrepresentative sample, considering society's focus on mind–body medicine, the use of alternative practices by people living with mental illness should be further investigated.

Occupational Therapy Practice

To be wellness focused, the occupational therapy profession must define how it can effectively meet the needs of the people it serves on all dimensions, including physical, mental, environmental, emotional, social, and spiritual. This focus requires divergence from our medical-model roots. Professional education needs to include health promotion principles and an understanding of the public health model. The profession should gain a clearer understanding of wellness, health promotion, and social determinants of health, and occupational therapists are encouraged to develop and expand their professional roles into community health and wellness. Advanced occupational therapists are challenged to examine their own lifestyles and the lifestyles of the people they serve to fulfill the mandate of a health-oriented society. Occupational therapists have valuable skills to contribute, and they should engage in applied scientific inquiry to examine the efficacy and cost-effectiveness of wellness and health promotion guidelines.

Occupational therapists are in an ideal position to create opportunities for people living with mental illness to fully realize a lifestyle centered on wellness. Occupational therapists can expand their roles in wellness promotion into arenas such as coaching, systems consultation, developing and directing community wellness initiatives, assisting the growing numbers of senior citizens in their new roles as retirees, and seeking consultant positions in the corporate United States.

The University of Southern California (USC) has created the Lifestyle Redesign process (see www.ot.usc.edu/programs). Lifestyle Redesign is the process of acquiring health-promoting habits and routines on the basis of an underlying occupational science foundation. Principles such as occupational self-analysis, module structure, and group process are integral components of the process. The Lifestyle Redesign approach draws on a variety of strategies identified in evidence-based literature relevant to the specific area being addressed. The USC Well Elderly Study demonstrated that Lifestyle Redesign can enhance the health and quality of life of older adults and reduce health care costs (Mandel, Jackson, Zemke, Nelson, & Clark, 1999). Lifestyle Redesign programs and services are focused on weight loss, lifestyle risk assessment, pain management, college students, multiple sclerosis, assisted living, creating a healthy work life, and life coaching.

The USC Occupational Therapy Faculty Practice offers the Continuous Lifestyle Redesign approach, which is appropriate for many diagnoses including Parkinson's disease, hypertension, fibromyalgia, hypercholesterolemia, multiple sclerosis, chronic fatigue, chronic pain, diabetes, repetitive stress disorder, and arthritis. Because lifestyle change is a comprehensive process and takes time and consistency, the treatment approach is often structured for long-term intervention. Fazio (2008) published the second edition of *Developing Occupation-Centered Programs for the Community,* which offers perspectives on the development of occupation-centered programs in the community.

Summary and Conclusion

That health is a complex phenomenon and occupational therapy is in an ideal position to assume a leadership role in the arena of health promotion and wellness is clear. This chapter presents a broad range of ideas regarding health promotion and wellness that are congruent with the profession's philosophy, are client centered and occupation based, and recognize how context affects performance. The chapter also examines the social determinants of health, health promotion, and public health initiatives and specifically the health concerns of people living with serious forms of mental illness. The health promotion principles and Wellness Model it proposes have important implications for occupational therapy practice. Occupational therapists are ideally suited to recognize how economic and social conditions affect health and to design educational strategies to empower people to assume responsibility for their own lifestyle habits.

Occupational therapy's client-centered model will foster and support the people we serve in their efforts to exert control over their health and well-being, as they define them. Significant roles exist for occupational therapy in terms of addressing the stigma regarding mental illness and seeking mental health services. It is important for occupational therapists to incorporate shared decision-making models into practice and continue to view the people they serve holistically through the lens of wellness (viewing them as being composed of the eight dimensions of wellness described in Chapter 15). Finally, pioneers at USC have embraced health promotion approaches for many years and have both developed and researched Lifestyle Redesign, which is a clear practice model for professionals working with people living with chronic health conditions.

References

Biddle, S., Fox, K., & Boutcher, S. (Eds.). (2000). *Physical activity and psychological well-being.* London: Routledge.

Bodenheimer, T., Lorig, K., Holman, H., & Grumbach, K. (2002). Patient self-management of chronic disease in primary care. *JAMA, 288*(19), 2469–2475.

Brown, C., Goetz, J., Van Sciver, A., Sullivan, D., & Hamera, E. (2006). A psychiatric rehabilitation approach to weight loss. *Psychiatric Rehabilitation Journal, 29*(4), 267–273.

Brown, S. (2006). Schizophrenia, weight gain, and atypical antipsychotics. *British Journal of Psychiatry, 188*(2), 191–192.

Brown, S., & Chan, K. (2006). A randomized controlled trial of a brief health promotion intervention in a population with serious mental illness. *Journal of Mental Health, 15*(5), 543–549.

Bruce, B., Lorig, K., & Laurent, D. (2007). Participation in patient self-management programs. *Arthritis Rheumatology, 57,* 851–854.

Bussema, E., & Nemec, P. (2006). Effective teaching. *Psychiatric Rehabilitation Journal, 29,* 315–317.

Center for Mental Health Services. (2005). *Building bridges: Mental health consumers and primary care representatives in dialogue.* Rockville, MD: Substance Abuse and Mental Health Services Administration, Center for Mental Health Services.

Copeland, M. E. (1997). *Wellness recovery action plan.* Brattleboro, VT: Peach Press.

Copeland, M. (2001). Wellness recovery action plan: A system for monitoring, reducing, and eliminating uncomfortable or dangerous physical symptoms or emotional feelings. *Occupational Therapy in Mental Health, 17*(3/4), 127–150.

Costa, D. (2008, August 25). Facilitating health literacy. *OT Practice, 13*(15), 13–16, 18.

Deegan, P. (2005). The importance of personal medicine: A qualitative study of resilience in people with psychiatric disabilities. *Scandinavian Journal of Public Health, 33,* 1–7.

Deegan, P. (2006). Shared decision making and medication management in the recovery process. *Psychiatric Services, 57*(11), 1636–1639.

del Vecchio, P. (2008). *SAMHSA's shared decision-making (SDM): Making recovery real in mental health care project.* Retrieved from http://download.ncadi.samhsa.gov/ken/msword/ SDM_fact_sheet_7-23-2008.doc

Druss, B. (2007). *The health and wellness of mental health consumers.* Retrieved May 16, 2009, from www.mentalhealthamerica.net/fall_policy_conference/Ben_Druss.pdf

Enger, C., Weatherby, L., Reynolds, R. F., Glasser, D. B., & Walker, A. M. (2004). Cardiovascular disease and schizophrenia serious cardiovascular events and mortality among patients with schizophrenia. *Journal of Nervous and Mental Disease, 192,* 19–27.

Faulkner, G., & Carless, D. (2006). Physical activity in the process of psychiatric rehabilitation: Theoretical and methodological issues. *Psychiatric Rehabilitation Journal, 29*(4), 258–266.

Fazio, L. (2008). *Developing occupation-centered programs for the community* (2nd ed.). Englewood Cliffs, NJ: Prentice Hall.

Hutchinson, D., Gagne, C., Bowers, A., Russinova, Z., Skrinar, G., & Anthony, W. (2006). Framework for health promotion services and for people with psychiatric disabilities. *Psychiatric Rehabilitation Journal, 29,* 241–250.

Institute of Medicine. (2004). *Health literacy: A prescription to end confusion.* Washington, DC: National Academies Press. Retrieved January 13, 2010, from www.iom.edu/?id=32784

Joukamaa, M., Heliövaara, M., Knekt, P., Aromaa, A., Raitasalo, R., & Lehtinen, V. (2006). Schizophrenia, neuroleptic medication, and mortality. *British Journal of Psychiatry, 188,* 122–127.

Kessler, R., Berglund, P., Demler, O., Jin, R., & Walters, E. (2005). Lifetime prevalence and age-of-onset distributions of *DSM–IV* disorders in the National Comorbidity Survey Replication (NCS-R). *Archives of General Psychiatry, 62*(6), 593–602.

Kessler, R., Chiu, W., Demler, O., & Walters, E. (2005). Prevalence, severity, and comorbidity of twelve-month *DSM–IV* disorders in the National Comorbidity Survey Replication (NCS–R). *Archives of General Psychiatry, 62*(6), 617–627.

Koyanagi, C. (2004). *Get it together: How to integrate physical and mental health care for people with serious mental disorders.* Washington, DC: Bazelon Center for Mental Health Law.

Leas, L., & McCabe, M. (2007). Health behaviors among individuals with schizophrenia and depression. *Journal of Health Psychology, 12*(4), 563–579.

Lieberman, J., Stroup, T., McEvoy, J., Swartz, M., Rosenheck, R., Perkins, D., et al. (2005). Effectiveness of antipsychotic drugs in patients with chronic schizophrenia. *New England Journal Medicine, 353*(12), 1209–1223.

Lorig, K., Hurwicz, M., Sobel, D., Hobbs, M., & Ritter, P. (2004). A national dissemination of an evidence-based self-management program and process evaluation study. *Patient Education Counseling, 59*(1), 69–79.

Mandel, D., Jackson, J., Zemke, R., Nelson, L., & Clark, F. (1999). *Lifestyle redesign: Implementing the Well Elderly Study.* Bethesda, MD: American Occupational Therapy Association.

Manderscheid, R., & del Vecchio, P. (2008). Moving toward solutions: Responses to the crisis of premature death. *International Journal of Mental Health, 37*(2), 3–7.

Mauer, B. (2003). *Behavioral health/primary care integration models, competencies, and infrastructure.* Rockville, MD: National Council for Community Behavioral Healthcare.

Meltzer, H. (2005). Focus on metabolic consequences of long-term treatment with olanzapine, quetiapine, and risperidone: Are there differences? *International Journal of Neuropsychopharmacology, 8*(2), 153–156.

Mental Health America. (2007). *Position Statement 16: Health and wellness for people with serious mental illnesses.* Retrieved July 13, 2007, from www.mentalhealthamerica.net/go/position-statements/16

Nasrallah, H., Meyer, J., Goff, D., McEvoy, J., Davis, S., Stroup, T., et al. (2006). Low rates of treatment for hypertension, dyslipidemia, and diabetes in schizophrenia: Data from the CATIE schizophrenia trial sample at baseline. *Schizophrenia Research, 6*(1–3), 15–22.

National Alliance on Mental Illness. (n.d.). *Hearts and minds.* Retrieved September 3, 2008, from www.nami.org/template.cfm?section=Hearts_and_Minds

National Association of State Mental Health Program Directors. (2007). *Tobacco-free living in psychiatric settings: A best practices toolkit to promote wellness and recovery.* Retrieved September 14, 2008, from www.nasmhpd.org

National Institute for Mental Health in England. (2005). *Mental health promotion in primary care.* Leeds, England: Author. Retrieved from www.iimhl.com/IIMHLUpdates/MHP-TOOLKIT_FINAL-a.pdf

National Institute of Mental Health. (2008). *The numbers count: Mental disorders in America.* Retrieved May 26, 2009, from www.nimh.nih.gov/health/publications/the-numbers-count-mental disorders-in-America/index.shtml

Osborne, H. (2005). *Health literacy from A to Z: Practical ways to communicate your health message.* Sudbury, MA: Jones & Bartlett.

Parks, J., Svendsen, D., Singer, P., Foti, M., & Mauer, B. (2006, October). *Morbidity and mortality in people with serious mental illness* (Tech. rep.). Retrieved September 14, 2008, from www.nasmhpd.org/general_files/publications/med_directors_pubs/Technical%20Report%20on%20Morbidity%20and%20Mortaility%20-%20Final%2011-06.pdf

President's New Freedom Commission on Mental Health. (2003). *Achieving the promise: Transforming mental health care in America* (Final Report, DHHS Pub. No. SMA–03–3832). Rockville, MD: Author. Retrieved May 26, 2009, from www.mentalhealthcommission.gov/reports/FinalReport/toc.html

Richardson, C., Faulkner, G., McDevitt, J., Skrinar, G., Hutchinson, D., & Piette, J. (2005). Integrating physical activity into mental health services for persons with serious mental illness. *Psychiatric Services, 56,* 324–331.

Robert Wood Johnson Foundation Smoking Cessation Leadership Center. (2008). *Mental health.* Retrieved October 21, 2008, from http://smokingcessationleadership.ucsf.edu/MentalHealth.html

Russinova, Z., Wewiorski, N., & Cash, D. (2002). Use of alternative health care practices by persons with serious mental illness: Perceived benefits. *American Journal of Public Health, 92,* 1600–1603.

Swarbrick, M. (1997, March). A wellness model for clients. *Mental Health Special Interest Section Quarterly, 20,* 1–4.

Swarbrick, M. (2006). A wellness approach. *Psychiatric Rehabilitation Journal, 29,* 311–314.

Swarbrick, M., Hutchinson, D., & Gill, K. (2008). The quest for optimal health: Can education and training cure what ails us? *International Journal of Mental Health, 37*(2), 69–88.

Unutzer, J., Schoenbaum, M., Druss, B., & Katon, W. (2006). Transforming mental health care at the interface with general medicine: Report for the president's commission. *Psychiatric Services, 57,* 37–47.

U.S. Department of Health and Human Services. (2000). *Healthy People 2010: Understanding and improving health* (2nd ed.). Washington, DC: U.S. Government Printing Office.

U.S. Department of Health and Human Services. (2005). *The Surgeon General's call to action to improve the health and wellness of persons with disabilities.* Rockville, MD: U.S. Department of Health and Human Services, Public Health Service, Office of the Surgeon General.

Ussher, M., Stanbury, L., Cheeseman, V., & Faulkner, G. (2007). Physical activity preferences and perceived barriers to activity among persons with severe mental illness in the United Kingdom. *Psychiatric Services, 58,* 405–408.

Wilkinson, R., & Marmot, M. (2003). *Social determinants of health: The solid facts* (2nd ed.). Geneva: World Health Organization Regional Office for Europe.

Williams, J., Ziedonis, D., Speelman, N., Vreeland, B., Zechner, M., Rahim, R., et al. (2005). *Learning about healthy living: Tobacco and you manual.* Trenton: New Jersey Division of Mental Health Services.

CHAPTER 4

Evidence-Based Practice: Conducting and Understanding Evidence-Based Reviews

Robert W. Gibson, PhD, OTR/L;
Mariana D'Amico, EdD, OTR/L, BCP;
and Lynn Jaffe, ScD, OTR/L

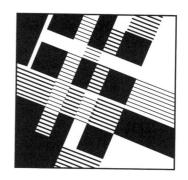

Learning Objectives

After reading this material and completing the examination, readers will be able to

- Identify the components of evidence-based clinical decision making;

- Identify how to transform a clinical question or problem into a person–population–problem, intervention–prognostic factor, comparison intervention, and outcome (PICO) question;

- Identify search terms to complete an evidence-based search of the literature and determine how they can best be used;

- Identify the strength of evidence discussed in research studies; and

- Recognize how evidence is organized into critically appraised papers (CAPs) and critically appraised topics (CATs) to support intervention decisions.

This chapter is designed to acquaint you with the process of finding and evaluating evidence to support the advanced practice and interventions discussed in the remainder of this self-study. It will also assist you in sharing evidence-based information by developing your own evidence-based reviews. As you read the chapter and complete the learning activities, you will become acquainted with a model of evidence-based practice (EBP); learn how to generate evidence-based questions; become familiar with evidence-based resources; and find evidence, organize it, and assess its value.

The practice of medicine in general and occupational therapy specifically have increasingly called for clinical decision making and practice that is grounded in and substantiated by evidence. *Evidence-based medical practice* has been defined as the "conscientious, explicit, and judicious use of current best evidence in making decisions about the care of individual clients. The practice of evidence-based medicine means integrating individual clinical expertise with the best available external clinical evidence from systematic research" (Sackett, Rosenberg, Gray, Haynes, & Richardson, 1996, p. 71). The occupational therapy profession's embrace of evidence-based medicine can be seen in the recurring Evidence-Based Practice Forum in the *American Journal of Occupational Therapy* from 1999 through 2004 and a variety of publications including works by Taylor (2007), Dunn (2008), and Law and MacDermid (2008). In addition, the American Occupational Therapy Association (AOTA) and the American Occupational Therapy Foundation (AOTF), with funds from the Agency for Healthcare Research and Quality, cosponsored an international EBP conference (AOTA, 2004; Coster, 2005).

It is no surprise to most occupational therapists that the efficacy of many traditional occupational therapy interventions, especially those used in mental health practice, are not well substantiated by research. Although this lack of evidence presents a challenge, it also provides an opportunity and some might say an obligation for occupational therapists working in mental health, especially those with experience, to begin to rectify this absence. Despite the perception that limited evidence supports many occupational therapy interventions, a wide array of mental health research literature does exist. Within that research literature, many studies can provide support for occupational therapy clinical decision making and practice. Therefore, knowing how to effectively search for existing research, evaluate it, and use it to support practice decisions is important.

Some of you who are completing this chapter may have experience with EBP, and others may be unfamiliar with this approach to clinical care. For those occupational therapists who are familiar with EBP, this chapter can serve as a review. You are encouraged to read the chapter and review the resources, especially the online resources. Bookmark these resources in your Internet browser for future use. This chapter can also serve as a prompt for you to complete some evidence-based reviews of your own. If, however, you are unfamiliar with the topic of EBP, this chapter and the accompanying resources will serve as a step-by-step introduction to EBP and provide you with the opportunity to develop the skills necessary to begin using evidence effectively in your clinical practice.

Model of Evidence-Based Practice

Often when clinicians first hear about EBP, they immediately think of research studies and their findings. In the early literature about EBP, research evidence was often singularly prioritized in the clinical decision-making process. Over time, this prioritization has changed, and EBP proponents have refined the way in which various types of evidence can be used most effectively in practice. Haynes, Devereaux, and Guyatt (2002) represented the process of evidence-based decision making with the model found in Figure 4.1. This model of evidence-based decision making is composed of four elements: (1) the client's clinical state and the circumstances or clinical setting, (2) the client's preferences and actions, (3) the research evidence, and (4) the provider's clinical expertise. The *client's clinical state and circumstances* include all the diagnostic information and the available intervention resources. The *client's preferences* include the client's values, prior experience, aversion to risk, family resources, and other unique attributes. *Research evidence* includes the results of systematic observations of clinical and laboratory studies. This model differs from other

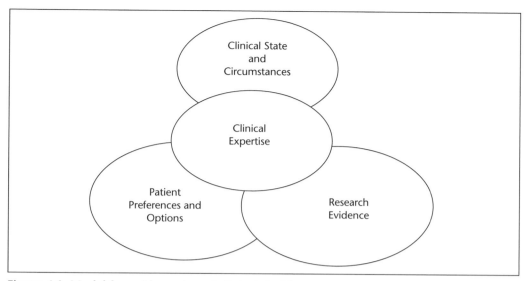

Figure 4.1. Model for evidence-based clinical decisions.

Source. From "Clinical Expertise in an Era of Evidence-Based Medicine and Patience Choice," by R. B. Haynes, P. J. Devereaux, and G. H. Guyatt, 2002, *Vox Sanguinis, 83*(Suppl. 1), p. 384. Copyright © 2002 by John Wiley & Sons. Used with permission.

approaches to evidence-based decision making because *clinical expertise* assumes an integrating role, balancing information from each of the three previously described components to reach a unified and practical intervention approach that best addresses the client's needs in the current intervention context. To be successful, this model of EBP relies heavily on the clinical expertise of advanced occupational therapists. In this model, evidence does not replace experience or expertise; rather, the two are used together along with client preferences to achieve excellent client-centered care.

The remainder of this chapter will take you through the steps of creating an evidence-based question, finding evidence to answer your question, demonstrating ways to organize and evaluate evidence, and applying your evidence to practice. The steps in this process are modeled by developing and answering an evidence-based mental health practice question. We suggest that you follow along and replicate the process with a question of your own.

Creating an Evidence-Based Question

EBP begins with a well-formed question that encapsulates the specific population or clinical problem and the range of choices or interventions being considered. Evidence-based medicine generally uses one of four archetypical questions that address all aspects of health research. These questions can be used to help determine the best therapy, diagnosis or screening process, etiology, and prognosis of a specific illness. Feeling that these questions did not adequately address the evidence needs of occupational therapists, Tickle-Degnen (1999) proposed the use of three types of questions more relevant to occupational therapy practice. Specifically, these questions address finding descriptive information about health conditions, determining the appropriateness and quality of assessments, and evaluating the effectiveness of interventions. The writing of EBP questions has been formalized. The format for evidence-based questions

Box 4.1. Three Forms of an Evidence-Based Question

	PICO			
	Population–Person	Intervention	Comparison intervention (if applicable)	Outcome
Terms:	Adults with schizophrenia	Skills training	A comparison intervention was not selected.	Increased ability to manage homemaking tasks
Descriptive question:	What is the percentage of adults with schizophrenia who are able to complete homemaking tasks independently?			
Assessment question:	Which is a reliable, valid, and relevant assessment of homemaking task skills for an adult with schizophrenia?			
Intervention question:	For adults with schizophrenia, is skill training an effective method for achieving independence in homemaking tasks?			

is referred to by the abbreviation *PICO* (*p*erson–population–problem, *i*ntervention–prognostic factor, *c*omparison intervention, and *o*utcome). Substituting the specific information relevant to your question for each component begins to focus your search for information. The PICO format works best for evidence-based questions evaluating interventions; however, the format can be modified to find descriptive and evaluative information. Box 4.1 provides an example of an evidence-based question written out in the three different forms suggested by Tickle-Degnan (1999). Multiple resources, listed at the end of this chapter under Web Resources, are available that describe this process in more detail.

Take some time to practice developing PICO questions. Begin with a clinical question that you would like to address. Identify whether this question is focused on descriptive information about an illness or condition, some aspect of an assessment, or the efficacy of an intervention. The example described in this chapter focuses on an intervention question, but the process is generally the same for the other two types of questions. First, state the problem and the specific clinical population that you are interested in. Second, list the specific intervention or interventions you want to know about. Third, if you are comparing two interventions, list the alternative intervention. Fourth, state the intended outcome, such as a change in behavior or level of accomplishment or success. Once your question has been developed and refined, you are ready to begin the search for evidence. Throughout this lesson, the following evidence-based question is used as an example: For adults with schizophrenia, is skill training an effective method for achieving independence in homemaking skills?

Finding Evidence

Before the advent of the Internet, therapists' search for evidence was often limited to the references on their shelves or the books and journals they could access at a local library. The range of information was limited; however, the process of gathering evidence seemed manageable. With the advent of the Internet and an increasing number of online medical resources, the amount of medical information and evidence available to health care practitioners and consumers has grown phenomenally. Now you can choose a topic of interest and search for it on the Internet, and a plethora of related and unrelated information is listed on your computer screen in seconds. Although the search for evidence is now much easier, extensive review is needed to identify the information's legitimacy, quality, and relevance and get to the articles or research of importance. The strength of the evidence you use to support practice is important. Peer-reviewed research and publications are considered more trustworthy and should serve as the basis for your decision making. When these are not available, you may need to use other, less reliable sources such as expert opinion. A good starting point is to limit the amount of citations and abstracts that needs to be reviewed by considering both the search terms you will use and the places you will search. Searching for scholarly information on the Web is a skill that can be improved with both planning and practice.

Basic Search Strategies

Carefully choosing search terms allows you to find the most relevant research with the least amount of distracting or unnecessary information. Search engines specifically designed for literature searches often provide three typical approaches to searching: by journal, author, or key words. If you are familiar with the literature, you may know of journals that frequently publish research on the topic of interest or you may know of a particular researcher who has written extensively on it. If so, the journal and author approaches will get you started but may sacrifice comprehensiveness and not gather all the research pertinent to your question.

The first place to look for key words or search terms is in your PICO question. Your PICO question identified the population or diagnostic group and the interventions of interest. These terms can serve as your initial search terms. You can refine these terms further by converting them to medical subject headings, or MeSH terms, their commonly used name. Note that not all electronic databases use MeSH terms.

The home page of the PubMed site (www.ncbi.nlm.nih.gov/pubmed/) offers access to the MeSH database and three brief training videos that detail how to convert your topic of interest into MeSH search terms. MeSH search terms can be combined using conjunctions such as *and, or,* and *not. And* used in the phrase "schizophrenia and substance abuse" should produce a list of references that contain both search terms. If, however, you used *or* as the conjunction, references that use either search term would be listed. In the example "schizophrenia not substance abuse," *not* is used to exclude articles that relate to substance abuse. Advanced search features allow you to use check boxes to further limit your search to a specific sex or age of participants, language, or type of research. You can also limit the number of articles retrieved by limiting the range of publication, such as in the past 5 or 10 years. If you are uncertain how much literature is available, begin your search using the broadest categories. If this search produces more than 100 articles, explore ways to limit your search by increasing the number of *search parameters,* or restrictions that you can impose on your search to make it more focused, such as type of research, number of years, or specific journals. If, however, your search reveals few or unrelated articles, reexamine your search terms, revise or expand them, and decrease the limits on the search. Your goal in adjusting your search parameters is to develop a list of articles that you can review one at a time to determine their relevance to your research question. This number will vary by search topic and your willingness to review retrieved articles. A good number to aim for is usually between 10 and 20 citations. Once you have a list of citations, begin to review the titles and abstracts, discarding those that are irrelevant to your question.

Additional Search Strategies

Once you have found some research articles on your topic of interest, you can use these articles to identify additional or related search terms. You can also review the reference lists of these articles to identify other related articles. Searching from multiple perspectives such as topic, MeSH heading, journal, and author will make it more likely that you will find the information you are looking for. Although there is no way to know for certain that you have found all the relevant research on a specific topic, when the same references keep coming up in your searches, it is safe to assume that you have found the core research on this topic and you can move on to the next step in the process. The following search terms were used for the example question, "For adults with schizophrenia, is skills training an effective method for achieving independence in homemaking tasks?": *schizophrenia, adults, skills training, independent living, home management,* and *evidence.*

Places to Search

The preceding example demonstrated a PubMed search, but many other search engines and databases are available, including EBSCOhost, ProQuest, Ovid, and LexisNexis. Collections of literature include the Cumulative Index to Nursing and Allied Health Literature (CINAHL), Education Resources Information Center (ERIC), PsycINFO (for psychology literature), the Cochrane Collaboration, and the Sociological Collection, to name but a few. Many of these sources require subscriptions, but they are usually accessible in a college library. PubMed, however, is a freely available database. Search engines specific to each library and library system also allow for database searches. Many college libraries will allow public access for an hour at a time. Note that many journals embargo online access to full-text articles or journals for 6 months to a year, even if you are a paid subscriber. You might have access to the abstract but not to the whole article, which may be available for purchase through the publisher (e.g., Elsevier Science, Walters Kluwer, Wiley InterScience).

In addition to the databases listed earlier, many occupational therapy–specific resources are now available on the Web. The resource list at the end of this chapter lists some Web sites, electronic mailing lists, and discussion groups that may be population or diagnosis specific. These sites will often include lists of articles, books, or other Web sites that contain valuable resources. AOTA provides evidence-based services that can be accessed from its Web site. From www.aota.org, choose the Practitioners link and then choose Evidence-Based Practice and Research, which will take you to helpful EBP information. You can also access OT Search, a fee-based search engine. OT Search will allow you to search the AOTF's Wilma West Library. Another wonderful free site for high-quality information and access to other databases is www.otseeker.com. This site is a joint effort by two Australian universities to make available evidence-based data for use by practitioners, and it includes links to databases such as the Physiotherapy Evidence Database (www.pedro.fhs.usyd.edu.au/), or as it is commonly known, PED*ro,* and to other occupational therapy resources.

One final note about searches: It is important to keep a detailed record of your search strategy, including terms, search engines used, and results, for future use such as updating a search or if you intend to create a systematic review on a topic that you would like to share or publish. This information on where and how you searched contributes to the reliability and validity of your work. At the end of your search, you will have either a stack of printed research articles or electronic PDFs saved in a folder on your computer.

We searched OT Search with the term *schizophrenia*. OT Search only allows the use of one search term at a time. That search yielded 292 resources from 1911 through 2008. To make the number of articles manageable and relevant to our question, we limited the years of our search to 2004 to 2008, which produced 35 articles. We repeated the search using EBSCOhost. This search was conducted using all the search terms listed earlier and a 10-year time span (1998–2008). This search yielded 27 references from four databases (Psychology and Behavioral Sciences Collection, CINAHL, Academic Search Complete, and Research Library). An additional search using just CINAHL, again with the same terms and 10-year time span, yielded 28 references. Results from the different databases can vary widely. It is important to consider the focus of the literature in a particular database when making a choice. The next step will be to organize and evaluate this research to help you answer your PICO question.

Organizing and Evaluating Evidence

We recommend that you use a three-ring binder to organize the paper copies of articles you have found. Now that many journal articles are available in PDF form, however, we suggest that you consider using Zotero to organize them. Zotero is a free, open-source bibliographic program that runs in the Firefox Web browser. It will hold and link references, documents, pictures, and snapshots of Web pages and search for source articles. Its features, such as notes, internal search, and organization, will work offline, although in the online mode you have more functionality. Full documentation and video tutorials are on the Zotero Web site. There is also a plug-in for integrating your collection with Microsoft Word. Begin by downloading the Mozilla Firefox browser from www.mozilla.com/en-US/firefox/all.html, and then add in Zotero from www.zotero.org

Depending on the results of your search, you may now have many articles that present with a variety of research designs, quality, and outcomes. It is important to use the most rigorous research available to help answer your PICO question. Evaluating evidence has become increasingly standardized, and several research rating systems now exist. Members of the Centre for Evidence-Based Medicine at the University of Oxford were the first to create a simple scale of evidence levels that depicted quality of evidence by study design. This classification has been modified, updated, and enhanced by colleagues around the world to make the classifications applicable to various health disciplines (Law & MacDermid, 2008). This system of levels of evidence is frequently depicted as a pyramid (see Figure 4.2), with the most rigorous study design at the top and decreasing strength of evidence as you move toward the base. The evidence pyramid in Figure 4.2 is reflective of the ratings typically used in medicine and applies solely to the type of research design. The levels depicted in the pyramid are often identified by the Roman numerals I through V, with I representing the strongest evidence and V the weakest. Although general agreement regarding the hierarchy of evidence exists, the use or labeling of the levels by Roman numerals will vary from rating system to rating system. Rating systems will sometimes further subdivide these categories by features of the study design

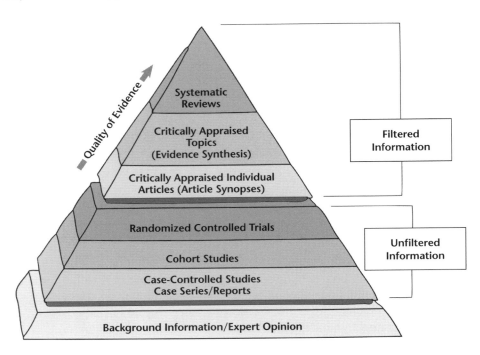

Figure 4.2. Evidence pyramid.

Source. From EBM Pyramid and EBM Page Generator. Produced by Jan Glover, Dave Izzo, Karen Odato, and Lei Wang. Copyright © 2006 by the Trustees of Dartmouth College and Yale University. All rights reserved. Retrieved from www. ebmpyramid.org/home.php. Used with permission.

or sample. Some evidence-based reviews often limit the research used to Levels I through III. For a more detailed description of each type of evidence, see Figure 4.3 and the University of Buffalo Web Resource link at the end of the chapter.

Note that within the various health professions, you may need to use different types or less rigorous sources of information to support clinical decision making and practice. Some areas of intervention may not have evidence at Levels I or II, so studies in Levels III through V become more important. Additionally, it is important to note the position of qualitative research. Quantitative approaches are prioritized within biomedical outcomes research. This type of research is conducted to predict and generalize about populations at large. Qualitative research is often not suitable to answer these types of questions and is therefore rated low in this context. Qualitative research can have greater strength than other types of research in other contexts or for other types of questions.

Qualitative research is derived from different theoretical perspectives than quantitative research (see Taylor, 2007, for a more complete discussion). Qualitative research evidence is best suited to answering questions examining meaning, experiences, and cultural aspects of behavior, and it can be appraised as to its contribution to evidence-based decision making; however, one must use a different approach from that with quantitative research. To judge qualitative research, one must first evaluate the research itself. How well is it designed and carried out? Does the presentation of the results leave you with many questions, or do you have a comprehensive picture of what was studied? In conjunction with this overview, one must

Level I: Systematic reviews, meta-analyses, randomized controlled trials

Level II: Two groups, nonrandomized studies (e.g., cohort, case-control)

Level III: One group, nonrandomized (e.g., before and after, pretest and posttest)

Level IV: Descriptive studies that include analysis of outcomes (single-subject design, case series)

Level V: Case reports and expert opinion that include narrative literature reviews and consensus statements

Figure 4.3. Levels of evidence.

Source. From "From the Desk of the Editor—State of the Journal," by S. Gutman, 2008, *American Journal of Occupational Therapy, 62,* p. 620. Copyright © 2008 by the American Occupational Therapy Association. Used with permission.

evaluate the research for trustworthiness (Taylor, 2007). Taylor (2007) described four components of trustworthiness: (1) credibility, (2) transferability, (3) dependability, and (4) confirmability. *Credibility* refers to whether the researcher painted a true picture of the experience being studied. *Transferability* pertains to whether the results can be expanded or applied to other settings or groups. Establishing transferability is the responsibility of the person attempting to use the research. The researcher's responsibility is to provide sufficient detail and description to allow the reader to make connections between the research and its possible applications. *Dependability* refers to the consistency of the data. The methods should be clearly explained, including how the data were collected and analyzed. *Confirmability* pertains to the processes the researcher used to reduce bias in collecting and analyzing the data. The last step is to evaluate how relevant the research is to your question. Are there similarities between the settings, patient needs, or problems into which the research is providing insight? The more overlap there is, the more the research can contribute to your evidence-based decision making.

Realizing that clinicians tend to have little time to keep up with the burgeoning literature available to them, many health disciplines have created critically appraised papers (CAPs) and critically appraised topics (CATs) to help health care providers remain up to date with the current evidence without having to read all of the research. The CAP is a structured summary or table of a quantitative or qualitative research article. This synopsis typically contains the article citation; a brief description of the research design and sample; a rating of the design using the rating system described in Figure 4.3; and the methods, intervention, and outcome of the study. The CAT is a structured synthesis–summary of research articles on a specific topic. Similar to a CAP, a CAT contains a synopsis of the individual research articles but then goes further to weigh the evidence from multiple studies and conclude whether support exists for a particular intervention approach and the strength of that support.

Two examples of CAPs are found in Boxes 4.2 and 4.3. A link to AOTA Guidelines for completing CAPs and CATs is located in the CAPS and CATS Resources section at the end of this chapter. Samples of occupational therapy–related CAPs and CATs can be found on the AOTA Web site, in the *Australian Occupational Therapy Journal,* and in other online resources listed at the end of this chapter.

Box 4.2. Example of a Critically Appraised Paper

Clinical Bottom Line
- Comprehensive empirically derived pharmacological and psychosocial treatment is associated with greater reductions in negative symptoms and minor psychotic episodes and in stabilizing positive symptoms than optimal pharmacotherapy and problem-oriented case management alone for patients with recent-onset schizophrenia.
- Comprehensive treatment doubled the proportion of cases with excellent 2-year clinical outcomes, but 47% of cases remained in need of continuing treatment for their persisting symptoms and/or disability or risk of recurrence.

Clinical Population Recent-onset schizophrenia

Four-part question (PICO)
For adults with schizophrenia, is skill training an effective method for achieving independence in homemaking tasks?

Study

Citation
Grawe, R. W., Falloon, I. R. H., Widen, J. H., & Skogvoll, E. (2006). Two years of continued early treatment for recent-onset schizophrenia: A randomized controlled study. *Acta Psychiatrica Scandinavica, 114,* 328–336.

Critical Appraisal

Threats to internal validity	Present (Yes/No)	Comments
Random allocation	Yes	
Concealed allocation	No	
Intention to treat analysis	Yes	
Long enough treatment/follow-up	Yes	
Blinding	Yes	Outcomes rater was blinded
Groups equal at baseline	Mostly	Integrated treatment group had higher Global Assessment of Functioning (GAF) at beginning
Attrition less than 20%	Just	
Other threats		

Evidence level? I (AOTA)

Subjects
50 participants with recent-onset schizophrenia; 30 in IT group, 20 in standard treatment (control) group

Intervention/Method
Standard treatment. ST patients received regular clinic-based case management with antipsychotic drugs, supportive housing and day care, crisis inpatient treatment at one of two psychiatric hospitals, rehabilitation that promoted independent living and work activity, brief psychoeducation, and supportive psychotherapy.

Integrated treatment. IT patients were treated by a multidisciplinary team that was independent of the ST program. Pharmacotherapy and case management was similar to ST with a low caseload (patient–staff ratio approximately 1:10). In addition, IT cases received structured family psychoeducation, cognitive–behavioral family communication and problem-solving skills training, intensive crisis management provided at home, and individual cognitive–behavioral strategies for residual symptoms and disability.

Treatment in both groups was goal and problem oriented.

Results
Fewer hospital admissions in IT group and 53% vs. 25% better outcomes ($p < .05$); better adherence to psychosocial treatment in IT (97%) than ST (70%) group; improvements noted in positive and negative symptoms better in IT.

Additional Comments
IT group had a significantly higher baseline GAF score than the ST group ($t = 2.3$, $df [1, 4] = 48$, $p < .05$), but otherwise the study groups did not differ in any respect.

This was a 2-year study supporting a flexible, individualized approach to intervention that included pharmacotherapy and psychosocial treatments.

Box 4.3. Example of a Critically Appraised Paper (CAP) Using the American Occupational Therapy Association's (AOTA's) CAP Format

Citation: Grawe, R. W., Falloon, I. R. H., Widen, J. H., & Skogvoll, E. (2006). Two years of continued early treatment for recent-onset schizophrenia: A randomized controlled study. *Acta Psychiatrica Scandinavica, 114,* 328–336.	

	COMMENTS
LEVEL OF EVIDENCE	I (AOTA)
RESEARCH OBJECTIVE/ QUESTION	To determine the benefits of continued integrated biomedical and psychosocial treatment for recent-onset schizophrenia.
DESIGN ☒ RCT ☐ Cohort ☐ Single Case ☐ Before–After ☐ Case Control ☐ Cross Sectional	Two group random-controlled study; part of the International Optimal Treatment multisite project.
SAMPLING PROCEDURE ☐ Random ☐ Controlled ☐ Consecutive ☒ Convenience	
SAMPLE $N = 50$; mean age = 25.4; male $n = 31$, female $n = 19$; ethnicity, Norwegian	50 participants with recent-onset schizophrenia; 30 in IT group, 20 in ST (control) group

PARTICIPANT CHARACTERISTICS 18–35 years old	*Medical Diagnosis/Clinical Disorder* Recent-onset schizophrenia	*OT Treatment Diagnosis* Recent-onset schizophrenia		

OUTCOMES	*Measures*	*Reliability*	*Validity*	*Outcome—*	*Outcome—*
	Target psychotic symptoms; Brief Psychiatric Rating Scale; Global Assessment of Functioning (GAF)	Y/N Not addressed	Y/N Not addressed	OT terminology	ICIDH–2 terminology

INTERVENTION				
Description		*Who Delivered*	*Setting*	*Frequency/Duration*
Standard treatment. ST patients received regular clinic-based case management with antipsychotic drugs, supportive housing and day care, crisis inpatient treatment at one of two psychiatric hospitals, rehabilitation that promoted independent living and work activity, brief psychoeducation, and supportive psychotherapy. Integrated treatment. IT patients were treated by a multidisciplinary team that was independent of the ST program. Pharmacotherapy and case management was similar to ST with a low caseload (patient–staff ratio approximately 1:10). In addition, IT cases received structured family psychoeducation, cognitive–behavioral family communication and problem-solving skills training, intensive crisis management provided at home, and individual cognitive–behavioral strategies for residual symptoms and disability.		ST hospital outpatient services or local community general health services IT multidisciplinary team (not specified)	Community	ST not specified IT tailored to needs of patient; began with weekly hour-long sessions for 2 months, then at least one session every 3 weeks for 1st year; one session a month during 2nd year.

RESULTS	IT group had a significantly higher baseline GAF score than the ST group ($t = 2.3$, $df[1, 4] = 48$, $p < .05$), but otherwise the study groups did not differ in any respect. Fewer hospital admissions in IT group and 53% vs. 25% better outcomes ($p < .05$); better adherence to psychosocial treatment in IT (97%) than ST (70%) group; improvements noted in positive and negative symptoms better in IT group.

CONCLUSIONS
 Biases
   Attention
   Masking/blinding
   Contamination
   Co-intervention
   Dropouts
	Outcomes rater was masked. IT group had higher GAF at baseline. Similar low attrition rate for both groups.

Note. This is an abbreviated version of an AOTA CAP Worksheet.

Evaluating Your Search Results

Using the methods we have described, you can now organize, evaluate, and synopsize the research articles you found in response to your PICO question. As you read through the articles, sort them into three groups: one consisting of research articles specifically related to your PICO question, one consisting of articles that provide background or additional information related to your question, and one consisting of unrelated articles. As you read the research articles, you will want to summarize the information. These summaries can range from more formal and detailed CAPs or evidence tables to less structured notes. To learn more about CAPS, review some of the completed CAPs found in the Web resources at the end of this chapter and the two completed CAP examples in Boxes 4.2 and 4.3. Although the information included in CAPs is fairly standardized, the format and presentation can vary significantly, and each format has its own strengths and weaknesses, as can be seen in Boxes 4.2 and 4.3. The format you choose will be influenced by your own preferences and the purpose of the CAP.

If you are unfamiliar with the description of the types of research designs, consult a research text or check online for additional information. It is important that you evaluate what the researcher did as you review a study and complete the CAP. Did the researcher use appropriate measurement tools, were the study procedures valid and reliable, and were there missing participants? You can consult numerous online resources to assist you in further evaluating research. An excellent example can be found at the Centre for Evidence-Based Medicine's Web site (www.evidence-based-medicine.co.uk).

You can also summarize your reading in an evidence table. See Table 4.1 for an example using the AOTA evidence table. Each line of the table contains a different article. Evidence tables contain less detail than CAPs but still contain all of the pertinent research information.

After you have completed CAPs or an evidence table for the articles that you have read, it is time to compile the results of your review. Again, there are many ways to do this; this chapter describes two methods. Table 4.2 contains the Level III and higher results from the CINAHL search discussed earlier. This table provides a quick visual overview of the types and strength of the research found, including two meta-analyses, three CATs, two randomized controlled trials, and one cohort study. We did not include the one qualitative and three background articles in the table. This table makes it readily apparent that most of the research used to address the PICO question is the strongest type of evidence, Level I.

The second approach is to make a more detailed summarization table (Table 4.3) that lists each of the studies, the evidence level, and then whether the study provided supporting or contradictory evidence. Studies can be listed in order of the strength of their evidence. Then check the boxes to note whether the study supports, opposes, or is inconclusive regarding your PICO question. We used some of the same articles in Table 4.3 as in Table 4.2. After reviewing the information presented in such a table, you can write a summary of your results. When evaluating support for an intervention, remember to consider both the strength and the rigor of a study and its level of evidence. A limited number of well-done studies generally outweighs a larger number of studies that use less rigorous methods.

The next step in this process would be to write up your review in the form of a CAT. A CAT is now a common way to share a review of research examining

Table 4.1. Evidence Table

Author/Year	Study Objectives	Level/Design/ Participants	Intervention and Outcome Measures	Results	Study Limitations	Implications for Occupational Therapy
Grawe, Falloon, Widen, & Skog-voll (2006)	Evaluate benefits derived from continued integrated bio-medical and psychosocial intervention for recent-onset schizophrenia.	(Level 2) Randomized controlled study 50 people with schizophrenia	Standard treatment (ST). ST patients received regular clinic-based case management with antipsychotic drugs, supportive housing and day care, crisis inpatient treatment at one of two psychiatric hospitals, rehabilitation that promoted independent living and work activity, brief psychoeducation, and supportive psychotherapy. Integrated treatment (IT). IT patients were treated by a multidisciplinary team that was independent of the ST program. Pharmacotherapy and case management was similar to ST with a low caseload (patient–staff ratio approximately 1:10). In addition, IT cases received structured family psychoeducation, cognitive–behavioral family communication, and problem-solving skills training, intensive crisis management provided at home, and individual cognitive–behavioral strategies for residual symptoms and disability. Measures: Target Psychotic Symptoms; Brief Psychiatric Rating Scale; Global Assessment of Functioning.	IT group was superior to ST in reducing negative symptoms and minor psychotic episodes and in stabilizing positive symptoms but did not reduce hospital admissions or major psychotic recurrences. More IT patients had better 2-year outcomes than ST patients.	Difficulties in recruiting large numbers of recent-onset cases reduced the power of the study, and therefore the results of this study should be interpreted with caution. Major psychotic episodes and hospital readmissions did not differ in the two intervention conditions.	Occupational therapy skills and knowledge appear to be beneficial in the long-term functional outcome for people with schizophrenia on an ongoing basis.

Source. From "Evidence-Based Practice Forum—AOTA's Evidence-Based Literature Review Project: An overview," by D. Lieberman and J. Scheer, 2002, *American Journal of Occupational Therapy, 56,* 344–349. Copyright © by the American Occupational Therapy Association. Used with permission.

the effectiveness of an intervention. A CAT includes the steps described previously but goes further in the depth of analysis and synthesis of information and usually involves a large number of articles. Links to examples of CATs can be found in the resource list at the end of this chapter. Many opportunities exist to publish CATs either in print or electronically.

You are now at the end of the review process. Did the evidence you found provide an answer to your PICO question? Answers are not always as definitive as one might like; however, make a statement that summarizes what you found. Was there evidence to support the effectiveness of an intervention that was weak because it had not been evaluated with the most rigorous methods? Was there good evidence of the effectiveness of an intervention that was not applied to the population you are specifically interested in? Was there evidence that supported a different approach? Was the evidence generally weak and not really provide support for a change in practice?

Regardless of the outcome, draft a summary of your conclusion and share it with a colleague or present it as part of a department in-service or colloquium. Ask

Table 4.2. Results of Cumulative Index to Nursing and Allied Health Literature Search

Level of Evidence	Study Design and Methodology of Selected Articles	No. of Articles Selected
I	Systematic reviews (0), meta-analyses (2), randomized controlled trials (2), critically appraised topics (3)	7
II	Two groups, nonrandomized studies (e.g., cohort, case-control; 1)	1
III	One group, nonrandomized (e.g., before and after, pretest and posttest)	0
Total		8

Table 4.3. Summarization Table

Study Citation	Level	Supports Use of Intervention	Results Inconclusive	Does Not Support Use of Intervention
Anzai et al. (2002)	I	X Supports use of skills training but not specific to homemaking.		
Grawe, Falloon, Widen, & Skogvoll (2006)	II	X Supports use of psychosocial intervention.		
Kopelowicz, Zarate, Gonzales Smith, Mintz, & Liberman (2003)	I	X Supports use of skills training but not specific to homemaking.		

for questions and comments regarding your findings. Your peers' questions and comments will alert you to where you may need additional information and provide you with important feedback on your research.

What Does This Tell Me About My Practice? What Should I Do?

The last step in an evidence-based review is to apply the results to your practice. Thinking back to the opening discussion of the use and types of evidence, you should remember that the application of evidence must take into account the client's perspectives, awareness of the environment, and what it can support. It is important to ask yourself questions such as these: Is there enough evidence that your approach to intervention should be changed? Will this change be appropriate for the clients to whom you generally provide service? Is the environment, both physical and social, amenable to the changes necessary to implement this approach to intervention? Do you have the necessary resources or training to begin this approach? Are the theories that support the intervention consistent with those that you use in your practice?

If sufficient evidence of an intervention's effectiveness exists, begin to make the changes necessary to provide your patients with the most effective care. If you are going to change the way you practice, it is necessary to create a plan not only to implement the change but also to collect data for future outcome analysis. In this way, you can document outcomes of the intervention changes you have implemented. This process provides you with an opportunity to conduct clinical research at a practical level and to contribute to your profession's body of knowledge.

After tasting the victory of researching evidence, revising practice, and collecting outcomes data, the search for evidence and the generation of evidence from one's practice can become a fulfilling part of one's daily practice. In this manner, therapists continue to grow and provide benefits for their clients through the process of lifelong learning with practical application and evidence to support the beneficence and viability of occupational therapy.

Efforts from AOTA to support EBP began in 1998 (Lieberman & Scheer, 2002). From this initial effort, a variety of evidence-based support materials are now available on the AOTA Web site. The link to this portion of the AOTA Web site can be found in the resource section at the end of this chapter.

An important part of the effort to develop evidence-based materials to support practice is the Evidence-based Academic Partnerships. AOTA now works collaboratively with occupational therapy education faculty and, in some instances, graduate students to develop evidence-based reviews. Some of the most recent reviews have been on topics important to therapists who work in mental health. These reviews include the completed evidence-based review of interventions for people with substance use disorders by Stoffel and Moyers (2004), the forthcoming CAT that examines effective occupational therapy interventions to support and maintain participation and performance in paid and unpaid employment of people with mental illness (see Chapter 6 for information from this CAT), and a CAT that is examining the effectiveness of occupation-based interventions for people with significant behavioral health problems.

It is our hope that this introduction to the use and development of EBP information will encourage you to contribute to the growing body of intervention evidence in occupational therapy.

Acknowledgments

We acknowledge Peter Shipman, MLIS, assistant professor and outreach librarian at the Medical College of Georgia, for his assistance.

References

American Occupational Therapy Association. (2004). *International Conference on Evidence-Based Occupational Therapy: Summary report.* Retrieved September 5, 2008, from www.aota.org/Educate/Research/39451.aspx

*Anzai, N., Yoneda, S., Kumagai, N., Nakamura, Y., Ielguchi, E., & Liberman, R. (2002). Training persons with schizophrenia in illness self-management: A randomized controlled trial in Japan. *Psychiatric Services, 53*(5), 545–547.

Coster, W. (2005). International Conference on Evidence Based Practice: A collaborative effort of the American Occupational Therapy Association, the American Occupational Therapy Foundation, and the Agency for Healthcare Research and Quality. *American Journal of Occupational Therapy, 59,* 356–358.

Dunn, W. (2008). *Bringing evidence into everyday practice: Practical strategies for healthcare professionals.* Thorofare, NJ: Slack.

*Grawe, R. W., Falloon, I. R. H., Widen, J. H., & Skogvoll, E. (2006). Two years of continued early treatment for recent-onset schizophrenia: A randomized controlled study. *Acta Psychiatrica Scandinavica, 114,* 328–336.

Haynes, R. B., Devereaux, P. J., & Guyatt, G. H. (2002). Clinical expertise in the era of evidence-based medicine and patient choice [Editorial]. *Vox Sanguinis, 83*(Suppl. 1), 383–386.

*Kopelowicz, A., Zarate, R., Gonzalez Smith, V., Mintz, J., & Liberman R. P. (2003). Disease management in Latinos with schizohprenia: A family-assisted, skills training approach. *Schizophrenia Bulletin, 29*(2), 211–227.

---

*Reference is cited in an evidence table but not in the main text of the chapter.

Law, M., & MacDermid, J. (Eds.). (2008). *Evidence-based rehabilitation: A guide to practice* (2nd ed.). Thorofare, NJ: Slack.

Lieberman, D., & Scheer, J. (2002). AOTA's Evidence-Based Literature Review Project: An overview. *American Journal of Occupational Therapy, 56,* 344–349.

Sackett, D., Rosenberg, W., Gray, M., Haynes, B., & Richardson, S. (1996). Evidence-based medicine: What it is and what it isn't. *British Medical Journal, 312,* 71–72.

Stoffel, V. C., & Moyers, P. A. (2004). An evidence-based and occupational perspective of interventions for persons with substance-use disorders. *American Journal of Occupational Therapy, 58,* 570–586.

Taylor, M. C. (2007). *Evidence-based practice for occupational therapists* (2nd ed.). Oxford, England: Blackwell.

Tickle-Degnen, L. (1999). Evidence-based practice forum—Organizing, evaluating, and using evidence in occupational therapy practice. *American Journal of Occupational Therapy, 53,* 537–539.

Web Resources

American Occupational Therapy Association. Click on the Educators–Researchers tab, then on the Evidence-Based Practice Resource Directory link. Contains evidence briefs, CATs, and CAPS. www.aota.org/Educate/Research.aspx (members only)

Bandolier glossary of research and statistical terms. www.medicine.ox.ac.uk/bandolier/glossary.html

Institute for Research in Extramural Medicine, one of five research institutes of the VU University Medical Center, Amsterdam, the Netherlands. Their activities predominantly deal with research in primary care and public health, focusing on chronic diseases and aging. www.emgo.nl/

National Registry of Evidence-Based Programs and Practices, a service of the Substance Abuse and Mental Health Services Administration. www.nrepp.samhsa.gov/

OT Seeker, a database of abstracts of systematic reviews and randomized control trials at www.otseeker.com/. www.otevidence.info/images/Introduction.pdf

U.S. Department of Health and Human Services, Substance Abuse and Mental Health Services Administration. *A Guide to Evidence-Based Practices (EBP) on the Web* for the public; includes links for substance abuse prevention, substance abuse intervention, mental health intervention, and prevention of mental health disorders; can also be searched by age group. www.samhsa.gov/ebpWebguide/index.asp

University of Buffalo, Health Sciences Library. *Evidence Based Health Care: A Guide to the Resources.* Includes an introduction to evidence-based practice, a glossary of terms, information on subject headings, and links to databases. http://libweb.lib.buffalo.edu/dokuwiki/hslwiki/doku.php?id=ebhc_guide

University of Rochester Medical Center, Milner Library. *Nesbit Guide to Evidence-Based Resources.* A collection of links, organization, tutorials, systematic reviews, critically appraised topics, and related Web sites. www.urmc.rochester.edu/hslt/miner/digital_library/evidence_based_resources.cfm

University of Texas Health Science Center at San Antonio, Academic Center for Evidence-Based Practice. Basic information about evidence-based practice, plus links to multiple resources. www.acestar.uthscsa.edu/Learn_model.htm

CAPS and CATS Resources

American Occupational Therapy Association. (2008). *How to use the CATs and CAPs.* Retrieved February 12, 2010, from www.aota.org/educate/research/catsandcaps/howtousethecatsandcaps.aspx

McCluskey, A. (2003). *CATS: Occupational therapy critically appraised topics.* Sydney, New South Wales, Australia: University of Western Sydney. Retrieved February 12, 2010, from www.otcats.com/topics/index.html

New York Academy of Medicine. (n.d.). *About the EBM Resource Center Web page.* Retrieved February 12, 2010, from www.nyam.org/fellows/ebhc/eb_about.html

Occupational Engagement and Psychiatric Conditions

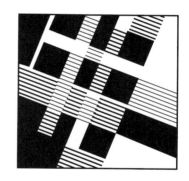

CHAPTER 5

Occupational Engagement of Children and Youth With Mental Illness

Renee Watling, PhD, OTR/L, and
Sarah Nielsen, MMGT, OTR/L

Learning Objectives

After reading this material and completing the examination, readers will be able to

- Identify symptoms indicative of mental health conditions in children and youth,
- Identify mental health conditions common among children and youth,
- Recognize factors that place a child at risk for developing mental illness,
- Recognize biomedical approaches used to treat symptoms of mental illness in children and youth, and
- Delineate the impact of various mental health conditions on the occupational performance of children and youth.

This chapter discusses the characteristics, prevalence, and biomedical approaches to managing mental health disorders that have onset in childhood and adolescence, the impact that mental health dysfunction can have on a child's occupational performance, risk factors for mental illness in children, and practice arenas for occupational therapists working with children and youth with mental illness. The chapter identifies medications that are likely to be encountered when working with this population, although the recommended medications change frequently. Because of its focus on biomedical interventions, the chapter does not include treatment techniques specific to occupational therapy; see Chapter 9 for a discussion of occupational therapy intervention for children and youth with mental health conditions.

Although the chapter presents diagnostic conditions as distinct categories, recent data have suggested that comorbidity of conditions among children and youth is more common than singular diagnoses (Jensen & Weisz, 2002). Occupational therapists should keep this pattern in mind when reviewing referrals for service and formulating evaluation and intervention plans for children and youth.

During the roughly 20 years of childhood and adolescence, children are expected to achieve specific developmental milestones, form secure attachments, establish healthy relationships, and develop effective coping skills. However, mental, emotional, and behavioral problems can affect the way young people think, feel, and behave and interfere with their success in daily life. Such problems are stressful for the child and family, and when left untreated, mental health disorders in youth can lead to school failure, drug use, violence, and even suicide (Substance Abuse and Mental Health Services Administration [SAMHSA], 2003a).

Mental health disorders in children and youth are more common than most people realize. Recent estimates have suggested that at any one time, as many as one in five children and adolescents may have a mental health disorder that requires treatment (SAMHSA, 2003a).

Affective Disorders

Depression

Description of Disorder

People once believed that depression did not occur in childhood. Today, experts agree that severe depression can occur at any age. In fact, studies have shown that at any point in time, 2 of every 100 children may have major depression and as many as 9 of every 100 adolescents may be affected (SAMHSA, 2008), which equates to approximately 10% to 15% of the child and adolescent population at any given time displaying some symptoms of depression (American Association of Child and Adolescent Psychology [AACAP], 2008), with about 5% of children ages 9 to 17 receiving the diagnosis.

Children with *major depressive disorder* may experience feelings of sadness, diminished interest in activities, declining performance at school, social isolation, extreme sensitivity to rejection or failure, and a self-defeating attitude (SAMHSA, 2003d; U.S. Department of Health and Human Services [DHHS], 1999). The symptoms of depression in children vary with the age of the child (Sadock & Sadock, 2004). Young children often exhibit withdrawal, sad appearance, poor self-esteem, and somatic complaints. In later adolescence, symptoms include pervasive loss of pleasure, sense of hopelessness, delusions, and severe psychomotor retardation. Symptoms of depression that occur across age groups include depressed or irritable mood, lack of energy or motivation, changes in appetite and sleep patterns, difficulty concentrating, and suicidal ideation.

Effect on Occupational Performance

Major depression in children and adolescents typically lasts from 7 to 9 months and can have serious effects leading to school failure, alcohol or other drug use, and even suicide. A family history of depression increases the chances that a child or adolescent may develop depression. Once a young person has experienced major depression, he or she is at risk of experiencing another depressive episode within the next 5 years. Estimates have suggested that 20% of children who experience and recover from depression relapse within 2 years, and 70% relapse within 5 years (Geller, Zimmerman, Williams, Bolhofner, & Craney, 2001; Sadock & Sadock, 2004). Moreover, 20% to 40% of adolescents with depression eventually develop bipolar disorder (DHHS, 1999; Dopheide, 2006).

Occupational performance in children and youth with depression can be considerably impaired. The depression affects motivation, energy level, and desire, resulting in a general lack of participation in activities the child previously found meaningful and enjoyable. A marked decrease may be seen in performance of activities of daily living (ADLs), educational activities, work tasks, play and leisure, and social participation. In addition, a lack of fulfillment of role responsibilities and participation in routines may occur as a result of the general passivity characteristic of depression.

Interventions

A comprehensive review (Kaslow & Thompson, 1998) of the effectiveness of psychosocial interventions for depression identified cognitive–behavioral therapy (CBT) characterized by a minimum of 12 sessions of group intervention involving training in social skills, assertiveness, relaxation, imagery, and cognitive restructuring as "probably effective" treatment methods. A second CBT approach that used training in coping skills was deemed "probably efficacious," and a more recent review revealed that CBT in conjunction with the antidepressant fluoxetine was the most effective treatment (Dopheide, 2006).

Dysthymia

Description of Disorder

Dysthymic disorder is characterized by occurrence of almost daily depressed mood for at least 1 year. This condition is more chronic but less severe than major depression. Dysthymia is seen in approximately 13% of adolescents and is characterized by low energy, sleep or appetite disturbances, and low self-esteem (Sadock & Sadock, 2004). The person may maintain many of his or her ADLs, such as personal care; however, the symptoms can be severe enough to interfere with fulfilling life role responsibilities (DHHS, 1999). The mean age of onset for dysthymic disorder in youth is 10 to 13 (Nobile, Cataldo, Marino, & Molteni, 2003). A dysthymic period in children and adolescents typically lasts for around 4 years (Kovacs, Obrosky, Gatsonis, & Richards, 1997; Sadock & Sadock, 2004). Research has shown that 70% of youth who demonstrate dysthymia eventually experience an episode of major depression, 13% experience bipolar disorder, and 15% go on to experiment with substance abuse (Kovacs, Akiskal, Gatsonis, & Parrone, 1994; Nobile et al., 2003; Sadock & Sadock, 2004).

Effect on Occupational Performance

The impact of dysthymic disorder on occupational performance is somewhat less than that of depression. Youth with dysthymia tend to maintain performance of ADLs and general participation in school and social events. However, chronic depressed mood can have an impact on motivation, energy, and desire to participate. In addition, emotional regulation may be affected, which can impede the social interactions needed for fulfillment of roles and social participation (Nobile et al., 2003). Social difficulties associated with dysthymia tend to persist beyond recovery from the condition (Klein, Lewinsohn, & Seeley, 1997).

Interventions

Treatment of dysthymia is similar to that for depression and includes CBTs and pharmacological interventions.

Bipolar Disorder

Description of Disorder

Bipolar disorder, also known as *manic–depressive illness,* is a brain disorder characterized by mood swings that alternate or cycle between periods of mania and depression. Bipolar disorder in youth is usually first manifested as a depressive episode. The first manic features may be suspended for a few months or even a few years (DHHS, 1999). In children, the cycles can be rapid, with the cycling sometimes occurring more than once in a single day (SAMHSA, 2005). The depressive phases are characterized by the traditional symptoms of depression, as described earlier. In contrast, the manic phases are characterized by high energy, confidence, and feelings of being special. Excessively elevated moods; periods of high, goal-directed activity; racing thoughts; erratic sleep patterns; and excessive involvement in extreme activities may also be present. Manic episodes can be especially problematic if the child's ideas about his or her capabilities become exaggerated or delusional. In adolescents, a lack of inhibition and overconfidence can lead to risky behavior, including fast driving, promiscuity, and general disorganization and recklessness (DHHS, 1999).

Bipolar disorder is estimated to affect at least 750,000 children in the United States (SAMHSA, 2005). Age of onset varies, and the disorder can occur in children as young as age 4 (Birmaher et al., 2009). A family history of bipolar disorder is a predisposing factor, as is a history of depression in adolescence. However, bipolar disorder among children and youth can be difficult to recognize and diagnose because its symptoms can be mistaken for those of other conditions (SAMHSA, 2005).

Effect on Occupational Performance

The impact of bipolar disorder on occupational performance fluctuates with the mood shifts. During phases of depression, when energy and motivation are low, the child is more likely to be passive and withdrawn, engaging less in daily activities. During manic episodes, occupational performance may be impaired in very different ways. Excessive energy and activity can make it difficult for the child to focus or maintain attention, demonstrate self-control, and see an activity through to completion. The child may begin projects that he or she does not finish, approach tasks in a chaotic fashion, and be unable to organize him- or herself to sustain engagement. The lack of inhibition can impede social interaction because of poor judgment and disregard for socially appropriate behavior. For example, children in a manic phase often become intensely focused on certain books or series of books that then dominate their activities and conversations to the point that they are unable to engage in activity or conversation on other topics. The swings between depressive and manic periods can be extremely difficult for people close to the affected child because the mood swings are unpredictable and the behaviors irrational.

Interventions

Recommended treatment for bipolar disorder includes both psychotherapeutic interventions and pharmacologic treatment. A natural fit for occupational therapists may be the recommended psychotherapeutic interventions (AACAP, 2007b), including educating the client and family, individual therapy to support psychological development and skill building for personal and social success, and educational or vocational supports to maximize success in school and employment. Medications include mood stabilizers (e.g., lithium, valproate) and antipsychotic agents (e.g., haloperidol, risperidone, clozapine; AACAP, 2007b). In addition, enrollment in a system of care may be recommended. A *system of care* is a network of community-based services and supports that coordinate with each other to meet the needs of children and families experiencing the effects of mental illness (SAMHSA, 2005). Effectiveness measures of systems of care for children and youth with bipolar disorder have indicated that service recipients show improvement in emotional and behavior functioning, including reduced conflicts with others, fewer contacts with the juvenile justice system, and improvements in academic-related activities.

Anxiety Disorders

Generalized Anxiety Disorder

Description of Disorder

Chronic excessive fear, worry, and uneasiness are common symptoms of anxiety. When these manifestations persist for long periods and substantially interfere with a person's ability to engage in daily life activities or be productive, an anxiety disorder may be present. *Generalized anxiety disorder* is characterized by extreme worry about everyday life events and occurrences (AACAP, 2007a). The worry causes feelings of tension and self-consciousness. Anxiety disorders have a combined prevalence that is higher than that of all other mental health disorders associated with childhood and adolescence (DHHS, 1999; Roberts, Roberts, & Xing, 2007). Estimates have suggested that 6% to 20% of 9- to 17-year-old youths have an anxiety disorder (AACAP, 2007a). Anxiety disorders include phobias, generalized anxiety disorder, obsessive–compulsive disorder (OCD), posttraumatic stress disorder (PTSD), and separation anxiety disorder.

Risk for anxiety disorders in children and youth is thought to be related to the person's temperament (SAMHSA, 2003b). Shyness and withdrawal in unfamiliar situations may be the first signs of risk for an anxiety disorder. A recent investigation of mental health conditions in preschoolers suggested that although fewer than 1% of preschoolers demonstrate obvious signs of generalized anxiety disorder, the actual prevalence of anxiety among preschoolers may be masked by disorders such as oppositional defiant disorder (ODD) and attention deficit hyperactivity disorder (ADHD; Lavigne, LeBailly, Hopkins, Gouze, & Binns, 2009). Researchers have suggested that ages 6 to 8 may be a window on the likelihood that a child will develop an anxiety disorder because during this period children typically show a decrease in fears related to darkness and imaginary creatures and an increase in anxiety about school performance and social relationships. Excessive anxiety during this time may possibly be a warning sign for later development of an anxiety disorder (SAMHSA, 2003b).

Effect on Occupational Performance

Children with anxiety disorders may experience disruptions in occupational performance because of preoccupation and worry about the source of anxiety. Fear of or worry about the unknown may prevent the child from participating in new situations. Concerns about being embarrassed or failing at a task can lead to frequent school absences, lack of social participation, and perfectionist tendencies (SAMHSA, 2003b). Other impairments may include low self-esteem, impaired social relationships, reduced play and leisure participation, and diminished role performance. In addition, children with anxiety disorders are often unsure of themselves and constantly seek approval and reassurance about their performance and their anxieties (American Psychiatric Association [APA], 2000). The child's anxiety also has an impact on the family. The child may resist daily tasks such as going to school or an appointment or refuse social participation such as attending family events or going to a restaurant for dinner.

Interventions

Treatment for anxiety disorders typically involves CBT aimed at modifying the way the child thinks and behaves about the situations that cause feelings of anxiousness, training in relaxation techniques, using biofeedback to control stress and muscle tension, and medications (SAMHSA, 2003b). In addition, parent training in strategies to support the child is often used. Pharmacological management of anxiety disorders includes selective serotonin reuptake inhibitors (SSRIs).

Obsessive–Compulsive Disorder

Description of Disorder

OCD occurs in approximately 1% of children and up to 2% of adolescents (Gilbert & Maalouf, 2008) and is characterized by recurrent obsessions or compulsions severe enough to cause severe distress, usually begins in adolescence or young adulthood. The obsessions are often unrealistic or irrational and characterized by recurrent and persistent thoughts, impulses, or images that cause the young person marked anxiety and distress. The compulsions are repetitive behaviors such as hand washing, hoarding, or arranging and rearranging things or mental acts such as counting or avoiding to the degree that they interfere with productivity (SAMHSA, 2003b). Often, the behaviors are performed in an effort to prevent the obsessive thoughts or make them go away (National Institute of Mental Health [NIMH], 2008c). Frequently, the young person recognizes that the thoughts or behaviors are irrational; however, the pattern becomes ritualistic and is difficult to stop. Research based on studies of first-degree relatives and twins has demonstrated a strong familial link in OCD (Gilbert & Maalouf, 2008).

Effect on Occupational Performance

OCD can have a considerable impact on occupational functioning. The obsessive–compulsive behaviors interfere with the child's ability to perform the normal routine, function in an academic setting, participate in social activities, or engage in relationships (AACAP, 2001). The child often feels shame and embarrassment about the OCD behaviors and may fear the stigma of being labeled with a mental illness.

Case Example of Adolescent With Obsessive–Compulsive Disorder

Sarah, a 16-year-old high school sophomore, is the last person in her family to leave the house in the morning. When preparing to leave, she repeatedly checks the coffee maker and toaster to make sure that they are unplugged, and then she goes through a routine of getting her coat and backpack from the closet, putting them on just so, placing her key in the lock and taking it out to make sure the key fits, turning the key in the lock with the door open to make sure it will operate the lock, and going halfway down the front steps, then returning to the front door to ensure that it is locked. Sarah has received many demerits for being late to school and is at risk for failing her first-hour course because of missing classes while checking on things at home.

Interventions

Treatment for OCD includes both psychotherapy and pharmacology. Psychotherapy often includes a type of CBT called *exposure therapy*, in which the person, with the guidance of a trained professional, works on becoming desensitized by facing the situations that he or she finds fearful (NIMH, 2006a).

Posttraumatic Stress Disorder

Description of Disorder

Although *PTSD* has traditionally been thought to be a disorder experienced by adults, research has shown that it is an appropriate diagnosis for some children who have experienced severe abuse or witnessed a horrific event. Other triggers for PTSD among children are living through a disaster, experiencing sexual abuse, or being a victim of or witnessing violence (SAMHSA, 2003b). Reliving the event through memories, flashbacks, and other troublesome thoughts is common in PTSD, and as a result, the child may try to avoid anything that he or she associates with the trauma. The child may also experience difficulty sleeping or become agitated if startled (SAMHSA, 2003b).

Research estimates have suggested that 14% to 43% of children have experienced at least one traumatic event and that PTSD may be diagnosed in 3% to 15% of these girls and 1% to 6% of these boys (AACAP, 2008a). Rates of PTSD correlate with the type of trauma experienced. Estimates have suggested that as many as 35% of youth witnessing community violence and 100% of children exposed to parental homicide or sexual assault may be diagnosed with PTSD (Hamblen, 2007).

Effect on Occupational Performance

PTSD presents differently in children at different stages of development and affects occupational performance in accordance with those stages. Very young children may exhibit symptoms of generalized fear, separation anxiety, and sleep disturbance that can interfere with patterns of engagement, social participation, and role performance. Play and leisure are affected when play scenarios take on themes of the traumatic event. In addition, children may regress in previously acquired developmental skills, such as toilet training (Hamblen, 2007). Elementary school–age children frequently develop the belief that warning signs predicted the trauma and that if they remain alert enough they will recognize warning signs and be able to avoid future traumatic events (Hamblen, 2007). Preoccupation with noticing warning signs can impede a child's engagement in all areas of occupation and interfere with performance patterns. For example, a child may constantly scan the room for potential threats, causing him or her to miss instructions for a task or interference with participation in group work activities. Adolescents are likely to incorporate aspects of the trauma into their daily lives, including reenactment of the traumatic situation, and may demonstrate impulsive and aggressive behaviors.

Interventions

Treatment for PTSD typically involves a cognitive–behavioral approach to psychotherapy in which the child talks about the traumatic event and learns anxiety management techniques and correction of inaccurate trauma-related thoughts (Silva et al., 2003). Another effective treatment for PTSD in youth includes play therapy, with some common forms being release play therapy and child-centered play therapy (Ogawa, 2004). Parent training is a key aspect of treatment. Research has shown that better parental coping and parental support for the child with PTSD leads to better child functioning (Hamblen, 2007).

Disruptive Behavior Disorders

Attention Deficit Hyperactivity Disorder

Description of Disorder

For a child to be diagnosed with *ADHD,* at least six symptoms of inattention or six hyperactive and impulsive behaviors must be present for at least 6 months (APA, 2000). In addition, the symptoms must be present before age 7 and must result in significantly impaired academic, social, or occupational functioning in at least two settings (APA, 2000). Although hyperactivity and fleeting attention are not uncommon in children, such behaviors occur with greater frequency and intensity among children with ADHD. Attention deficits may not be apparent until children enter school, at which time inability to sustain mental effort, complete schoolwork, and follow through on instructions becomes problematic for the child's success in required daily activities. Three types of ADHD exist: predominantly inattentive type, predominantly hyperactive-impulsive type, and combined type (Centers for Disease Control and Prevention, 2005).

Recent data have estimated that ADHD affects approximately 8.4% of children ages 6 to 17 (Pastor & Reuben, 2008). These statistics reflect a 3% annual increase between the years 1997 and 2006; youth ages 12 to 17 showed the greatest increase in incidence. Boys are twice as likely as girls to receive the diagnosis.

Effect on Occupational Performance

Occupational performance in children with ADHD can be significantly affected by the lack of attention and hyperactivity characteristic of the disorder. Distractibility interferes with completing tasks; impulsivity can infringe on the rights of others; and fidgeting and restlessness can be disruptive to others and impede the child's ability to focus. Completing homework can be especially difficult because of disorganization, lack of attention to detail, and difficulty focusing attention. Children with ADHD often fail to write down or remember relevant information; lose attention while retrieving needed materials, resulting in a deficient or inappropriate set of objects; and have difficulty organizing space and materials, compounding their challenges in completing tasks.

Interventions

Treatment of ADHD relies heavily on parent involvement, appropriate educational placement and supports, and pharmacology. Behavioral strategies, including systematic contingency management, are a primary component of intervention for children with ADHD. Both parents and teachers who have regular contact with children with ADHD should be thoroughly trained in these methods and in how to strategically exert high levels of environmental control. In addition, training children in problem-solving, social, and self-management skills can support success in daily activities. Pharmacology for ADHD typically includes stimulants, with the most commonly used medications being methylphenidate and dextroamphetamine (NIMH, 2008b).

Oppositional Defiant Disorder

Description of Disorder

ODD is characterized by an ongoing pattern (at least 6 months) of negative, hostile, and defiant behaviors typically directed toward authority figures. Common behaviors include openly defying adult direction, blaming others for one's own actions, refusal to comply with adult requests and rules, deliberately annoying others, mean and hateful talk, and temper tantrums. In addition, the person is often angry and resentful (APA, 2000; AACAP, 1999). Estimates have suggested that approximately 2% to 16% of all school-age children have ODD (Sadock & Sadock, 2004). Occurrence before puberty is more common in boys, but after puberty occurrence is similar between genders. The disorder is more common in adolescents between ages 13 and 16. Onset can occur as early as age 4 and continues to steadily increase through adolescence with a median age of onset of 12 years (Nock, Kazdin, Hiripi, & Kessler, 2007). Child-centered risk factors seem to be high reactivity, difficulty being soothed, and high motor activity. External risk factors include marital discord, disrupted child care, and inconsistent or unsupervised child rearing. ODD is associated with increased risk for other mental disorders during childhood (Burke, Loeber, Lahey, & Rathouz, 2005).

Effect on Occupational Performance

Occupational performance of children and youth with ODD is disrupted by their pervasive hostility and lack of cooperation with authority. These disruptive behaviors can cause significant difficulties with fulfilling family roles, participating in social situations, building healthy and productive relationships, engaging in productive activity such as school or work, and participating in cultural contexts (DHHS, 1999).

Case Example of Child With Oppositional Defiant Disorder

Stefan is a 9-year-old boy enrolled in a third-grade classroom. His teacher states that Stefan often has difficulty focusing on his schoolwork, following directions given to the class, and finishing assignments. He constantly fidgets with his clothing and does not sit still in his chair. When the teacher addresses his behaviors in class, Stefan becomes verbally defensive and accusatory, often stating that the teacher is being unfair. Stefan is sent to the principal's office a minimum of 4 times per week for disrespecting the teacher's authority and not complying with stated classroom expectations. His negativity and oppositional social interactions have resulted in a lack of functional peer relationships, declining school participation and performance, and reduced engagement in family and community activities.

Interventions

Treatment of ODD is similar to that for conduct disorder and includes parent training programs that teach behavior management skills, individual psychotherapy focused on anger management strategies, CBT to assist in problem solving, and social skills training to improve peer interaction skills (AACAP, 1999; DHHS, 1999; Sadock & Sadock, 2008). Pharmacological interventions have not been shown to be consistently effective for managing ODD.

Conduct Disorder

Description of Disorder

Conduct disorder is characterized by repeated violations of the personal or property rights of others (SAMHSA, 2003c) in addition to violations of the basic expectations of society. The diagnosis is given when symptoms are serious and persist for 6 months or longer. Symptomatic behaviors include aggression that harms or threatens other people or animals, destruction of property, theft, deceitfulness, truancy and other serious rules violations, and precocious sexual activity (AACAP, 2000; SAMHSA, 2003c). The main difference from ODD is that the disruptive behavior violates the rights of others.

Conduct disorder occurs in up to 10% of youth ages 9 to 17 (AACAP, 2008a) and is more common in boys than in girls. Incidence of the disorder in boys peaks around age 10. For girls, incidence increases between the ages of 10 and 16. Because conduct disorder is defined by cultural expectations, the ages and incidences are expected to vary among cultural groups. Risk for conduct disorder is increased by such factors as neglect, abuse or violence, harsh or punitive parenting, separation from parents with an insufficient replacement caregiver, crowding, lack of social competence, and poverty (Sadock & Sadock, 2008; SAMHSA, 2003c). Generally, aggressive behavior in young children ages 4 to 5 is believed to be an early warning sign of an emerging disruptive behavior disorder (DHHS, 1999). ODD in children is sometimes a precursor to conduct disorder (APA, 2000)

Effect on Occupational Performance

Youth with conduct disorder usually have little concern for others and repeatedly violate the rules of society. Poor self-regulation can lead to impulsive behavior that conflicts with societal norms. The intrusive and destructive behaviors can impede occupational performance in the domains of education, work, play, and social participation. Performance at school often lags behind what is expected for the young person's age or IQ (DHHS, 1999). Young people with conduct disorder may shirk expectations associated with familial roles and develop habits and routines that are contrary to those generally accepted in the cultural and social contexts in which they interact. The offenses associated with conduct disorder often grow more serious over time. The following case example portrays conduct disorder's impact on the occupational performance of a youth.

Case Example of Child With Conduct Disorder

Felipe is in seventh grade. He is regularly late for classes, does not turn in homework or participate in learning activities, and is inattentive. Felipe regularly has verbal outbursts in class, begins arguments with other students, and has been caught defacing school property. He has been picked up by the police for truancy and is suspected of being involved in a residential burglary.

Interventions

Treatment for conduct disorder can be particularly challenging because of the uncooperative attitudes and distrust of adults that are commonly exhibited. Correlational studies have shown that the behavior and attributes of 3-year-old children are predictive of aggression in the same children when they are ages 8 to 13 (Morrell & Murray, 2003; Raine, Reynolds, Venables, Mednick, & Farrington, 1998). Therefore, treatment for conduct disorder should begin as soon as symptoms are recognized. Treatment varies with the severity of the behaviors and may include behavior therapy and pharmacology. Two intervention methods have been identified as well established: (1) a manualized parent training program that instructs parents in operant conditioning methods for rewarding desirable behaviors and punishing undesirable behaviors and (2) a videotape modeling program for parents (DHHS, 1999). In addition, providing high-intensity case management through multisystemic treatment, training the child in problem-solving strategies, enrolling the child in youth-focused community-based interventions, and instructing the child in anger management techniques can be helpful (Karnik & Steiner, 2007; SAMHSA, 2003c).

Schizophrenia

Description of Disorder

Schizophrenia is an uncommon but serious mental illness in children. Symptoms include hallucinations, withdrawal from others, and distorted sense of reality (AACAP, 2004). Additional symptoms are delusional or disordered thoughts, inability to experience pleasure, confusing television or dreams with reality, and having paranoid thoughts that people are out to get one (AACAP, 2004). Although schizophrenia affects only approximately 1 in 40,000 young people under age 12, it has been documented in children as young as 5 (NIMH, 2006b). Retrospective data have shown that most children who develop schizophrenia demonstrated delays in language, transient symptoms of pervasive developmental delay (e.g., rocking, posturing, hand flapping), and uneven motor development during infancy and early childhood (Mental Health America, 2007). Onset of schizophrenia most often occurs in late adolescence for males (mean age = 18) and early adulthood for females (mean age = 25; AACAP, 2008a). The symptoms and behavior of children and adolescents with schizophrenia may change slowly over time. Signs of the disorder that may emerge during adolescence include becoming more shy or withdrawn, talking about strange fears and ideas, seeming to be in one's own world, and saying things that do not make sense (AACAP, 2004). Additional symptoms include change in friends, irritability, sleep problems, and a decrease in academic functioning (NIMH, 2006b).

Effect on Occupational Performance

Occupational performance can be substantially impaired in children and youth with schizophrenia. The distorted sense of reality directly impairs the person's cognitive skills and can cause him or her to neglect performance of ADLs, fulfillment of roles as family member and student, and engagement in functional play and leisure activities. Time and energy may be directed to irrelevant or unimportant tasks. Shyness or general withdrawal behaviors can impair relationships and lead to lack of social participation.

Interventions

Schizophrenia is a lifelong disease that can be controlled but not cured (AACAP, 2004). A combination of individual and family therapy, medication, and specialized programs often make up the treatment of childhood schizophrenia (AACAP, 2004). Antipsychotic medications such as chlorpromazine, haloperidol, perphenazine, and fluphenzine are the first choice for treating schizophrenia's psychotic symptoms. However, side effects such as rigidity, persistent muscle spasms, tremors, and restlessness can occur. Newer atypical antipsychotics such as clozapine, risperidone, and olanzapine are also possibilities; however, each medication also has associated side effects, and some must be closely monitored for potential threats to the person's well-being (Mental Health America, 2007).

Autism Spectrum Disorders

Description of Disorders

Autism spectrum disorders (ASDs) is the name given to a group of related disorders in which the child has deficits in communication, impaired social interaction, and restricted and repetitive patterns of behavior and interests (APA, 2000; Filipek et al., 1999). ASDs are neurobiological disorders that impair mental, emotional, and behavioral capacities in approximately 1 in 100 children (CDC, 2009; Kogan et al., 2009). Although symptoms and severity vary widely, early signs of ASDs include lack of social smile by age 6 months; lack of joint attention by 9 months; failure to babble, reach, or wave by 12 months; no single words by 16 months; and no two-word combinations by 24 months (Johnson, Myers, & Council on Children With Disabilities, 2007). Diagnosis of ASDs is behavioral in nature because no specific medical tests for the condition exist. Diagnostic criteria specify that symptoms must be present by age 3. However, diagnosis can occur reliably as early as age 2 (Lord et al., 2006).

Effect on Occupational Performance

The broad range of deficits present in ASDs has implications for occupational performance in all areas. Among the most problematic issues are poor regulation of behavior, communicative and social deficits, rigidity, restricted interests, and lack of adaptive behaviors. Inability to communicate and emotional unresponsiveness impair relationships with family members and acquaintances. Impulsiveness and destructive behavior can interfere with participation in academic, community, and other social contexts. Children with ASD typically have delayed acquisition of self-care skills and often have restricted play skills. Sleep problems are common, as are food allergies or a restricted range of foods the child is willing to eat. Many children with ASDs also have mental retardation, which affects learning and independent functioning.

Interventions

Effective treatment for ASDs has its roots in behavioral methods, with early, intensive, and comprehensive services giving the best prognosis. Research has suggested that treatment should consist of frequent, highly structured, interactive sessions that focus on helping the child with an ASD to develop new skills, become more adaptive and flexible, and develop effective strategies for managing unusual or disruptive behaviors (AACAP, 2008b; Johnson et al., 2007). Services should include parent training in managing the child's behaviors and helping the parents to cope with the challenges of raising a child with an ASD (Mental Health America, 2006). Pharmacological treatment is sometimes recommended for the child with autism to help reduce problematic aggressive behaviors or address sleep irregularities. Some medications used with this population are risperidone, olanzapine, and SSRIs (NIMH, 2008a).

Risk Factors and Contextual Influences

Mental health disorders in youth are influenced by both biology and environment. Biological factors, such as prenatal exposure to alcohol, drugs, and tobacco; low birthweight; genetics; chemical imbalances; and damage to the central nervous system, place young children at risk for developing mental health disorders (DHHS, 1999). A family history of mental illness increases the likelihood that a child will develop a mental health disorder or other health condition. This increased risk may be from genetic predisposition or because a parent's mental illness can drastically impair his or her ability to care for the child, resulting in significant neglect and the possibility of central nervous system damage. Such damage can result in a chronic health condition or impaired sensory processing, poor behavioral regulation, and ineffective coping abilities of the child. Chronic health problems in a child can lead to secondary emotional problems, including disordered interests, motivation, and play as well as emotional and behavioral problems (DHHS, 1999).

Environmental factors, such as poverty, extreme stress, deprivation, abuse, exposure to violence, and loss of an important person also can influence a young person's mental health status. In fact, several childhood conditions have been linked to environmental factors. Conduct disorder and antisocial personality disorder have been associated with severe parental discord, parent psychopathology, overcrowding, and large family size (DHHS, 1999). Economic hardship has been linked to behavioral disorders among children of parents who demonstrate stress-related mental health problems or child abuse (DHHS, 1999). Other environmental risk factors include caregiver disability, crime rate in the child's community, and social isolation. A variety of relational situations also can increase risk for mental illness; among those are family stress related to cultural and social issues and a destructive or damaging parent–child relationship.

Occupational Therapy

Occupational therapists can be key players in meeting the needs of children and youth with mental illness. Evaluation of occupational performance can determine the child's skills, challenges, and the contextual and environmental factors that influence behavior and performance (American Occupational Therapy Association [AOTA], 2008b). Intervention services help the child learn social skills, develop self-regulatory abilities, and develop strategies for supporting attention, organization, and stress management. In addition, occupational therapists work with the child, parents, teachers, and other service providers to develop strategies and programs to support the child's successful participation in meaningful occupations (AOTA, 2008a). Occupational therapists also work to promote wellness and prevent mental illness by helping children and youth build interaction skills, reduce bullying and school violence behaviors, improve organizational and sequencing abilities, and build competence in peer relationships.

Occupational therapists provide assessment and intervention services to young people with mental health disturbances in a variety of settings and contexts. Hospitals, private therapy clinics, public and private schools, and early education centers are common practice settings for occupational therapists. In keeping with current trends for bringing mental health services to clients rather than having clients come to a specialized location, occupational therapists are increasingly providing services through community-based programs such as mental health treatment centers, domestic violence and homeless shelters, and day care settings (AOTA, 2008a). In addition, private practices specializing in occupational therapy addressing the needs of children and youth with mental health issues are growing (AOTA, 2008b).

An overarching theme of service provision for children and youth with mental illness is working toward recovery (SAMHSA, 2008). *Individual recovery* is defined according to each person's characteristics and condition. For some, recovery includes living a fulfilling and productive life despite disability, and for others recovery focuses on the reduction or remission of symptoms (Gray, 2005). Occupational therapy services often use personal adaptation, environmental modification, and skill building to improve the functioning of their clients with mental illness (AOTA, 2008a; Champagne, 2005; Gray, 2005).

Contextual influences of the educational and social community also affect children's mental well-being. Factors include experiences of success and failure and acceptance or rejection, resistance or compliance with peer pressure, and perceived and imposed roles within various contexts and social structures. Additional factors related to developmental progression and adjusting to new life stages also have bearing on young people's mental health and well-being and should be attended to by occupational therapists.

Children and youth are members of families, school communities, peer groups, and other social networks. As such, children are dependent on their communities to ensure that their needs are met in a way that supports healthy lifestyles and wellness, including mental health. Parents are crucial in the success of any program aimed at children and youth. Families and communities, working together, can help meet the needs of children and adolescents with mental disorders.

References

American Academy of Child and Adolescent Psychiatry. (1999). *Children with oppositional defiant disorder* (Facts for Families No. 72). Washington, DC: Author. Retrieved from www.aacap.org/cs/root/facts_for_families/children_with_oppositional_defiant_disorder

American Academy of Child and Adolescent Psychiatry. (2000). *Conduct disorder* (Facts for Families No. 33). Washington, DC: Author. Retrieved from www.aacap.org/cs/root/facts_for_families/conduct_disorder

American Academy of Child and Adolescent Psychiatry. (2001). *Obsessive–compulsive disorder in children and adolescents* (Facts for Families No. 60). Washington, DC: Author. Retrieved from www.aacap.org/cs/root/facts_for_families/obsessivecompulsive_disorder_in_children_and_adolescents

American Academy of Child and Adolescent Psychiatry. (2004). *Schizophrenia in children* (Facts for Families No. 49). Washington, DC: Author. Retrieved from www.aacap.org/cs/root/facts_for_families/schizophrenia_in_children

American Academy of Child and Adolescent Psychiatry. (2007a). Practice parameter for the assessment and treatment of children and adolescents with anxiety disorders. *Journal of the American Academy of Child and Adolescent Psychiatry, 46,* 267–283.

American Academy of Child and Adolescent Psychiatry. (2007b). Practice parameter for the assessment and treatment of children and adolescents with bipolar disorder. *Journal of the American Academy of Child and Adolescent Psychiatry, 46,* 107–125.

American Academy of Child and Adolescent Psychiatry. (2008a). *Child and adolescent mental illness and drug abuse statistics.* Retrieved February 13, 2008, from www.aacap.org/cs/root/resources_for_families/child_and_adolescent_mental_illness_statistics

American Academy of Child and Adolescent Psychiatry. (2008b). *The child with autism* (Facts for Families No. 11). Washington, DC: Author. Retrieved from www.aacap.org/cs/root/facts_for_families/the_child_with_autism

American Occupational Therapy Association. (2008a). *Mental health in children and youth: The benefit and role of occupational therapy* [Fact sheet]. Bethesda, MD: Author. Retrieved from www.aota.org/Practitioners/Resources/Docs/FactSheets.aspx

American Occupational Therapy Association. (2008b). Occupational therapy practice framework: Domain and process (2nd ed.). *American Journal of Occupational Therapy, 62,* 625–683.

American Psychiatric Association. (2000). *Diagnostic and statistical manual of mental disorders* (4th ed., text rev.). Washington, DC: Author.

Birmaher, B., Axelson, D., Strober, M., Gill, M. K., Yang, M., Ryan, N., et al. (2009). Comparison of manic and depressive symptoms between children and adolescents with bipolar spectrum disorders. *Bipolar Disorders, 11,* 52–62.

Burke, J. D., Loeber, R., Lahey, B. B., & Rathouz, P. J. (2005). Developmental transitions among affective and behavioral disorders in adolescent boys. *Journal of Child Psychology and Psychiatry, 46,* 1200–1210.

Centers for Disease Control and Prevention. (2005). *What is attention deficit/hyperactivity disorder (ADHD)?* Retrieved August 14, 2008, from www.cdc.gov/ncbddd/adhd/what.htm

Centers for Disease Control and Prevention. (2009). Prevalence of autism spectrum disorders—Autism and Developmental Disabilities Monitoring Network, United States, 2006. *MMWR, 58*(SS–10), 1–20.

Champagne, T. (2005). Expanding the role of sensory approaches in acute psychiatric settings. *Mental Health Special Interest Section Quarterly, 28*(1), 1–4.

Dopheide, J. A. (2006). Recognizing and treating depression in children and adolescents. *American Journal of Health-System Pharmacy, 63,* 233–243.

Filipek, P. A., Accardo, P. J., Baranek, G. T., Cook, E. H., Jr., Dawson, G., Gordon, B., et al. (1999). The screening and diagnosis of autistic spectrum disorders. *Journal of Autism and Developmental Disorders, 29,* 439–484.

Geller, B., Zimmerman, B., Williams, M., Bolhofner, K., & Craney, J. L. (2001). Bipolar disorder at prospective follow-up of adults who had prepubertal major depressive disorder. *American Journal of Psychiatry, 158,* 125–127.

Gilbert, A. R., & Maalouf, F. T. (2008). Pediatric obsessive–compulsive disorder: Management priorities in primary care. *Current Opinion in Pediatrics, 20*(5), 544–550.

Gray, K. (2005). Mental illness in children and adolescents: A place for occupational therapy. *Mental Health Special Interest Section Quarterly, 28*(2), 1–3.

Hamblen, J. (2007). *PTSD in children and adolescents*. Retrieved May 15, 2008, from www.ncptsd.va.gov/ncmain/ncdocs/fact_shts/fs_children.html

Jensen, A. L., & Weisz, J. R. (2002). Assessing match and mismatch between practitioner-generated and standardized interview–generated diagnoses for clinic-referred children and adolescents. *Journal of Consulting and Clinical Psychology, 70,* 158–168.

Johnson, C. P., Myers, S. M., & Council on Children With Disabilities. (2007). Identification and evaluation of children with autism spectrum disorders. *Pediatrics, 120,* 1183–1215. doi: 10.1542/peds.2007-2361

Karnik, N. S., & Steiner, H. (2007). Evidence for interventions for young offenders. *Child and Adolescent Mental Health, 12,* 154–159.

Kaslow, N. J., & Thompson, M. P. (1998). Applying the criteria for empirically supported treatments to studies of psychosocial interventions for child and adolescent depression. *Journal of Clinical Child Psychology, 27,* 146–155.

Klein, D. N., Lewinsohn, P. M., & Seeley, J. R. (1997). Psychosocial characteristics of adolescents with a past history of dysthymic disorder: Comparison with adolescents with past histories of major depressive and non-affective disorders, and never mentally ill controls. *Journal of Affective Disorders, 42,* 127–135.

Kogan, M. D., Perrin, M., Ghandour, R. M., Singh, G. K., Strickland, B. B., Trevathan, E., et al. (2009). Prevalence of parent-reported diagnosis of autism spectrum disorder among children in the US, 2007. *Pediatrics, 124,* 1–9.

Kovacs, M., Akiskal, H. S., Gatsonis, C., & Parrone, P. L. (1994). Childhood-onset dysthymic disorder: Clinical features and prospective naturalistic outcome. *Archives of General Psychiatry, 54,* 613–623.

Kovacs, M., Obrosky, D. S., Gatsonis, C., & Richards, C. (1997). First-episode major depressive and dysthymic disorder in childhood: Clinical and sociodemographic factors in recovery. *Journal of the American Academy of Child and Adolescent Psychiatry, 36,* 777–784.

Lavigne, J. V., LeBailly, S. A., Hopkins, J., Gouze, K. R., & Binns, H. J. (2009). The prevalence of ADHD, ODD, depression, and anxiety in a community sample of 4-year-olds. *Journal of Clinical Child and Adolescent Psychology, 38,* 315–328.

Lord, C., Risi, S., DiLavore, P. S., Shulman, C., Thurm, A., & Pickles, A. (2006). Autism from 2 to 9 years of age. *Archives of General Psychiatry, 63,* 694–701.

Mental Health America. (2006). *Factsheet: Autism*. Retrieved July 11, 2008, from www.mentalhealthamerica.net/go/autism

Mental Health America. (2007). *Factsheet: Schizophrenia in children*. Retrieved May 15, 2008, from www.mentalhealthamerica.net/go/information/get-info/schizophrenia/schizophrenia-in-children

Morrell, J., & Murray, L. (2003). Parenting and the development of conduct disorder and hyperactive symptoms in childhood: A prospective longitudinal study from 2 months to 8 years. *Journal of Child Psychology and Psychiatry, 44,* 489–508.

National Institute of Mental Health. (2006a). *Anxiety disorders* (NIH Pub. No. 06–3879). Bethesda, MD: Author. Retrieved from www.nimh.nih.gov/health/publications/anxiety-disorders/nimhanxiety.pdf

National Institute of Mental Health. (2006b). *Schizophrenia* (NIH Pub. No. 06–3517). Bethesda, MD: Author. Retrieved from www.nimh.nih.gov/health/publications/schizophrenia/index.shtml

National Institute of Mental Health. (2008a). *Autism spectrum disorders, pervasive developmental disorders*. NIH Publication No. 08–5511. Bethesda, MD: U.S. Department of Health and Human Services. Retrieved February 10, 2010, from www.nimh.nih.gov/health/publications/autism/nimhautismspectrum.pdf

National Institute of Mental Health. (2008b). *Mental health medications*. Bethesda, MD: Author. Retrieved January 17, 2009, from www.nimh.nih.gov/health/publications/mental-health-medications/nimh-mental-health-medications.pdf

National Institute of Mental Health. (2008c). *Obsessive–compulsive disorder*. Retrieved July 10, 2008, from www.nimh.nih.gov/health/topics/obsessive-compulsive-disorder-ocd/index.shtml

Nobile, M., Cataldo, G. M., Marino, C., & Molteni, M. (2003). Diagnosis and treatment of dysthymia in children and adolescents. *CNS Drugs, 17,* 927–946.

Nock, M. K., Kazdin, A. E., Hiripi, E., & Kessler, R. C. (2007). Lifetime prevalence, correlates, and persistence of oppositional defiant disorder: Results from the National Comorbidity Survey Replication. *Journal of Child Psychology and Psychiatry, 48,* 703–713.

Ogawa, Y. (2004). Childhood trauma and play therapy intervention for traumatized children. *Journal of Professional Counseling: Practice, Theory, and Research, 32,* 19–29.

Pastor, P. N., & Reuben, C. A. (2008). Diagnosed attention deficit disorder and learning disability: United States, 2004–2006. *Vital Health Statistics, 10*(237).

Raine, A., Reynolds, C., Venables, P. H., Mednick, S. A., & Farrington, D. P. (1998). Fearlessness, stimulation-seeking, and large body size at age 3 years as early predispositions to childhood aggression at age 11 years. *Archives of General Psychiatry, 55,* 745–751.

Roberts, R. E., Roberts, C. R., & Xing, Y. (2007). Rates of *DSM–IV* psychiatric disorders among adolescents in a large metropolitan area. *Journal of Psychiatric Research, 41,* 959–967.

Sadock, B. J., & Sadock, V. A. (2004). *Kaplan and Sadock's concise textbook of clinical psychiatry* (2nd ed.). Philadelphia: Lippincott Williams & Wilkins.

Sadock, B. J., & Sadock, V. A. (2008). *Kaplan and Sadock's concise textbook of clinical psychiatry* (3rd ed.). Philadelphia: Lippincott Williams & Wilkins.

Silva, R. R., Cloitre, M., Davis, L., Levitt, J., Gomex, S., Ngai, I., et al. (2003). Early intervention with traumatized children. *Psychiatric Quarterly, 74,* 333–347.

Substance Abuse and Mental Health Services Administration. (2003a). *Child and adolescent mental health.* Retrieved July 9, 2008, from http://mentalhealth.samhsa.gov/child/childhealth.asp

Substance Abuse and Mental Health Services Administration. (2003b). *Children's mental health facts: Children and adolescents with anxiety disorders.* Retrieved March 20, 2008, from http://mentalhealth.samhsa.gov/publications/allpubs/CA-0007/default.asp

Substance Abuse and Mental Health Services Administration. (2003c). *Children's mental health facts: Children and adolescents with conduct disorder.* Retrieved May 15, 2008, from http://mentalhealth.samhsa.gov/publications/allpubs/CA-0010/default.asp

Substance Abuse and Mental Health Services Administration. (2003d). *Major depression in children and adolescents.* Retrieved May 15, 2008, from http://mentalhealth.samhsa.gov/publications/allpubs/CA-0011

Substance Abuse and Mental Health Services Administration. (2005). *Children's mental health facts: Bipolar disorder.* Retrieved March 20, 2008, from http://mentalhealth.samhsa.gov/publications/allpubs/sma05-4058/

Substance Abuse and Mental Health Services Administration. (2008, May 13). *The NSDUH Report: Major depressive episode among youths aged 12 to 17 in the United States: 2004 to 2006.* Rockville, MD: Author.

U.S. Department of Health and Human Services. (1999). *Mental health: A report of the Surgeon General.* Rockville, MD: U.S. Department of Health and Human Services, Substance Abuse and Mental Health Services Administration, Center for Mental Health Services & National Institute of Mental Health. Retrieved November 17, 2009, from www.surgeongeneral.gov/library/mentalhealth/home.html

CHAPTER 6

Occupational Engagement of Adults With Mental Illness

*Onda Bennett, PhD, OTR/L, and
Dana W. Logsdon, MS, OTR/L*

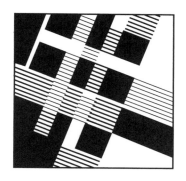

Learning Objectives

After reading this material and completing the examination, readers will be able to

- Recognize the course of severe and persistent mental illness (SPMI) and its effects on areas of occupation of work and education,

- Identify models of intervention that support recovery for adults with SPMI in the areas of work and education,

- Identify evidence that supports models of intervention in the areas of work and education for people with SPMI, and

- Identify the role of occupational therapy in the delivery of services to people with SPMI.

This chapter focuses on programs or services that are of particular importance in enabling people with severe and persistent mental illness (SPMI) to participate in the occupational areas of work and education. Occupational therapy has an integral role in the complex and developing service system to facilitate people's engagement in these essential areas of occupation. The chapter provides a brief description of the system supporting people with SPMI; a review of the literature in these important areas; and an in-depth description of day programs, skill training, vocational programs, educational programs, and volunteerism. Research supporting work and educational programs as effective interventions is drawn from a recent evidence-based review conducted as part of the American Occupational Therapy Association (AOTA) Evidence-Based Practice Project (AOTA, 2008).[1] This research provides up-to-date evidence for work and educational programs. In addition, the chapter provides a

---

[1] The evidence-based review was initiated as part of an Inquiry Team made up of faculty and students in 2006–2007. Student participants were Dana W. Logsdon, Anita Nolan, and Meghan Whitaker.

description of occupational therapists' roles and a discussion of what advanced practice occupational therapists can do in the future to facilitate the development of occupational therapy as a central factor in the recovery of people with SPMI.

Severe and Persistent Mental Illness

According to the National Institute of Mental Health (NIMH; 2008), serious mental illness affects a subpopulation of 6% of adults. *Serious mental illness* is a term that generally applies to mental illnesses that interfere in some way with social functioning. Approximately half of people with a severe mental illness are identified as being even more seriously affected by mental illness (NIMH, 2008). Such adults are considered to have SPMI, which includes schizophrenia; bipolar disorder; and severe forms of depression, panic disorder, and obsessive–compulsive disorder.

The current understanding of mental disorders points to multidimensional etiology of serious mental illness (U.S. Department of Health and Human Services [DHHS], 1999). Biological, genetic, psychosocial, emotional, and environmental issues have all been implicated in the ongoing progression of a serious mental illness. Exacerbation and remission of debilitating symptoms, including the negative symptoms seen in schizophrenia (blunted affect, apathy, alogia, anhedonia, attentional impairment) and other severe psychological and social deficits, are the hallmark of SPMI and underscore its debilitating effects in every area of functioning.

The typical course of an SPMI would begin with a long-term or repeated hospitalization (1–3 months) in which the primary intervention would be aimed at decreasing symptoms through medical approaches (DHHS, 1999). In addition, a multidisciplinary team would provide a thorough evaluation of the client's functional level and the network of services needed for community placement. In hospital settings in which occupational therapy services are provided, occupational therapists play an integral role in providing evaluation and intervention in functional and cognitive areas that might indicate the level of services and intervention that would eventually be required in the community. The focus of the hospital stay is to evaluate and prepare the person for a return to the community. When needed community supports are not provided, many people continue on a course of exacerbation and remission of symptoms and loss of functional ability. Although the family may be actively involved early in the process, a series of rehospitalizations may ensue and the person with SPMI may lose the family and other social support networks, vocational or educational opportunities, and functioning needed to support independent living. The service system has grown up around the overwhelming needs of a person with SPMI.

The serious and debilitating effects of SPMI lead to innumerable costs in both personal and economic areas over a lifetime. Intrusive psychiatric symptoms, low levels of social and occupational functioning, and a lack of independent living skills point to the need for a comprehensive system of services that will facilitate recovery to lessen the personal, economic, and social costs of SPMI. The National Institute of Mental Health (2008) has indicated that 15% of the burden of disease in established market economies is the result of serious mental illness. This issue alone should catapult services to people with SPMI to the forefront of health care issues. However, a history of pessimism about the chances for recovery of the person with SPMI has resulted in a concomitant lack of funding and community support. This problem continues, but recently hoped-for changes have occurred.

Although the historical view posits that people with SPMI have a severe disorder with little chance of symptomatic or functional recovery, a growing body of recent evidence is less pessimistic, indicating that recovery can indeed occur with appropriate intervention provided as early as possible and comprehensive, well-coordinated, and continuous services fully integrated into the community. This comprehensive service system would include programs and services geared toward the development of skills and supports in the social, daily living, and vocational–educational areas and a system of medical services and case management.

Service System

Over the past 3 decades, a service system for people with SPMI has evolved into an array of programs focused on providing supports and improving the functioning of people with SPMI in specific environments. Although recognition that there is hope for improved functioning in the community has grown, the service system has been described as being in disarray (President's New Freedom Commission on Mental Health, 2003) and as, at least in some part, a cause of the continued dysfunction of adults with mental illness. The service system frequently provides interventions that range from medical management and intervention to rehabilitation, but a lack of coordination across service systems and discontinuity within systems exists. Most recently, the Recovery Model has provided a foundation for services. Recovery of a person with SPMI implies a long-term, multidimensional process with the outcome of meeting one's potential for growth, healing, and community integration (President's New Freedom Commission on Mental Health, 2003). Contrary to historical beliefs, mental health professionals now have a strong and shared belief in the potential for positive outcomes in all areas of community living for people with SPMI.

Occupational therapy services, as with all mental health services over the past 2 decades, have undergone major changes as the paradigm for services has shifted from hospital to community and from medical model to rehabilitation and, more recently, to the Recovery Model. Occupational therapy has typically followed those shifts in a slow and methodical way, with little recognition of the major role therapists might play in the recovery of people with SPMI. Occupational therapy's involvement and the evidence supporting its role have been spotty at best, and occupational therapy's involvement in mental health practice has continued to decline (Brown et al., 2006). The recovery paradigm is only now being integrated as a transformational process for the mental health service system (President's New Freedom Commission on Mental Health, 2003). Medical, counseling, and case management services are provided, although in many instances they are not coordinated to provide effective supports for optimal functioning of people with SPMI. These services are designed to meet people's needs for opportunities to engage in the community and acquire the skills required to be successful and satisfied in daily living, vocation, or education. Interventions designed to facilitate the recovery process focus on the person, the environment, and their interaction.

The belief that intervention should be authentic and provided in the client's community has led to the development of a system of community-based programs.

A proliferation of psychosocial programs, skill training initiatives, housing options, and vocational and educational programs offer expanded roles for occupational therapy and its unique contributions to meeting the needs of people with SPMI living in the community.

Although the number of occupational therapists working in mental health is in decline, the need for occupational therapy's unique skills with this population will continue to expand from interventions focusing on the individual and family to those focusing on the service system or community. Using their skills to facilitate the development of vocational and educational outcomes, occupational therapists can be an integral part of the recovery process for people with SPMI.

Occupational therapy's fit with both the Recovery Model and community-based practice is evident. Occupational therapists assist people with serious mental illness and their families with meeting role responsibilities through a process of evaluation and intervention that considers the complex interactions among client, context, environment, and the client's occupations. Occupational therapy recognizes that those interactions result in the effective performance of occupations in context. For people with SPMI, developing the skills and obtaining the supports necessary for productive living are at the core of their ability to thrive in their preferred community setting.

This chapter focuses on the services that are of particular importance to people with SPMI for their participation in the occupations of paid and unpaid employment. Included in paid and unpaid employment are work, education, and volunteerism. Those areas of occupation are addressed by various parts of the system, including day programs, case management initiatives, various supported and sheltered work or educational programs, and in-home services. The program models, described in the next section, include a variety of combinations of interventions with many names, including assertive community treatment, clubhouse models, intensive case management, sheltered employment, supported employment, and other vocational and educational programs. Occupational therapy's role has been varied and context dependent but does include assessment, intervention, and consultation with the person, program, community, or system of services. Occupational therapy interventions, with their focus on the person, the environment, and their interaction, are a good fit with the emerging models focused on recovery. To explore that role fully, the chapter examines day programs and skill training that are precursors to targeted vocation- and education-specific programs. Finally, the chapter presents a discussion of vocational and educational initiatives designed to meet the needs of people with SPMI.

Program Overview

In the 1970s, community support programs were developed to complement the more established community mental health system. These programs provided varying levels of structure, support, supervision, and medical treatment or rehabilitation to maintain or rehabilitate people with SPMI. Community support services funded day programs, case management, transportation, housing, and a variety of other programs to maintain the recently deinstitutionalized patients in the community. The development of the programs resulted in an array of models designed to teach skills and provide the supports necessary to ensure the community tenure (and later success and satisfaction in daily living, vocational, and residential areas) for the person with SPMI.

The development of psychiatric rehabilitation as a model for skill training had a great impact on the development of day programs. This model focused on teaching skills and providing supports based on behavioral concepts and learning theory. The mission of psychiatric rehabilitation was to "help persons...improve their functioning with the least amount of ongoing professional supervision" (Anthony, Cohen, Farkas, & Gagne, 2002, p. 2). Boston University's Center for Psychiatric Rehabilitation, under the direction of William Anthony, designed and implemented a comprehensive training program and developed protocols and programs for staff providing services to people with SPMI. The information was disseminated through training programs, publications, and research. Frequent and ongoing research by the psychiatric rehabilitation movement has looked into the efficacy of using the model for people with SPMI. The center has provided resources, training, and models for development of services based on best practice and that are foundational to the recovery movement (for further information on the Center for Psychiatric Rehabilitation, go to www.bu.edu/cpr/). Occupational therapy is closely identified with the model's foundation of skill training, behavioral concepts, and learning theory.

The next section focuses on the variety of models developed over the past 3 decades. These models were used to provide services thought to best offer successful and satisfying outcomes to clients in their specific communities. Although psychiatric rehabilitation and its core elements were foundational to many models, the programs were context dependent and based on the philosophy or vision of the staff who worked in them. Differences in experience, professional orientation, and vision led to a variety of designs for the delivery of services.

Although individual differences were evident in programs, note that most effective programs shared common elements. They provided some type of psychosocial intervention or rehabilitation and skill training, and they frequently provided medical management, case management, and counseling services to clients and their families. In addition, a vocational component was integral to many, although not all, of these programs. This array of services, housed in the community, was frequently referred to as *psychosocial programs.*

The evidence supports the efficacy of psychosocial programs that include the common elements of rehabilitation, medical and case management, counseling, and vocation (Mueser et al., 2004). Randomized clinical trials have shown that participation in psychosocial programs resulted in fewer and shorter hospitalizations and had a moderate impact on symptomatology (Dilk & Bond, 1996; Penn & Mueser, 1996; Scot & Dixon, 1995). In addition, evidence supported that such programs had better vocational outcomes and lower recidivism (Bond & Dincin, 1986; Cook & Jonikas, 1996). The effectiveness of psychosocial programs continues to improve with the strengthening of their common elements and with increasing depth and complexity of the supports and rehabilitation provided in context.

The next section provides an overview of several of the major program models that have been implemented to meet the outcome of successful performance in the community. Performance areas and performance skills are addressed in these programs, both with and without occupational therapists providing that service. Paid and unpaid employment—including work, education, and volunteerism—are frequently integral components of these programs and are described in that context.

Program Models

Psychoeducational Model

The psychoeducational model was initially described in 1980 by Anderson, Hogarty, and Reiss. It focused primarily on the educational methods that would teach living skills (Cara & MacRae, 2005). People would attend classes and be given ample opportunities to apply and practice skills both in the day program and at home. Occupational therapists developed life skills programs or groups that included areas such as goal setting, stress management, budgeting, social skills training, and other instrumental activities of daily living (IADLs; Scaffa, 2001). In addition, occupational therapists provided consultation to programs developing curricula that could be used by other professionals in the program to develop skills. Today's day programs include many aspects of the psychoeducational model; however, few, if any, use this model exclusively to meet the variety of needs of people with SPMI.

Clubhouse Model

Fountainhouse was the first clubhouse model, and it served as the exemplar for club-type treatment settings (Beard, Propst, & Malamud, 1982). Clubhouse models are run by mental health consumers, called *members,* who are expected to be responsible participants in the club. They prepare the food and participate in the transitional work program and in the social aspects of the clubhouse environment. Work programs in clubhouses range from in-house cleaning, cooking, and administrative duties to transitional employment opportunities. (Transitional employment is described later in the chapter.) The philosophy is that all members need to work and be a part of a social support system, and the clubhouse provides those opportunities.

In the clubhouse model, occupational therapists can participate in both clinical and administrative roles. They might function as a program manager or a case manager. They might design and implement groups or participate in vocational assessment and planning (Urbanak, 1995). A significant role for occupational therapy would be in the development of transitional work and vocational programming (which are discussed later in this chapter).

Assertive Community Treatment

The assertive community treatment (ACT) model (also called Program for Assertive Community Treatment [PACT]) originated in 1972 in Madison, Wisconsin, in response to the deinstitutionalization of adult patients with a long-term history of SPMI from a state hospital (Allness & Knoedler, 1998). The patients had multiple needs for treatment, rehabilitation, and intensive support services to survive in the community. The ACT program provided a mobile transdisciplinary team of mental health professionals who provided those services to their clients in their homes, at their jobs, or in social settings (Allness & Knoedler, 1998).

The core service in this model is an enhanced case management program. The purpose of case management is to coordinate service delivery and to ensure continuity and integration of services for people with SPMI. Because of ACT's intensity and cost, it is typically used with people who are at high risk of hospitalization or who are "high users" of services. ACT case managers are engaged in coordinating and locating services and in more intensive rehabilitation and clinical care. When occupational therapy services are available, case managers work closely with the occupational therapist and client to ensure that the client's stated vocational and functional outcomes are being met. Moreover, occupational therapists easily fill the role of case manager in these programs.

The occupational therapist on this team contributes to the evaluation of rehabilitative needs and provides ongoing rehabilitation services in place. Each client has an individualized plan that would help with structuring his or her day; the client would participate in a vocational rehabilitation process and structured leisure. The services are provided in authentic settings with the necessary training and support of the PACT team.

Research has demonstrated that assertive community intervention and similar models of intensive case management are effective. Programs such as PACT appear to help clients to increase daily task functioning, residential stability, and independence and to reduce their hospitalizations (Borland, McRae, & Lycan, 1989; Rosen, Mueser, & Teesson, 2007). They also promote continuity of outpatient care and increase community tenure and residence stability (Bond, McGrew, & Fekete, 1995; Lehman, 1998; Stein & Test, 1980). No clear evidence exists as to which ACT program components have these effects, but recent evidence has pointed to occupational therapists' ability to engage the client, continuity in staff, and caseload size as important factors (Chinman, Allende, Bailey, Maust, & Davidson, 1999; Salkever et al., 1999). In addition, some evidence has indicated that the good results are not maintained after discharge from the ACT program (Allness & Knoedler, 1998), suggesting a need for continued support in the community.

Skill Training

Skill training is a generic term used to describe a variety of interventions that produce improvement in specific individual competencies for daily living, which may include social skills, ADL and IADL skills, vocational skills, interpersonal skills, and any other ability one might require to be successful and satisfied in context. Most day programs will claim that skill training is integral to their program, but few use skill training alone in the treatment of people with a severe mental illness. Occupational therapists can serve as the designer and implementer of these interventions; however, many professionals claim skill training in their repertoire of interventions.

A developing body of research on different types of skill training has shown promising results. Evidence from multiple randomized control trials has supported the use of highly structured manual-driven treatment programs that combine social skills and daily living skill training to improve independent living skills (Anzai et al., 2002; Kopelowicz, Wallace, & Zarate, 1998; Liberman et al., 1998; Patterson et al., 2003, 2005, 2006). Two meta-analyses (Corrigan, 1991; Dilk & Bond,

1996) found that general social skills training programs enhanced skill acquisition. A more recent meta-analysis by Pilling et al. (2002) did not find a difference between social skills training focusing only on interpersonal skills and comparison interventions. However, Torres, Mendez, Merino, and Moran (2002) demonstrated improved social functioning when combining social skills training, psychomotor skills training, occupational therapy, and a problem-solving board game. Some evidence has emerged supporting more focused social skills training, such as that tailored to the work environment (Mueser et al., 2005; Tsang & Pearson, 2001). The evidence points to occupational therapists' expertise in skill training and daily living skills being essential to effective services for adults with SPMI; however, more research is needed.

Evidence examining the effectiveness of programs related to homemaking and IADL skills is promising but limited. Duncombe (2004) found significant improvements in cooking skills in a randomized control trial examining cooking skills training in context. Although cooking skills improved, the study did not show a difference between the context of the intervention (home or clinic). A study by Brown, Rempfer, and Hamera (2002) supported grocery shopping skills training to improve the acquisition of independent living skills.

A paucity of evidence supports general life skills training exclusive of social skills training. A Cochrane Database systematic review (Robertson, Connaughton, & Nicol, 1998) found that the available evidence supporting life skills training programs focused on independent functioning in daily living was inconclusive when compared with traditional rehabilitation, described as recreation, art, and occupational therapy. Few studies have examined skills training derived from a theory or model. However, Schindler (2005) found improvements in social roles, task skills, and interpersonal skills in a nonrandomized controlled trial examining participants of the Role Development Program, an individualized theory-based intervention program. Considering occupational therapy's key role in life skills training and the scarcity of evidence to support the efficacy of these approaches, it is essential that occupational therapists begin to write and research on these topics. Robertson et al. (1998) noted in their review of the research on life skills programs: "Considering that there is next to no evidence that life skill training programs are of value, it is questionable whether recipients of [this] care should be put under pressure to attend such programmes" (p. 6).

Services Specific to Employment

Work is extremely important to the process of recovery and is a strong contributor to feelings of living normally (Deegan, 1988; Leete, 1989). This occupational area has been an integral part of the service system and is frequently integral to programs for people with SPMI. As with skill training and support programs, vocational and educational services are delivered through a continuum of settings that provide varying levels of structure, support, and supervision. In the development of this continuum, a progression from institutional or staff-centered programs to client-centered, community-based services has occurred. Recognition of the need for a close relationship among consumer, family, employer, and mental health professionals in planning and providing vocational services to produce successful vocational outcomes is growing. This ongoing, changing paradigm has led to the development of a variety of programs that will support, train, and place people with SPMI in vocational settings.

Two primary models exist in the provision of vocational services. Scaffa (2001) referred to them as the *Place-and-Train Model* and the hierarchical *Train-and-Place Model*. The Train-and-Place Model focuses on teaching vocational skills in a sheltered work or day program and then attempts to place the person in a work setting. Sheltered workshops have been the traditional settings for the Train-and-Place Model. In these settings, occupational therapists might provide evaluation, group or individual work in any variety of skills needed for vocations, and work adjustment training. Although sheltered workshops are part of the array of vocational services, they are associated with institutional facilities. The settings are believed to tend to increase dependency on the service system and therefore are not in favor for use with people with SPMI.

The Place-and-Train Model is based on the "Choose–Get–Keep" Model pioneered by psychiatric rehabilitation (Anthony et al., 2002). In this model, the client chooses a job path ("choose"), and the advocate works with the client to find ("get") an appropriate job and might provide skill training or support on the job as needed by a job coach or other support staff. Necessary support is then provided to help the client keep the job ("keep"). The Train-and-Place Model is also integral to the clubhouse model, in which the client is put into a work adjustment unit where he or she receives initial assessment and vocational training. The models are reflected in the program settings typically associated with vocational services. As in the development of day programs, a variety of named vocational programs have been established for people with SPMI and others, including consumer-operated businesses, transitional employment, and supported employment.

Consumer-Operated Businesses

Consumer-operated businesses are a part of many clubhouse program models. These businesses are run by the consumer and typically provide a service (e.g., lawn maintenance, housekeeping, small coffee shops). Consumers earn various levels of pay. Staff provide help with community contacts and work assignments and may do the work of the business. Occupational therapists might develop and monitor work evaluations and work adjustment programs. They may recommend programmatic or individual site accommodation (Scaffa, 2001).

Transitional Employment

Transitional employment (TE) involves having a job in a normal place of employment that pays the prevailing wage and allows job coaching on site for a predetermined period of time. TE's purpose is to give people an opportunity to practice their work and social skills in preparation for full-time employment (Davidson, Harding, & Spainol, 2006). The job itself belongs to the program, and people must give it up at the end of a specified time period. The program guarantees that the position will be filled at all times, decreasing the risk to employers. Evidence seems to support that, given opportunity, support, and time, people with SPMI can perform effectively in a job. TE gives the needed support and training to allow the person with SPMI to transition to the worker role. Occupational therapists could be managers of the TE program or job coaches. Additionally, occupational therapists are important in completing task analyses and task and environmental modifications that support the person in the work setting (Urbanak, 1995).

Supported Employment

According to Anthony and Blanch (1987), supported employment (SE) is the preferred method of vocational rehabilitation intervention for people with SPMI. SE, referred to by Anthony et al. (2002) as the Individual Placement and Support (IPS) Model, is defined as "a part-time or full-time competitive paid job, averaging at least 20 hours per week in an integrated work setting where contact with nondisabled people regularly occurs and with support services provided for more than 18 months" (Anthony et al., 2002, p. 250). After evaluation, the client is placed in a job with a job coach. The coach works with the employer to train the client and make accommodations if needed. The coach is available to help the client with difficulties with the job or by supporting daily living functions. The coach works closely with other mental health professionals to support and assess any issues that might interfere with job performance. Occupational therapists contribute to performance assessment, the job-matching process, and the development of accommodations.

Strong evidence exists for SE–IPS's efficacy in leading to employment of people with severe mental illness. Two strong studies, a systematic review and a meta-analysis (Crowther, Marshall, Bond, & Huxley, 2001; Twamley, Jeste, & Lehman, 2003) have reported positive results for SE–IPS programs when compared with other vocational rehabilitation programs. In addition, research has supported SE's effectiveness in helping people with SPMI to obtain competitive employment and stay employed over time (Cook et al., 2005).

Supported Education

Supported education was initially developed for people returning to school. A variety of support-type programs were developed that ranged from onsite support provided by the educational system to current developments in mobile teams to help people return to any postsecondary education setting (Sullivan, Nicolellis, Danley, & MacDonald-Wilson, 1993). These programs provide people with an opportunity to attend a real educational program as regular students integrated into the school

According to Danley, Sciarappa, and MacDonald-Wilson (1992), people with SPMI do not require intensive on-campus support to succeed; rather, they need support to meet the social and emotional demands of school. A variety of models are available that show potential to provide those supports. For example, the self-contained classroom is composed of only people with SPMI, who attend a class with a specialized curriculum (Unger, Danley, Kohn, & Hutchinson, 1987). Programs that encourage attendance in a regular classroom with support from mental health service staff also exist (Sullivan et al., 1993). In a third model, people with SPMI attend regular classes and receive onsite support from education staff (Furlong-Norman, 1990).

Good evidence for supported education is emerging. A 1998 randomized control trial (Collins, Bybee, & Mowbray, 1998) found positive results in its comparison of three different supported education models. All three models showed increases in enrollment in school or vocational education programs. More recent studies (Gutman, 2008; Gutman et al., 2007; Hutchinson, Anthony, Massaro, & Rogers, 2007) have reported significant improvement in life skill areas such as time management and basic writing skills as well as gains in employment status or enrollment in educational programs.

Volunteer Work

Volunteer work has been used for work adjustment or to establish a productive life role for a person living with mental illness. Volunteer programs have been used extensively by occupational therapists in clinical areas to provide "work therapy" or meaningful activities for clients who choose not to work. Successful volunteer projects help the person practice skills but also, as Tryssenar (1998) noted, provide opportunities to contribute to society. Little research has been done on volunteer work's effectiveness in leading people with SPMI to work or providing them with a sense of efficacy.

Case Example

John came to the Horizons Program from his most recent stay at Western State Hospital. He has had five hospitalizations over the past 10 years, all a result of reported noncompliance with or ineffective medication regimes. He had a spotty work record, interrupted by his hospitalizations. His brother transported him to Horizons and stated that his parents could no longer provide a residence for John because they were experiencing health problems and could no longer cope with his frequent regressions.

John's consistent goal has been to obtain a steady job. Because he attended college for two semesters when he was 18, he believed he could become a doctor if only he were provided the supports he needs to return to school. However, he stated that he was ready to do any job right now just to "get some cash and my own place." After some discussion with his case manager, John decided to try the Horizon House, which would provide a residence, and work in its transitional employment program. The occupational therapist and John completed an occupational profile that indicated occupational performance deficits in cognitive skills related to organizing, prioritizing, and multitasking. He has a strong to desire to return to the student or worker role but has poor work habits reinforced over time as a result of his symptom exacerbations. Poor medication management has also affected his role participation. The activity demands of premed college-level classes will require strong organizational skills, study habits, and time management.

John quickly became oriented to the clubhouse routine and was able to participate in the daily government meetings. He completed his chores with little supervision but continued to have some difficulty following instructions from his supervisor in the gardening work program, and he was occasionally late for his work assignment. The occupational therapist provided social skills training and some cognitive assists to help John attend to his supervisor's instructions and arrive at work on time. He successfully participated in the gardening program and was referred for TE in an area lab. The therapist went with John for the first few days of his lab position. Working with the job coach, she was able to provide John with the support he needed to get to work on time and maintain effective working relationships with his supervisor and coworkers.

While John worked on developing and then maintaining his skills at work, the occupational therapist worked with him one evening a week to explore educational opportunities that might fit his needs. He explored the various medical professions, what the jobs entailed, their educational requirements, and the resources he would need to attend college. John used his experiences at work and at Horizon House to arrive at a fairly accurate assessment of his skills and abilities to participate in an educational setting. During his explorations, John decided he did not want to be a doctor because the educational requirements were too stringent and he was not willing to devote the time needed. However, he really liked his job at the lab and thought he might like to become a lab technician so that he could apply for a job where he had his TE placement. He and his occupational therapist began to explore community colleges that offered lab technician associate's degrees.

During this time, John stopped taking his medication and had an altercation with his supervisor at work. He was admitted to Western's county hospital for 1 week and returned to Horizon House. He returned to his TE and completed the placement. John was one of several Horizon transitional housing residents who wished to return to school, and the counselor in the community college disabilities office (an occupational therapist) was interested in working with the Horizon team to develop supported education. John and several others applied to the college and were accepted into the New Horizons Supported Education Program. He met with his peers and the occupational therapist and counselor from the disabilities office daily during the first few weeks of class and then weekly for the first year. The sessions provided information and training in the skills needed to succeed in college. More important, the groups gave John an opportunity to gain support and feedback from his peers and professionals. John has completed his first year of school and is working in the lab for the summer to help pay his tuition. He is convinced that with Horizon's support, and if he keeps to his current medication program, he will graduate and work in the lab as a lab technician.

Conclusion

The second edition of the *Occupational Therapy Practice Framework: Domain and Process* describes occupational therapy's overarching aim as "supporting health and participation in life through engagement in occupation" (AOTA, 2008, p. 626). The development of services for people with SPMI with needs in the occupational areas of work and education is integral to this domain. As discussed, occupational therapists can provide services to the person and family and to programs and communities striving to collaborate with people with SPMI on supported but independent functioning in work and education through skill training, psychosocial programs, and specific vocational and educational programs. The occupational therapy process reflects best practice in rehabilitation and this service system when the work is within context and done collaboratively with clients to support health and participation in life through engagement in occupations.

The evidence has indicated that many programs demonstrated to be effective with people with SPMI in the area of paid and unpaid employment fit within the scope of occupational therapy practice. Structured skill-development programs; SE; and supported education emphasizing skill development, goal setting, and cognitive training result in increased participation in work and education. These interventions serve as the core of rehabilitation in community mental health and are within occupational therapy's scope of practice.

As effective services for people with SPMI are implemented, the system continues to move toward increased community integration. Evidence has supported that higher levels of service integration correlate with better vocational and psychosocial outcomes (Gold et al., 2006). New program models are attempting to have community stakeholders be part of the rehabilitation team. Structured day and vocational programs may become obsolete as the service system becomes an integral part of the community. The intrusive nature of any special programming puts up barriers to the success and satisfaction of people with SPMI. The person, family, and community—all of them stakeholders—must eventually work together toward a shared understanding of the problems faced by people in a recovery process. The future points to continued integration, with the professional acting as a facilitator of that process. Occupational therapists' unique understanding of the person, environment, and performance and the interaction of those key elements points to occupational therapists' central role in the development of this new paradigm for recovery.

References

Allness, D. J., & Knoedler, W. H. (1998). *The PACT model of community-based treatment for persons with severe and persistent mental illnesses: A manual for PACT start-up*. Arlington, VA: National Alliance for the Mentally Ill.

American Occupational Therapy Association. (2008). Occupational therapy practice framework: Domain and process (2nd ed.). *American Journal of Occupational Therapy, 62*, 625–683.

Anderson, C. M., Hogarty, G. E., & Reiss, D. J. (1980). *Schizophrenia and the family.* New York: Guilford.

Anthony, W. A., & Blanch, A. (1987). Supported employment for persons who are psychiatrically disabled: A historical and conceptual perspective. *Psychosocial Rehabilitation Journal, 11*(2), 5–23.

Anthony, W., Cohen, M., Farkas, M., & Gagne, C. (2002). *Psychiatric rehabilitation* (2nd ed.). Boston: Center for Psychiatric Rehabilitation, Boston University.

Anzai, N., Yoneda, S., Kumagai, N., Nakamura, Y., Ikebuchi, E., & Liberman, R. P. (2002). Training persons with schizophrenia in illness self-management: A randomized controlled trial in Japan. *Psychiatric Services, 53*(5), 545–547.

Bond, B. R., McGrew, J. H., & Fekete, D. M. (1995). Assertive outreach for frequent users of psychiatric hospitals: A meta analysis. *Journal of Mental Health Administration, 22*(1), 4–16.

Beard, J., Propst, R., & Malamud, T. (1982). The Fountain House Model of psychiatric rehabilitation. *Psychosocial Rehabilitation Journal, 5*(1), 47–53.

Bond, G. R., & Dincin, J. (1986). Accelerating into transitional employment in a psychosocial rehabilitation agency. *Rehabilitation Psychology, 31*(3), 143–155.

Borland, A., McRae, J., & Lycan, C. (1989). Outcomes of five years of continuous intensive case management. *Hospital and Community Psychiatry, 40*(4), 369–376.

Brown, C., Moyers, P., Haertlein Sells, C., Learnard, L., Mahaffey, L. M., Pitts, D. B., et al. (2006). *Report of the Ad Hoc Committee on Mental Health Practice in Occupational Therapy.* Unpublished report to the AOTA Board of Directors.

Brown, C., Rempfer, M., & Hamera, E. (2002). Teaching grocery shopping skills to people with schizophrenia. *OTJR: Occupation, Participation and Health, 22*(Suppl. 1), 90S–91S.

Cara, E., & MacRae, A. (2005). *Psychosocial occupational therapy: A clinical practice.* Albany, NY: Delmar.

Chinman, M., Allende, M., Bailey, P., Maust, J., & Davidson, I. (1999). Therapeutic agents of assertive community treatment. *Psychiatric Quarterly, 70*(2), 137–162.

Collins, M. E., Bybee, D., & Mowbray, C. T. (1998). Effectiveness of supported education for individuals with psychiatric disabilities: Results from an experimental study. *Community Mental Health Journal,34*, 595–613.

Cook, J. A., & Jonikas, J. A. (1996). Outcomes of psychiatric rehabilitation service delivery. In D. M. Steinwaachs & L. M. Flynn (Eds.), *Using client outcomes information to improve mental health and substance abuse treatment* (New Directions for Mental Health Services No. 71, pp. 33–47). San Francisco: Jossey-Bass.

Cook, J. A., Leff, H. S., Blyler, C. R., Gold, P. B., Goldberg, R. W., Mueser, K. T., et al. (2005). Results of a multisite randomized trial of supported employment interventions for individuals with severe mental illness. *Archives of General Psychiatry, 62,* 505–512.

Corrigan, P. W. (1991). Social skills training in adult psychiatric populations: A meta-analysis. *Journal of Behavior Therapy and Experimental Psychiatry, 22*(3), 203–210.

Crowther, R. E., Marshall, M., Bond, G. R., & Huxley, P. (2001). Helping people with severe mental illness to obtain work: Systematic review. *British Medical Journal, 322,* 204–208.

Danley, K. S., Sciarappa, K., & MacDonald-Wilson, K. L. (1992). *Choose–get–keep: Psychiatric rehabilitation approach to supported employment* (Vol. 53). San Francisco: Jossey-Bass.

Davidson, L., Harding, C., & Spainol, L. (2006). *Recovery from severe mental illnesses: Research evidence and implications for practice.* Boston: Center for Psychiatric Rehabilitation, Boston University.

Deegan, P. (1988). Recovery: The lived experience of rehabilitation. *Psychosocial Rehabilitation Journal, 11,* 11–19.

Dilk, M. N., & Bond, G. R. (1996). Meta-analytic evaluation of skills training research for individuals with severe mental illness. *Journal of Consulting and Clinical Psychology, 64*(6), 1337–1345.

Duncombe, L. W. (2004). Comparing learning of cooking in home and clinic for people with schizophrenia. *American Journal of Occupational Therapy, 58*(3), 272–278.

Furlong-Norman, J. (1990). *Supported education* [Special issue]. *Community Support Network News, 6*(3).

Gold, P. B., Meisler, N., Santos, A. B., Carnemolla, M. A., Williams, O. H., & Keleher, J. (2006). Randomized trial of supported employment integrated with assertive community treatment for rural adults with severe mental illness. *Schizophrenia Bulletin, 32,* 378–395.

Gutman, S. A. (2008). Supported education for adults with psychiatric disabilities. *Psychiatric Services, 59*(3), 326–327.

Gutman, S. A., Schindler, V. P., Furphy, K. A., Klein, K., Lisak, J. M., & Durham, D. P. (2007). The effectiveness of a supported education program for adults with psychiatric disabilities: The Bridge Program. *Occupational Therapy in Mental Health, 23*(1), 21–38.

Hutchinson, D., Anthony, W., Massaro, J., & Rogers, E. S. (2007). Evaluation of a combined supported computer education and employment training program for persons with psychiatric disabilities. *Psychiatric Rehabilitation Journal, 30*(3), 189–197.

Kopelowicz, A., Wallace, C. J., & Zarate, R. (1998). Teaching psychiatric inpatients to re-enter the community: A brief method of improving the continuity of care. *Psychiatric Services, 49*(10), 1313–1316.

Leete, E. (1989). How I perceive and manage my illness. *Schizophrenia Bulletin, 21,* 195–200.

Lehman, A. F. (1998). Vocational rehabilitation in schizophrenia. *Schizophrenia Bulletin, 21,* 645–656.

Liberman, R. P., Wallace, C. J., Blackwell, G., Kopelowicz, A., Vaccaro, J. V., & Mintz, J. (1998). Skills training versus psychosocial occupational therapy for persons with persistent schizophrenia. *American Journal of Psychiatry, 155*(8), 1087–1091.

Mueser, K. T., Aalto, S., Becker, D. R., Ogden, J. S., Wolfe, R. S., Schiavo, D., et al. (2005). The effectiveness of skills training for improving outcomes in supported employment. *Psychiatric Services, 56*(10), 1254–1260.

Mueser, K. T., Corrigan, P. W., Hilton, D. W., Tanzman, B., Schaub, A., Gingerich, S., et al. (2004). Illness management and recovery: A review of the research. *Focus, 2,* 324–347.

National Institute of Mental Health. (2008). *The numbers count: Mental disorders in America.* Retrieved August 19, 2008, from www.nimh.nih.gov/health/publications/the-numbers-count-mental disorders-in-America/index.shtml

Patterson, T. L., Bucardo, J., McKibbin, C. L., Mausbach, B. T., Moore, D., Barrio, C., et al. (2005). Development and pilot testing of a new psychosocial intervention for older Latinos with chronic psychosis. *Schizophrenia Bulletin, 31*(4), 922–930.

Patterson, T. L., Mausbach, B. T., McKibbin, C., Goldman, S., Bucardo, J., & Jeste, D. V. (2006). Functional Adaptation Skills Training (FAST): A randomized trial of a psychosocial intervention for middle-aged and older patients with chronic psychotic disorders. *Schizophrenia Research, 86,* 291–299.

Patterson, T. L., McKibbin, C., Tayler, M., Goldman, S., Davila-Fraga, W., Bucardo, J., et al. (2003). Functional Adaptation Skills Training (FAST): A pilot psychosocial intervention study in middle-aged and older patients with chronic psychotic disorders. *American Journal of Geriatric Psychiatry, 11*(1), 17–23.

Penn, D. L., & Mueser, K. T. (1996). Research update on the psychosocial treatment of schizophrenia. *American Journal of Psychiatry, 153,* 607–617.

Pilling, S., Bebbington, P., Kuipers, E., Garety, P., Geddes, J., Martindale, B., et al. (2002). Psychological treatments in schizophrenia: II. Meta-analyses of randomized controlled trials of social skills training and cognitive remediation. *Psychological Medicine, 32,* 783–791.

President's New Freedom Commission on Mental Health. (2003). *Achieving the promise: Transforming mental health care in America* (Final Report, DHHS Pub. No SMA–03–3832). Rockville, MD: Author.

Robertson, L., Connaughton, J., & Nicol, M. (1998). Life skills programs for chronic mental illness: Playing the train game. *Psychiatric Services, 53*(7), 799–801.

Rosen, A., Mueser, K. T., & Teesson, M. (2007). Assertive community treatment—Issues from scientific and clinical literature with implications for practice. *Journal of Rehabilitation Research, 44*(6), 813–825.

Salkever, D., Domino, M. E., Burns, B. J., Santos, A. B., Deci, P. A., Dias, J., et al. (1999). Assertive community treatment for people with severe mental illness: The effects on hospitalization use and costs. *Health Services Research, 34*(2), 577–601.

Scaffa, M. (2001). *Occupational therapy in community-based practice settings.* Philadelphia: F. A. Davis.

Schindler, V. P. (2005). Role development: An evidence-based intervention for individuals diagnosed with schizophrenia in a forensic facility. *Psychiatric Rehabilitation Journal, 28*(4), 391–394.

Scot, J. E., & Dixon, L. B. (1995). Psychological interventions for schizophrenia. *Schizophrenia Bulletin, 21*(4), 621–630.

Stein, L. I., & Test, M. A. (1980). Alternatives to mental hospital treatment: I. Conceptual mode, treatment programs, and clinical evaluation. *Archives of General Psychiatry, 37*(4), 392–397.

Sullivan, P., Nicolellis, D., Danley, K. S., & MacDonald-Wilson, K. (1993). Choose–get–keep: A psychiatric rehabilitation approach to supported education. *Psychosocial Rehabilitation Journal, 17*(1), 705–714.

Torres, A., Mendez, L. P., Merino, H., & Moran, E. A. (2002). Improving social functioning in schizophrenia by playing the train game. *Psychiatric Services, 53*(7), 799–801.

Tryssenar, J. (1998). Vocational exploration and employment and psychosocial disabilities. In F. Stein & S. K. Cutler (Eds.), *Psychosocial occupational therapy: A holistic approach* (pp. 351–374). San Diego: Singular.

Tsang, H. W., & Pearson, V. (2001).Work-related social skills training for people with schizophrenia in Hong Kong. *Schizophrenia Bulletin, 27*(1), 139–148.

Twamley, E., Jeste, D., & Lehman, A. (2003). Vocational rehabilitation in schizophrenia and other psychotic disorders: A literature review and meta-analysis of randomized controlled trials. *Journal of Nervous and Mental Disease, 191*(8), 515–523.

Unger, K. V., Danley, K. S., Kohn, L., & Hutchinson, D. (1987). Rehabilitation through education for young adults with long-term mental illness. *Hospital and Community Psychiatry, 42,* 838–842.

Urbanak, M. A. (1995). Yahara House: A community-based program using the Fountain House model. *Mental Health Special Interest Newsletter, 18*(1), 1–3.

U.S. Department of Health and Human Services. (1999). *Mental health: A report of the Surgeon General.* Rockville, MD: U.S. Department of Health and Human Services, Substance Abuse and Mental Health Services Administration, Center for Mental Health Services & National Institute of Mental Health. Retrieved November 17, 2009, from www.surgeongeneral.gov/library/mentalhealth/home.html

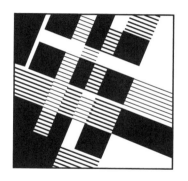

CHAPTER 7

Occupational Engagement of Older Adults With Mental Illness

Janie B. Scott, MA, OT/L, FAOTA, and
Lisa Mahaffey, MS, OTR/L

Learning Objectives

After reading this material and completing the examination, readers will be able to

- Identify evidence-based intervention resources and trends in geriatric mental health and substance abuse,

- Recognize geriatric mental health and substance abuse issues and their relation to participation in meaningful occupations,

- Delineate theoretical frameworks to draw from when assessing and planning intervention for the older adult diagnosed with mental illness or substance abuse,

- Determine effective intervention outcomes for older adults with mental illness on the basis of philosophies of recovery and resilience,

- Identify occupation-based components of caregiver education for older adults with mental illness, and

- Identify major legislation and resources that include older adults with mental illness.

Baby boomers are aging. Between 2018 and 2033, the number of people older than age 60 will double (Administration on Aging [AoA], 2009). The U.S. health care system is disjointed, and the signs and symptoms of mental illness manifested by older adults are often overlooked. This chapter describes issues and trends regarding the mental health and occupational engagement of older adults, including medication mismanagement, Alzheimer's disease, the mental health system of care, and legislation and regulations specifically addressing the needs of older adults with mental illness. Additionally, the chapter explores some of the social and cultural issues that affect this population and models of practice used by occupational therapy with older adults.

Overview

Background Data

Suicide among older adults occurs at a disproportionately high rate (National Institute of Mental Health [NIMH], 2003). In 2003, 12% of the population was older than 60; however, they accounted for 16% of all suicides. Even more alarming, 75% visited their primary care physician within a month of their suicide (NIMH, 2003). Additionally, two-thirds of people in long-term care facilities have a diagnosed mental illness and receive little effective care (McCurren, Dowe, Rattle, & Looney, 1999). Of community-dwelling older adults, 5% have a debilitating mental illness; that number increases to 13.5% for those actively engaged in the health care system (NIMH, 2003). Between 2% and 10% of community-dwelling older adults are either abusing or at risk for abusing substances (Bartels, Blow, Brockmann, & Van Citters, 2005), 11% have an anxiety disorder, 1% have bipolar disorder, and 1% are diagnosed with schizophrenia (U.S. Department of Health and Human Services, 1999).

Seven million people older than age 65 in the United States live with a diagnosable psychiatric illness. That number is expected to double. Older adults with psychiatric illness have lower quality of medical care, have higher mortality rates than those without psychiatric illness, and are more likely to be placed into nursing homes despite their ability to complete all self-care activities (Substance Abuse and Mental Health Services Administration [SAMHSA], 2004b).

That aging adults may need mental health or substance abuse (MH–SA) services is not a new concept. In *Achieving the Promise: Transforming Mental Health Care in America,* the President's New Freedom Commission on Mental Health's (2003) indicated that

> [o]lder adults are at risk of developing both depression and alcohol dependence for perhaps the first time in their lives. Mental illnesses have a significant impact on the health and functioning of older people and are associated with increased health care use and higher costs (p. 67).

As the number of older adults increases, so does the potential demand for MH–SA services. How to best deliver those services to a population who is typically concerned about the stigma attached to MH–SA care has become a focus of discussion and research. One example is the SAMHSA–sponsored Primary Care Research in Substance Abuse and Mental Health for the Elderly (PRISM–E) study exploring service delivery preferences of people with mental illness and substance abuse.

PRISM–E

The PRISM–E study, funded by SAMHSA, was a 6-year, multisite study that examined the outcomes for older adults who had or were at risk for mental illness, substance abuse, or both and were referred to MH–SA services either at enhanced specialty centers or in primary care settings. The models of care were developed and standards for care identified before the study's inception. The focus of the research "was to determine whether enhancements to, and standardization of, the care models improved access to treatment, outcome, and costs for patients, without mandating providers' conversion to standardized depression treatment algorithms or interventions" (Oslin et al., 2006, p. 947). The PRISM–E study involved collaboration among

SAMHSA's three centers (the Center for Mental Health Services, Center for Substance Abuse Prevention, and Center for Substance Abuse Treatment), the Department of Veterans Affairs, the Health Resources and Services Administration, and the Centers for Medicare and Medicaid Services (CMS). Many articles have been written analyzing PRISM–E and the benefits that the two different service delivery models had on study participants' reduction in symptoms.

PRISM–E researchers examined different components of service delivery for adults ages 65 and older living in the community. Bartels et al. (2004) explored "whether integrated mental health services or enhanced referral to specialty mental health clinics results in greater engagement in mental health/substance abuse services by older primary care patients." Oslin et al. (2006) examined the "relative effectiveness of two different models of care for reducing at-risk alcohol use among primary care patients aged 65 and older" (p. 954), and Krahn et al. (2006) reviewed "six-month outcomes for older primary care patients with depression who received different models of treatment" (p. 946).

Bartels et al. (2004) concluded that "older primary care patients are more likely to accept collaborative mental health treatment within primary care settings than in mental health and substance abuse specialty clinics" (p. 7). Krahn et al. (2006) found that for people without severe depression, the integrated system of care may offer better results; however, the outcomes for those with major depression were significantly better when their care was delivered through enhanced specialty centers. Oslin et al.'s (2006) efforts revealed that the outcomes for people who were considered at-risk drinkers and who entered a system of care (many refused screening and intervention) were comparable regardless of whether they used the integrated or enhanced system of care. Oslin et al.'s (2006, p. 957) work revealed "significant reductions in both quantity and frequency of drinking and binge drinking over six months." Early identification and treatment of people who are at-risk drinkers may help them curb their behaviors and potentially lead to a reduction in falls and other health- and socially related complications.

This chapter discusses how PRISM–E can inform and suggest opportunities for occupational therapists and occupational therapy assistants interested in community-based practice for older adults with MH–SA. Suffice it to say, many potential consumers of occupational therapy services will choose services near or within their primary care providers' offices.

Legislation, regulations, and trends all have an impact on the lives of older adults with MH–SA. This chapter outlines some of the policy initiatives that have a direct bearing on the people in this group and, in some cases, the caregivers who support them. The reference list provides direct links to this information.

Medication Mismanagement and Substance Abuse

Many adults will experience depression or chemical dependency for the first time in their later years. Several factors contribute to this late onset. One is increasing vulnerability to medication misuse. As people age, medications are increasingly used to manage pain, anxiety, and depression, and many of the medications used to treat these conditions can result in dependency, misuse, or accidental overdose. Older adults may combine alcohol with their medications—with dangerous results (Blow, Bartels, Brockmann, & Van Citters, 2004). Other factors, such as mild cognitive impairment or early memory loss, can cause older adults to forget whether they have taken their medications and to accidentally overdose. In 2004, SAMHSA developed a targeted campaign to address the increased incidence of accidental overdose. The campaign included educational materials geared to professionals and consumers in an effort to increase awareness of the dangers of interactions among prescription medications, over-the-counter medications, and alcohol (SAMHSA, 2004a).

The recent focus on falls prevention has highlighted another factor exemplifying the interaction between physical and mental health. Medication mismanagement or the side effects of commonly used medications are one of the risk factors for falls. Approximately one-third of people older than age 65 will fall in a given year. Although most falls result in only minor injuries, the fear of another, more devastating fall can interfere with a person's engagement in social or active life roles (Howland et al., 1993). Howland et al. (1993) interviewed 196 people in supported living situations about their fear of falling. Twenty-six percent said they were afraid of a fall in the next year; 35% said they avoided activities they would otherwise pursue because of their fear of falling; 4% said they did not socialize as a result of their fear; and 4% stated they would not walk alone (Howland et al., 1993). Other, smaller studies of community-dwelling older adults have drawn similar conclusions (Maki, Holiday, & Topper, 1991; Murphy & Isaacs, 1982; Tinetti, Speechley, & Ginter, 1988). Limiting participation in one's valued activities because of fear can lead to increasing levels of depression and social isolation. One could also assume that decreased participation in activity leads to an increasingly sedentary lifestyle and consequently to increased weakness, decreased balance and endurance, a greater tendency to fall, and other medical problems (CDC, 2008b; Peterson & Howland, 2003).

Alzheimer's Disease

Along with increased life expectancy, the prevalence of diseases related to memory and cognition has increased ("Rush Alzheimer's Disease Screening, Diagnosis, and Treatment," 2008). *Dementia* is listed in the *Diagnostic and Statistical Manual of Mental Disorders* (4th ed., text revision; American Psychiatric Association [APA], 2000) as the development of cognitive deficits including memory impairment, combined with other features such aphasia, agnosia, apraxia, and disturbance in executive function such as abstract thinking, planning and organization, and ability to manage complex behavior. The disease has an impact on affect and behavior and may manifest itself through anger, anxiety, or extreme sadness. When this happens, people can be successfully treated through mental health processes (APA, 2000). Several research studies have focused on the brain and dementia. Investigators at Rush Alzheimer's Disease Center in Chicago have two major research projects funded by the National Institute on Aging. One, the Memory and Aging Project, is a study of the risk factors for dementia ("Rush Alzheimer's Disease Screening, Diagnosis, and Treatment," 2008); the other is the Religious Orders Study, a study begun by David Snowdon in 1986 and later funded by the National Institute on Aging that has grown to a multidisciplinary research project (Snowdon, 2001). This study, which is funded through 2011, will provide information on the relationship between pathology of Alzheimer's disease and the cognitive changes in the brain. These longitudinal studies are looking at risk factors and methods for avoiding the onset of memory and cognitive diseases. One outcome of this research has been a resource center developed at Rush for people experiencing dementia. The center's primary goal is to provide resources to care providers of people with dementia to help them continue to live with dignity and purpose.

Mental Health System of Care for the Older Adult

Increasing health care costs and attempts to control them have affected the entire health care system. The effect has been to fragment and decentralize health care services. In the past, older people would continue to see the same physician they had had for years. That physician would be familiar with their medical history and would monitor and prescribe all of their medications. Specialization and reliance on managed care has resulted in older adults seeing several different doctors and specialists. Many people are now involved in primary care group practices in which the patient may rotate among doctors, nurse practitioners, and physician's assistants. The patient is less likely to form a close relationship with one primary care provider, reducing the likelihood that depression or other psychiatric symptoms will be detected and treated early. The system requires the older adult to seek psychiatric care outside of the primary care practice and, given the stigma attached to psychiatric care that remains prevalent with this age group, that is unlikely (*Olmstead v. L.C.*, 1999; SAMHSA, 2007).

Mental Health Legislation and Regulation

Chapter 17 contains a comprehensive discussion of legislation and policies that incorporate a focus on mental illness. The federal policy discussed in this chapter specifically addresses older adults with mental illness: the Supreme Court's *Olmstead* decision, the Older Americans Act of 1965, the White House Conference on Aging (WHCoA; 2005), Deficit Reduction Act of 2005, and the President's New Freedom Commission on Mental Health (2003).

Access to community-based mental health services is limited, particularly for seniors with severe or persistent mental illness. Deinstitutionalization in the early 1980s resulted in seniors with severe mental illness moving into nursing institutions. Nursing home institutionalization continues to be a common placement for older adults who cannot care for themselves because of mental health problems. Some relief resulted from the *Olmstead* decision in 1999 and the growing philosophy that mental health services should be provided in the least restrictive environment (e.g., the community).

Olmstead v. L.C.

The U.S. Supreme Court decision in the case *Olmstead v. L.C.* (1999) "held that unnecessary segregation of people in institutions is discriminatory and challenged States and communities to find appropriate alternatives for older adults with serious mental illness" (SAMHSA, 2004b, p. v). This decision mandates that community-based services be available to people with disabilities, including those with mental illness.

The *Olmstead* decision created opportunities for occupational therapy. Occupational therapists can assess clients' ability to perform activities of daily living (ADLs) and instrumental activities of daily living (IADLs) and safety for independent or supported living in the community. Occupational therapists and occupational therapy assistants can provide driving and community mobility assessments and interventions to clients institutionalized with mental illness who want to resume community living. Advocacy and education efforts can inform clients, families, and caregivers about the options under the act and encourage them to advocate to state and local aging and mental health agencies for funding for the community-based services that will allow older adults and those with disabilities to leave institutions or will help them avoid that level of care.

Older Americans Act of 1965

The Older Americans Act of 1965 is comprehensive legislation that emphasizes services that enable older adults to age in place. The Older Americans Act has many sections and titles; below is a brief summary of sections and titles of the Older Americans Act and its amendments of 2006 that specifically relate to older adults with MH–SA (AoA, 2006).

- *102(14)(D) Disease Prevention and Health Services.* This section addresses evidence-based health promotion programs, including alcohol and substance abuse reduction programs.
- *102(14)(G) Disease Prevention and Health Services.* This section provides for "screenings for the prevention of depression, coordination of community mental health services, provision of educational activities, and referral to psychiatric and psychological services" (AoA, 2009, p. 8).
- *201(f): Mental Health.* This section addresses "education about and prevention, detection, and treatment of mental disorders, including age-related dementia, depression, and Alzheimer's disease" (AoA, 2009).
- *202(a)(5).* This section encourages research and translation of research to practice focused on the needs of older adults, including those with mental illness.
- *205 and 214: Nutritional Services.* This section promotes nutrition and physical activity tied to maintaining or resuming a healthy lifestyle, including the needs of people with mental illness and people with substance abuse disorders (AoA, 2009).
- *Title III—Grants for States/Community Programs.* This title supports programs that provide in-home services and supports for families of people with Alzheimer's disease and other neurological conditions; access to mental health services; increasing awareness of community-based mental health services; grants for supportive services; and mental health screenings.
- *Title IV—Activities for Health Independence and Longevity.* This title makes grant funding available for graduate-level professional education for personnel who specialize in geriatric mental health; grants to multidisciplinary centers of gerontology; training and technical assistance to implement community-based mental health programs for older adults; and grants for mental screenings and interventions (AoA, 2009).
- *Part E—National Family Caregiver Support Program III–E.* This section recognizes the importance of family caregivers and provides assistance to support them. The 2006 amendments added language regarding caring for the person with Alzheimer's disease or a related dementia.

White House Conference on Aging Recommendations

The purpose of the WHCoA, which is required by law to occur every 10 years, is to make aging policy recommendations to the president and Congress and to assist the public and private sectors in promoting the dignity, health, independence, and economic security of current and future generations of older people.

Table 7.1 shows selected resolutions passed at the WHCoA, reflecting those that include mental health, substance abuse, and community-based programs that exemplify the range of services that advanced occupational therapy mental health practitioners can fill. Specific ways in which occupational therapists and occupational therapy assistants can become involved in the actualization of the selected recommendations are discussed in Chapter 11.

A copy of the WHCoA final report is available at www.whcoa.gov. This Web site also provides links to information related to the WHCoA recommendations and links to the U.S. Senate Special Committee on Aging, the AoA, the White House, and the U.S. government's official Web portal (www.USA.gov). No "one-stop-shopping" approach to learning how individual states have implemented the WHCoA recommendations is available. The most effective strategy for finding out about individual state implementation of the resolutions is to contact the governor's office, the state department on aging, or both.

Table 7.1. Selected 2005 White House Conference on Aging Resolutions

Rank	Resolution No.	Description
6	41	Support geriatric education and training for all health care professionals, paraprofessionals, health profession students, and direct care workers.
8	36	Improve recognition, assessment, and treatment of mental illness and depression among older Americans.
20	18	Encourage community designs to promote livable communities that enable aging in place.
25	56	Develop a national strategy for promoting new and meaningful volunteer activities and civic engagements for current and future seniors.
26	25	Encourage the development of a coordinated federal, state, and local emergency response plan for seniors in the event of public health emergencies or disasters.
29	46	Promote innovative evidence-based and practice-based medical and aging research.
32	48	Ensure appropriate recognition and care for veterans across all health care settings.
37	37	Prevent disease and promote healthier lifestyles by educating providers and consumers on consumer health care.
39	31	Apply evidence-based research to the delivery of health and social services as appropriate.
44	43	Ensure appropriate care for seniors with disabilities.
48	14	Expand opportunities for developing innovative housing designs for seniors' needs.
52	35	Enhance provider and consumer education about alcohol and substance abuse and appropriate treatment.

Source. White House Conference on Aging (2005).

Deficit Reduction Act of 2005

The Money Follows the Person (MFP) "rebalancing" initiative, which was included in the Deficit Reduction Act of 2005, is being implemented by CMS. This endeavor is also a part of former President George W. Bush's New Freedom Initiative (President's New Freedom Commission on Mental Health, 2003). MFP targets older adults and people with disabilities who live in long-term care settings and want to live in the community. States are allowed to make reforms that will change the long-term care systems. This cost-effective strategy benefits states and gives consumers greater control over their lives (CMS, 2006). MFP grants to states include services for people with mental illness.

Consumer choice is a key concept of MFP, as is the need to have community-based services conveniently available to meet consumer needs. The emphasis on translating evidence-based research into quality outcomes is hoped to improve service delivery, consumer satisfaction, and quality improvement. MFP provides most of the funding for transitioning people from nursing homes and into community settings and for the associated long-term care costs. Consumers' funds can be used for home health care, respite care, home modifications, personal care, and assistive devices (AoA, 2006). For details about the New Freedom Initiative, see Lipson et al. (2007) or CMS (2006).

New Freedom Commission on Mental Health

Former President George W. Bush established by Executive Order No. 13263 (2002) the President's New Freedom Commission on Mental Health. The order stated that

> [t]he mission of the Commission shall be to conduct a comprehensive study of the United States mental health service delivery system, including public and private sector providers, and to advise the President on methods of improving the system. The Commission's goal shall be to recommend improvements to enable adults with serious mental illness and children with serious emotional disturbances to live, work, learn, and participate fully in their communities. (p. 233)

The commission's final report, *Achieving the Promise: Transforming Mental Health Care in America* (President's New Freedom Commission on Mental Health, 2003), also encourages development of assistive technologies that support independent living for people with disabilities; development of transportation programs; and benefits protection when people begin working. The report provided definitions of *recovery* and *resilience* and encouraged orientation to this perspective when considering the needs of people with serious mental illness:

> *Recovery* refers to the process in which people are able to live, work, learn, and participate fully in their communities. For some individuals, recovery is the ability to live a fulfilling and productive life despite a disability. For others, recovery implies the reduction or complete remission of symptoms. Science has shown that having hope plays an integral role in an individual's recovery.

> *Resilience* means the personal and community qualities that enable us to rebound from adversity, trauma, tragedy, threats, or other stresses—and to go

on with life with a sense of mastery, competence, and hope. We now understand from research that resilience is fostered by a positive childhood and includes positive individual traits, such as optimism, good problem-solving skills, and treatments. Closely knit communities and neighborhoods are also resilient, providing supports for their members. (President's New Freedom Commission on Mental Health, 2003, p. 5)

Social and Cultural Issues

A consideration of the issues and trends regarding older adults' mental health and occupational engagement must include an acknowledgment of their social and cultural context. Occupational therapists must explore the physical environment, values, beliefs, and opportunities for work, rest, and leisure as well as elements of the social environment (American Occupational Therapy Association [AOTA], 2008).

Older adults are challenged by today's economy. Years ago, working-age adults planned for their retirement with a life expectancy of 10 to 15 more years. In 2009, people often live well into their 80s, 90s, or beyond; this longevity has a significant impact on people living on fixed incomes. These factors have resulted in older adults working more years than originally anticipated, giving up their homes and reluctantly moving in with their children, or seeking reverse mortgages. Relocation of one's home often reduces social engagement because the relocated senior loses his or her social network. The loss of familiar environments and cultural connections may result in depression or substance abuse if the adjustment to the changes is not successful. Additionally, many grandparents find themselves taking care of their grandchildren because the parents are both working or have their own challenges with mental illness or substance abuse.

Occupational therapists can be instrumental in advising the older employee and employer on how to modify the work environment and tasks to maintain efficiency. Redesigning job duties and establishing job-sharing possibilities may contribute to aging adults' physical and mental health. Occupational therapists and occupational therapy assistants can intervene with older adults in their caregiving roles by teaching energy conservation, stress management, money management, and resource coordination. Services can be delivered directly or through consultation.

Occupational Therapy and Older Adults With Mental Illness

Occupational therapists serve older adults in a variety of contexts. The most likely contexts are institutional settings such as hospitals, rehabilitation centers, and nursing homes. When mental health issues are the primary concern, occupational therapy intervention is delivered in community- and hospital-based programs dedicated to mental health and substance abuse treatment. However, a 1997 survey of Medicare beneficiaries revealed that at least 48% of respondents reported at least two chronic conditions and 21% reported five or more (Wolff, Starfield, & Anderson, 2002). Untreated depression is associated with increases in dementia, heart disease, diabetes, and possibly cancer (CDC, 2008a; Howland et al., 1993; Miller, Paschall, & Svendsen, 2006). Occupational therapists are likely to find that addressing older adults' occupational participation needs involves addressing the mental health aspects that interfere with recovery.

The second edition of the *Occupational Therapy Practice Framework* (AOTA, 2008) identified eight general areas of occupation: (1) ADLs, (2) IADLs, (3) rest and sleep, (4) education, (5) work (including volunteer work), (6) play, (7) leisure, and (8) social participation. Participation in all of those areas of occupation requires that the client meet a set of responsibilities (AOTA, 2008). For example, to successfully participate in volunteer work, a person must be able to get him- or herself up and ready by completing self-care routines and then traveling to the worksite. Duties include task completion, social interactions, exchange of information, and documentation; symptoms of mental illness can interfere with those responsibilities. Difficulty with cognitive processes, social isolation, lack of motivation, fearfulness, and anxiety all affect people's ability to meet their responsibilities. Many forms of mental illness have symptoms that directly affect people's ability to sleep or rest and appetite and self-care routines (APA, 2000). Increasingly, occupational therapists are focusing on the sensory processing factors that affect participation, such as increased sensory sensitivity with certain forms of dementia or the changes in ability to modulate arousal that come with depression or anxiety (Champagne, 2006). Occupational therapy's focus on participation prepares occupational therapists to create a unique role in treatment systems. Therapists can claim a particular expertise in function that is now the primary determinant of success in the Recovery Model used in community mental health systems (Auerbach, 2002; Pitts, 2001; SAMHSA, 2007). To assess a client's occupational performance and develop an intervention plan, the occupational therapist needs to understand the theories that guide occupational therapy practice for older adults with mental illness. This knowledge guides the clinical reasoning process.

Models of Practice for Clinical Reasoning

Several occupational therapy models can be used to frame treatment of the older adult with mental illness and substance abuse. One commonly used framework is the Cognitive Disability Frame of Reference (Allen, 1990), which equates the severity of a person's illness or disability to his or her capacity to learn, think, and engage in activity. This frame of reference has successfully been used to identify the progression of dementia in older adults by identifying the cognitive impairment and the remaining abilities that can be capitalized on to achieve maximum participation. An important component of the model assumes that severe disorders cannot be remediated by retraining or altering the thinking process. Occupational therapists use the model to help families, caregivers, and others adapt activities and modify the environment to improve both participation and safety.

Another learning theory model is Multi-Contextual Treatment (Brady, 1998). To benefit from this, the client must be able to process information and learn the components of the activities. Occupational therapy intervention requires knowledge of learning patterns and the understanding of task analysis and task breakdown. The goal is to break the task down into chunks that can be processed and learned more readily. For example, a woman presents for treatment of depression and is also recovering from a recent stroke. The therapist breaks down modified ADL tasks such as dressing with one flaccid arm, allowing her to practice and learn chunks of the task. The Motor Learning Theory (Adams, 1971; Jarus, 1994; Poole, 1991) assumes that learning and adaptation occur when a person repeatedly goes through an adaptive response. A good example is teaching someone with dementia to incorporate safety strategies, such as use of a walker, into his or her day by means of repeated auditory and visual reminders.

Several models of practice have occupational participation as the primary treatment outcome. Using an occupation-based practice model in any setting that includes older people allows occupational therapists and occupational therapy assistants to help clients understand their treatment or recovery as a process that reconnects them with a healthy lifestyle and valued life roles. One such model is the Person–Environment–Occupation Model (Law et al., 1996). This model is based on several assumptions, the most important being that the person is amenable and able to change in response to the environment. Another assumption is that the environment can be limiting, but it can also be easier to change than the person. The relationship between the model's three elements is translational and not easily separated. All three elements combined amount to occupational performance (Law et al., 1996; Law & Mills, 1998). Changes in the person are clearly noted in medical-based treatment of older people, but what was not always taken into account in their treatment is that environmental changes are inseparable from changes in occupation that inevitably occur.

Another occupation-based model is the Occupational Adaptation Model (Schkade & Schultz, 1993). This model identifies competence as a process of adaptation to performance. This lifelong process is affected by changes in physical or mental capacity to perform and participate, as well as emotional disability and life stressors. The number of changes that require adaptation accumulate and may overwhelm the older person's capacity to adapt. Changes include mental and physical health, human and nonhuman changes in the person's environment, and financial changes; even changes in technology can be overwhelming and increasingly more difficult to master.

The Model of Human Occupation (MOHO; Kielhofner, 2007) is based on systems theory, which states that a person is an open system, dynamic and responsive to the context in which he or she participates. MOHO is a client-centered theory that encourages teaching people to understand how they interact with their world and what factors affect the ability to interact and maintain a sense of mastery. MOHO considers the connection between mind and body, including understanding skills and skill development and the factors that affect them, as well as factors that affect motivation and desire for mastery. Multiple losses, including changes in cognitive and physical abilities, can alter performance patterns, for example, retirement from driving or work. The changes older adults experience affect their communication and performance skills and can seriously affect their motivation for continued mastery of their environment. Box 7.1 presents a case example of how those changes can affect occupational roles.

MOHO also helps one to understand the significant changes in the level of depression between community-dwelling older adults and older adults placed into long-term living facilities. Most long-term facilities offer little opportunity to engage in the life roles that give a sense of purpose or meaning. Although it is possible to engage in a few roles such as friend and, in some capacity, family, the level of engagement is based on the person's ability to find people with the same interests or understanding and their family's level of involvement. Other roles, such as

Box 7.1. Case Example: Nelly

Nelly came into the hospital after she made a costly mistake at her job. She is 76 years old and has held her job at a woman's dress shop for 42 years. She recently began to experience mild cognitive impairment, which has slowed her down physically and cognitively and caused her to make small but tolerable mistakes. The store owner recognized the changes in Nelly's ability to process information and had changed her responsibilities to accommodate her performance. Nelly also recognized the changes both in her processing of information and in her duties at the store. This recognition caused her to become significantly depressed. In her depression, she became more anxious and forgetful, and one day she overcharged a customer and then became angry when the customer pointed it out to her. The store owner recognized the value of having Nelly at her store, as a long-time worker and as a friend; however, she was concerned about Nelly's mental state.

The occupational therapist assigned to Nelly's care assessed her using MOHO and determined that the changes in her mental status affected several of her occupational roles. Patterns of social withdrawal and decreased attention to hygiene were detected. While Nelly was treated medically for depression and anxiety, she worked with the occupational therapist to discuss ways in which she could reengage in her roles despite her cognitive slowing. She was taught to use an organizer and agreed to allow the store owner to come by each morning before the store opened to go over her medications and check her mental status. Nelly was able to come to terms with her cognitive slowing and was able to recognize the connection between accepting help to maintain her role responsibilities and her mental status and her independence.

volunteering or caring for others or pets, are almost nonexistent in long-term facilities, leaving people with little meaningful activity or sense of purpose.

Mary Corcoran, in her AOTA online course on dementia, described the concept of excess disability (Corcoran, 2001), which is an important factor that must be considered in treatment with many older adults. She used the example of a broken wrist. If a young adult breaks a wrist, he or she understands that it will heal and that it will only be necessary to adapt to complete his or her daily responsibilities until that healing process is complete. When an older adult has a broken wrist, he or she may develop a fear of falling, leading to a decrease in participation, which in turn leads to decreased strength and endurance. Difficulty adapting to loss of ability and resistance to asking for help may in fact lead to a sense of helplessness. Nelly's depression may have been a response to her awareness of her mild cognitive impairment. Although mild cognitive impairment itself is not a reason for institutionalization, the symptoms of forgetfulness and decreased self-care that were part of the depression can be. Although Nelly's mild cognitive impairment cannot be resolved, she can be helped through occupational therapy to remain independent and engaged in her community.

A good understanding of development is important when working with the older adult. Erik Erikson identifies a stage of older adulthood characterized by wisdom, which he referred to as integrity versus despair (Erikson, 1959). According to Erikson, the older adult needs to look back over his or her life and come to terms with the choices and events that make up that life. The older adult with mental illness often focuses on his or her poor choices or negative situations. Developmental theory also helps therapists assess the client's stage in terms of the roles he or she occupies as an older adult (e.g., worker, volunteer, caregiver; Miller, 2001).

One occupational therapy theory that arises out of the developmental theories is sensory integration (Ayres, 1989; Fisher & Murray, 1991). Although primarily associated with pediatric occupational therapy, sensory integration is being increasingly recognized as relevant to adults (Champagne, 2006). Sensory integration is a theory of neurodevelopment that helps define behavior as a result of the person's neurological experience when interacting with the environment. One assumption of this theory is that sensory input is essential for healthy brain function and that integrated sensory responses adapt to environmental input and allow for appropriate responses. Another assumption is that people have an innate drive to alter their sensory integration to achieve adaptive responses (Ayres, 1989; Fisher & Murray, 1991). Given the dramatic changes in the older person's sensory organs, it makes sense to consider sensory integration theory when looking at function. Reduction in vision or hearing acuity may lead to social isolation and to a level of sensory deprivation.

Perception of sensory input may change, leading people to reject activities that in the past were a big part of their lives. For example, Henrietta, who had always been active with friends and family, began to avoid social gatherings because her hearing loss often led to embarrassing misinterpretations. Another example is Martin, who became resistive to taking showers because he claimed that the water hurt. The occupational therapist understood that this sensation was a manifestation of his tactile defensiveness. Sensory Modulation Theory (Champagne, 2006; Williams & Schellenberger, 1996) may allow for greater understanding of such behaviors as wandering, physical touch, rejection of personal care, and yelling.

Several learning theory perspectives that arose from psychology are used for the older adult who remains cognitively intact. Two common theories include behaviorism and cognitive–behavioral therapy (CBT; Bandura, 1977; Beck, 1993). Occupational therapy works well with behavioral theories from the perspective of teaching healthy engagement in meaningful or purposeful life roles. A connection exists between a person's self-perception and his or her engagement in the behaviors associated with meaningful activity. One older man was admitted to an inpatient unit after he was discovered driving into some dangerous areas of the city to buy cocaine. He initially started to use cocaine because it left him feeling more energetic, but it soon became an addiction. On further investigation, the occupational therapist noted that since this man's retirement, he felt as though he had no direction in his life and was useless. According to SAMHSA (2000), older adults are increasingly being treated for substance abuse and they are also responsive to treatment. The chemical dependency staff taught this man about cocaine and his addiction. The occupational therapy staff helped him develop meaningful occupations to structure his time. He learned that his negative beliefs about himself, lack of productive roles since retirement, and loss of social contacts contributed to his addiction. He chose to move into an assisted living facility where he could volunteer at a neighboring school and help the science teachers. He agreed that by engaging in activities that had meaning, he could regain a sense of pride in his abilities and accomplishments. Behaviorism and CBT have limited effects for people who have memory loss or other symptoms associated with dementia.

Several other models for intervention have come out of the work of neurology and social work that, when combined with occupational therapy–based models, can be extremely helpful in not only understanding behavior but even affecting changes in behavior that are more adaptive and result in a greater sense of happiness for the person with dementia.

According to Reisberg et al.'s (1999) Retrogenesis Theory, a person with Alzheimer's disease will regress through cognitive and physical developmental stages in approximately the same order and time frame as a baby develops from birth to about age 12. In other words, by watching how a person handles certain developmental milestones, one can make a guess as to where he or she is in the disease process. A couple of important distinctions exist, however. The last stage in which the person requires total care can last for a much longer period of time than it did for the infant. This phenomenon appears to apply strictly to Alzheimer's disease and not to other forms of dementia such as Pick's disease (Reisberg et al., 1999). What is helpful about this model is its implications for care and therapy. For instance, children are not able to manage utensils until about age 2 and must be much older to cut meat with a knife. Allowing people with Alzheimer's disease to use their fingers and, in fact, providing more finger foods can increase the amount they eat and still allow them the dignity and sense of control they get from feeding themselves. Although children who are new walkers tend to fall, most parents would try to set up the child's environment to allow for that behavior in the safest environment possible rather than restrict their opportunity to walk. Finding ways to encourage activity while reducing the risk of fall injury would allow people with Alzheimer's disease to meet their sensory needs and maintain the strength and flexibility needed to avoid increasing their risk of falls. Occupational therapists can work with clients and their families to create toileting schedules and identify sensory objects that are soothing and developmentally appropriate for this population.

Naomi Feil (2002) developed a model for communicating with confused older adults called Validation Therapy. Validation Therapy has several important assumptions that must be understood. Feil (2002) stated that although confused, this group of older adults must resolve the periods in their lives that are often emotionally laden and that this resolution is essential to maintaining a connection with the people around them. The job of the people around them is to help validate the feelings and thoughts associated with those times. However, confused older adults are also experiencing changes in their sensory systems that affect their ability to stay connected to reality. For instance, not being able to hear others in a group, combined with not being able to remember recent events, may cause people to retreat into their own memories. Feil (2002) stated that people with dementia do not experience time as linear; rather, they move back and forth in time, sometimes returning to a particular period over and over. This experience is further complicated when attention is focused on an unresolved emotional experience or may be a result of a memory sparked by a word, a song, or a visual or tactile cue. People who support someone during these emotional journeys can validate those feelings and help their resolution.

One nursing home resident asked to go home and, when restricted from leaving, would become angry and aggressive with whoever blocked his exit. One particular evening he was asked what was going on. He stated he needed to get home for his son's 10th birthday. In talking with his wife, the occupational therapist learned that in his life roles as family member, father, and spouse, one of his primary responsibilities was cooking. He had always done all the cooking for his family of eight children and was always home at 4:30 p.m. to begin that. The therapist also learned that he had missed his son's 10th birthday because of a work obligation and had not been able to forgive himself. Much of his negative behavior happened at 4:00 p.m. when he would once have set off home to assume his role as cook. What was called "sundowning" became much more understandable when his motivation was understood. By having him help the staff pass out trays to the other patients and allowing him to wait until all the others were taken care of before he was encouraged to eat, the staff was able to change his behavior, improve his level of anxiety and anger, and help him to accept where he was and maintain communication with the people he cared about.

Summary

Occupational therapists play a key role in understanding behavior and finding ways to intervene that help their clients maintain dignity, participation, and a sense of purpose. Life-altering events and treasured memories are always tied to a person's lifelong participation in occupation. Using this holistic approach when working with the older adult with mental illness allows for treatment that can result in continued satisfaction in occupation regardless of mental status.

References

Adams, J. A. (1971). A closed-loop theory of motor learning. *Journal of Motor Behavior, 3,* 111–150.

Administration on Aging. (2006). *Unofficial compilation of the Older Americans Act of 1965: As amended in 2006.* Retrieved April 18, 2008, from www.aoa.gov/AOARoot/AoA_Programs/ OAA/oaa_full.asp

Administration on Aging. (2009). *A profile of older Americans: 2009.* Retrieved January 22, 2010, from www.aoa.gov/AoARoot/Aging_statistics/Profile/2009/2.aspx

Allen, C. K. (1990). *Allen Cognitive Level test manual.* Colchester, CT: Worldwide.

American Occupational Therapy Association. (2008). Occupational therapy practice framework: Domain and process (2nd ed.). *American Journal of Occupational Therapy, 62,* 625– 683.

American Psychiatric Association. (2000). *Diagnostic and statistical manual of mental disorders* (4th ed., text rev.). Washington, DC: Author.

Auerbach, E. (2002). *An occupational therapist in an assertive community treatment program. Mental Health Special Interest Section Quarterly Newsletter, 25*(1), 1–2.

Ayres, J. (1989*). Sensory Integration and Praxis Test manual.* Los Angeles: Western Psychological Services.

Bandura, A. (1977). *Social learning theory.* Englewood Cliffs, NJ: Prentice Hall.

Bartels, S. J., Blow, F. C., Brockmann, L. M., & Van Citters, A. D. (2005). *Substance abuse and mental health among older Americans: The state of the knowledge and future directions.* Washington, DC: Substance Abuse and Mental Health Services Administration. Retrieved January 22, 2010, from www.samhsa.gov/OlderAdultsTAC/SA_MH_%20AmongOlder Adultsfinal10205.pdf

Bartels, S. J., Coakley, E. H., Zubritsky, C., Ware, J. H., Miles, K. M., Arean, P. A., et al. (2004). Improving access to geriatric mental health services: A randomized trial comparing treatment engagement with integrated versus enhanced referral care for depression, anxiety, and at-risk alcohol use. *American Journal of Psychiatry, 161,* 8.

Beck, A. T. (1993). Cognitive therapy: Past, present, and future. *Journal of Consulting and Clinical Psychology, 61,* 194–198.

Blow, F., Bartels, S. J., Brockmann, L. M., & Van Citters, A. D., for the Older Americans Substance Abuse and Mental Health Technical Assistance Center. (2004). *Evidence-based practices for preventing substance abuse and mental health problems in older adults.* Bethesda, MD: Substance Abuse and Mental Health Services Administration, Older Americans Substance Abuse and Mental Health Technical Assistance Center. Retrieved from www. samhsa.gov/OlderAdultsTAC/EBPCo-OccurringProblemssectionFINAL.pdf

Brady, F. (1998). A theoretical and empirical review of the contextual interference effect and the learning of motor skills. *Quest, 50*(3), 266–293.

Centers for Disease Control and Prevention. (2008a). *Falls among older adults: An overview.* Retrieved from www.cdc.gov/ncipc/factsheets/adultfalls.htm

Centers for Disease Control and Prevention. (2008b). *Preventing falls among older adults.* Retrieved from www.cdc.gov/ncipc/duip/preventadultfalls.htm

Centers for Medicare and Medicaid Services (2006). *Money follows the person grants.* Retrieved August 2009 from www.cms.hhs.gov/DeficitReductionAct/20_MFP.asp

Champagne, T. (2006). *Sensory modulation and environment: Essential elements of occupation. General handbook and reference* (2nd ed.). Southampton, MA: Champagne Conferences and Consultation. (Available from www.ot_innovations.com)

Corcoran, M. (Ed.). (2001). *Fundamentals of occupational therapy for individuals with dementia* (AOTA Online Course). Bethesda, MD: American Occupational Therapy Association.

Deficit Reduction Act of 2005, Pub. L. 109–171.

Erikson, E. (1959). *Identity and the life cycle.* New York: International University Press.

Exec. Order No. 13263, 3 C.F.R. 233 (2002).

Feil, N. (2002). *The validation breakthrough: Simple techniques for communicating with people with Alzheimer's-type dementia* (2nd ed.). Baltimore: Health Professions Press.

Fisher, A. G., & Murray, E. A. (1991). Introduction to sensory integration theory. In A. G. Fisher, E. A. Murry, & A. C. Bundy (Eds.), *Sensory integration theory and practice* (pp. 3–26). Philadelphia: F. A. Davis.

Howland, J., Peterson, E., Levin, W., Ried, L., Pordon, D., & Bak, S. (1993). Fear of falling among the community-dwelling elderly. *Journal of Aging and Health, 5,* 229–243.

Jarus, T. (1994). Motor learning and occupational therapy: The organization of practice. *American Journal of Occupational Therapy, 48,* 810–816.

Kielhofner, G. (2007). *A Model of Human Occupation: Theory and application* (4th ed.). Baltimore: Williams & Wilkins.

Krahn, D. D., Bartels, S. J., Coakley, E., Oslin, D. W., Chen, H., McIntyre, J., et al. (2006). PRISM–E: Comparison of integrated care and enhanced specialty referral models in depression outcomes. *Psychiatric Services, 57*(7), 946–953.

Law, M., Cooper, B., Strong, S., Stewart, D., Tigby, P., & Letts, L. (1996). The Person–Environment–Occupation model: A transactive approach to occupational performance. *Canadian Journal of Occupational Therapy, 63,* 9–23.

Law, M., & Mills, J. (1998). *Client-centered occupational therapy.* In M. Law (Ed.), *Client-centered occupational therapy* (pp. 1–18). Thorofare, NJ: Slack.

Lipson, D., Gruman, C., Schimmel, J., Colby, M., Denny-Brown, N., Peterson, S., et al. (2007). *Money follows the person demonstration grants: Summary of state MFP program applicants.* Retrieved from www.cms.hhs.gov/DeficitReductionAct/downloads/StateMFPGrantSummaries-All.pdf

Maki, M. E., Holiday, P. J., & Topper, A. K. (1991). Fear of falling and postural performance in the elderly. *Journals of Gerontology, Series A: Biological Sciences and Medical Sciences, 46*(A), M123–M131.

McCurren, C., Dowe, D., Rattle, D., & Looney, S. (1999). Depression among nursing home elders: Testing an intervention strategy. *Applied Nursing Research, 12,* 185–195.

Miller, B. J., Paschall, C. B., & Svendsen, D. P. (2006). Mortality and medical comorbidity among patients with serious mental illness. *Psychiatric Services, 57,* 1482–1487.

Murphy, J., & Isaacs, B. (1982). The post-fall syndrome: A study of 36 elderly patients. *Gerontology, 28,* 265–270.

National Institute of Mental Health. (2003). *Older adults: Depression and suicide facts* (NIH Pub. No. 03–4593). Washington, DC: U.S. Government Printing Office.

Office of the Press Secretary. (2002). *President's New Freedom Commission on Mental Health.* [Press release]. Retrieved from http://govinfo.library.unt.edu/mentalhealthcommission/20020429-2.htm

Older Americans Act of 1965, Pub. L. 89–73, 79 Stat. 218, 42 U.S.C. § 3001 *et seq.*

Olmstead v. L.C., 527 U.S. 581 (1999).

Oslin, D. W., Grantham, S., Coakley, E., Maxwell, J., Miles, K., Ware, J., et al. (2006). PRISM–E: Comparison of integrated care and enhanced specialty referral in managing at-risk alcohol use. *Psychiatric Services, 57*(7), 954–958.

Peterson, E., & Howland, J. (2003). Using cognitive behavioral strategies to reduce fear of falling: A matter of balance. *Journal of the American Society of Aging, 26*(4), 89–92.

Pitts, D. (2001). Assertive community treatment: A brief introduction. *Mental Health Special Interest Section Quarterly, 24*(1), 1–2.

Poole, J. (1991). Application of motor learning principles in occupational therapy. *American Journal of Occupational Therapy, 45,* 531–537.

President's New Freedom Commission on Mental Health. (2003). *Achieving the promise: Transforming mental health care in America* (Final Report, DHHS Pub. No. SMA–03–3832). Rockville, MD: Author. Retrieved from www.mentalhealthcommission.gov/reports/FinalReport/downloads/FinalReport.pdf

Reisberg, B., Franssen, E. H., Hasan, S. M., Monteiro, I., Boksay, I., Souren, L. E. M., et al. (1999). Retrogenesis: Clinical, physiologic, and pathologic mechanisms in brain aging, Alzheimer's, and other dementing processes. *European Archives of Psychiatry and Clinical Neuroscience, 249*(9), S28–S26.

Rush Alzheimer's disease screening, diagnosis and treatment. (2008). Retrieved July 2008 from www.rush.edu/rumc/page-1099611541603.html

Schkade, J. K., & Schultz, S. (1993). Occupational adaptation: An integrative frame of reference. In H. Hopkins & H. Smigh (Eds.), *Willard and Spackman's occupational therapy* (8th ed., pp. 87–91). Philadelphia: Lippincott.

Snowdon, D. (2001). *Aging with grace.* New York: Bantam Books.

Substance Abuse and Mental Health Services Administration. (2000). *Substance abuse among older adults: A guide for treatment providers. Treatment improvement protocol (TIP) 26* (DHHS Pub. No. SMA–05–4083). Rockville, MD: Author.

Substance Abuse and Mental Health Services Administration. (2004a). *As you age...A guide to aging, medicines and alcohol* (DHHS Pub. No. PHD–1082). Rockville, MD: Author.

Substance Abuse and Mental Health Services Administration. (2004b). *Community integration for older adults with mental illnesses: Overcoming barriers and seizing opportunities* (DHHS Pub. No. SMA–05–4018). Rockville, MD: Author.

Substance Abuse and Mental Health Services Administration. (2007). *Primary care research in substance abuse and mental health services for the elderly (PRISM–E).* Retrieved October 2, 2007, from www.samhsa.gov/aging/age_07.aspx

Tinetti, M. E., Speechley, M., & Ginter, S. F. (1988). Risk factors for falls among elderly persons living in the community. *New England Journal of Medicine, 319,* 1701–1706.

U.S. Department of Health and Human Services. (1999). *Mental health: A report of the Surgeon General* (Chapter 5). Rockville, MD: U.S. Department of Health and Human Services, Substance Abuse and Mental Health Services Administration, Center for Mental Health Services & National Institute of Mental Health. Retrieved January 22, 2010, from www.surgeongeneral.gov/library/mentalhealth/toc.html

White House Conference on Aging. (2005). *WHCoA Resolution vote tally.* Retrieved from www.whcoa.gov/about/resolutions/WCHoA_2005_Rank.pdf

Williams, M. S., & Schellenberger, S. (1996). *How does your engine run? A leader's guide to the Alert program for self-regulation.* (Rev. ed.). Lawrenceville, GA: Therapy Works.

Wolff, J. L., Starfield, B., & Anderson, G. (2002). Prevalence, expenditures, and complications of multiple chronic conditions in the elderly. *Archives of Internal Medicine, 162,* 2269–2276.

CHAPTER 8

Evaluation in Mental Health Occupational Therapy Advanced Practice

Deborah B. Pitts, MBA, OTR/L, CPRP, BCMH

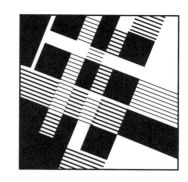

Learning Objectives

After reading this material and completing the examination, readers will be able to

- Recognize the contextualized and situated nature of occupational therapy and its impact on the evaluation process in mental health practice contexts;

- Identify macro-, meso-, and micro-level influences on the occupational therapy evaluation process in mental health contexts;

- Identify areas of best evidence for advanced occupational therapy practice in mental health contexts; and

- Recognize the political implications attendant in the occupational therapy evaluation process specific to mental health practice contexts.

Evaluation is a necessary first step in any professional practice, including health care practices such as occupational therapy. Advanced practice in the area of evaluation requires occupational therapists to deepen their entry-level understanding of the philosophical, theoretical, social, and political contexts within which they practice. Therapists need to stay current with the research documenting (1) the impact of psychiatric disability and adverse psychosocial circumstances on occupational engagement, (2) the role of occupation in facilitating health and participation in life for people with psychiatric disabilities, and (3) the most effective assessment tools or approaches for eliciting a comprehensive understanding of the client and his or her occupations and environments. Such knowledge is necessary so that the therapist and the client can collaboratively and effectively target interventions to support satisfying and successful participation. To make sense of occupational therapy evaluation as an advanced practice, this chapter frames evaluation as a contextualized–situated practice, as an evidence-based practice, and as a political practice. Each frame is presented as a way to facilitate the reflection on practice that is a necessary part of moving from being a novice therapist to an expert.

Evaluation as a Contextualized–Situated Practice

Making sense of occupational therapy evaluation practices requires occupational therapists to take account of the characteristics and dynamic interactions at and among the macro level (i.e., mental health system, state of the profession of occupational therapy), the meso level (i.e., particular practice settings), and the micro level (i.e., individual therapist interactions with particular people) of practice.

Macro-Level Influences

Changes in the philosophical and practical perspectives that guide how services are delivered within the mental health system, particularly the public mental health system, represent critical macro-level influences to which practitioners must respond. During the past 2 decades, the mental health delivery system has been called on to focus on resilience and recovery (Anthony, 1993; Jacobson & Curtis, 2000; President's New Freedom Commission on Mental Health, 2003; Substance Abuse and Mental Health Services Administration [SAMHSA], 2005; U.S. Department of Health and Human Services, 1999) and to adopt and implement evidence-based practices (EBPs) to support that resilience and recovery (Anthony, Rogers, & Farkas, 2003; Farkas, Gagne, Anthony, & Chamberlin, 2005; Ganju, 2003; Torrey et al., 2001).

Recovery, for people with a psychiatric disability, has come to be understood as satisfying and successful participation in meaningful life roles, even if symptoms persist (Bellack, 2006; Corrigan, Giffort, Rashid, Leary, & Okeke, 1999; Davidson et al., 2005; Jacobson & Greenley, 2001; Liberman, Kopelowicz, Ventura, & Gutkind, 2002; Rebeiro-Gruhl, 2005; Secker, Membrey, Grove, & Sebolm, 2002; Young & Ensing, 1999). Ralph (2000), in a review of the recovery literature, cited several definitions of *recovery* from consumer–survivor first-person accounts, including that of Patricia Deegan, an internationally respected consumer–survivor advocate:

> Recovery is a process, a way of life, an attitude, and a way of approaching the day's challenges. It is not a perfectly linear process. At times our course is erratic and we falter, slide back, regroup, and start again. The need is to meet the challenge of the disability and to reestablish a new and valued sense of integrity and purpose within and beyond the limits of the disability; the aspiration is to live, work, and love in a community in which one makes a significant contribution. (p. 6)

Rebeiro-Gruhl (2005) has argued that occupational therapy's practice philosophy and theoretical models and the intervention approaches that they inform are a good fit with this focus on recovery and resilience. She argued further that recovery, and the role of occupation in recovery, was articulated in the early literature on occupational therapy (Meyer, 1922). More recently, research on recovery and the occupational experiences of people with psychiatric disability has come from an international cadre of occupational therapy researchers (Bejerholm & Eklund, 2004; Chaffey & Fossey, 2004; Eklund, 2001; Eklund, Hansson, & Ahlqvist, 2004; Kennedy-Jones, Cooper, & Fossey, 2005; Krupa, 2004; Laliberte-Rudman, 2002;

Laliberte-Rudman, Yu, Scott, & Pajouhandeh, 2000; Lloyd & Waghorn, 2007; Mee & Sumsion, 2001; Mee, Sumsion, & Craik, 2004; Merryman & Riegel, 2007).

EBP is not without its critics (Cooper, 2003; Tanenbaum, 2005) and implementation challenges (Deane, Crowe, King, Kavanagh, & Oades, 2006; Goldman et al., 2001; Isett et al., 2007). EBPs have particularly been criticized with regard to the fit of resilience and recovery as a particularly individualized experience with the often protocol-driven process of EBPs (Davidson, O'Connell, Tondora, Styron, & Kangas, 2006; Farkas et al., 2005; Frese, Stanley, Kress, & Vogel-Scibilia, 2001; Ralph, Lambert, & Kidder, 2002). In spite of those criticisms, EBP initiatives are moving forward, for example, in committees in state governments determining "best practice." What counts for evidence in EBP has been in dispute, both within the larger health care environment and within mental health or behavioral health care (Frese et al., 2001; Ralph et al., 2002). Anthony et al. (2003) noted that the EBP level of evidence hierarchy prioritizes large randomized trials, and fewer studies of that magnitude exist for mental health interventions beyond medication trials.

Additional macro-level dynamics have influenced occupational therapy evaluation practices in the past several years:

- Structural shifts in how mental health services are delivered, specifically prioritizing the delivery of services in the natural environment (e.g., wrap-around services for children; supported employment, education, and housing for adults), the development of forced-treatment initiatives (e.g., involuntary outpatient commitment and community treatment orders; Allen & Smith, 2001; Swartz & Swanson, 2004), and an increase in the incarceration of people with psychiatric disability (Lamberti et al., 2001)
- Policy shifts regarding funding for mental health and occupational therapy services, particularly Medicaid and Medicare (e.g., the use of Medicaid funding to implement the Olmstead Community Integration initiative) and the use of systemwide outcome measures (e.g., National Outcomes Measures initiative with state departments of mental health; SAMHSA, n.d.)
- Changes in standards set by accrediting bodies, including the Joint Commission and the Commission on Accreditation of Rehabilitation Facilities (e.g., credentialing of allied health practitioners in hospitals)
- Increased interest in the impact of trauma and natural disasters (e.g., Hurricane Katrina, the 2004 Indian Ocean tsunami) on the health and welfare of the population at large, partnered with renewed interest in theoretical and developmental perspectives on attachment (Schultz-Krohn & Cara, 2000; Shore, 2001) for psychosocial adjustment and building resilience
- Demand from the mental health consumer community for full partnership in the delivery of mental health services, including the power to refuse care and to intentionally exit the mental health system without reprisal or the need for continued surveillance (Campbell, 1997; Honey, 1999; Mowbray, Moxley, & Collins, 1998; Salzer, 1997).

Given the current federal mandate, and in light of other macro-level influences, the focus of occupational therapy intervention in the mental health delivery system must be on promoting recovery and resilience for people with or at risk for psychiatric disability. The occupational therapy evaluation must then elicit information that facilitates an understanding of the client-, environment-, and occupation-specific resources and barriers that support or thwart the targeted outcomes identified by the client and his or her support system that optimize recovery and resilience.

Meso-Level Influences

At the meso level of particular practice settings, occupational therapy presence in inpatient psychiatric settings has a long tradition (Kielhofner & Burke, 1977; Meyer, 1922). That presence has at various times in occupational therapy's history been challenged (Fidler, 1991; Jackson, 1984), particularly given that accreditation bodies, such as the Joint Commission, do not identify occupational therapy as a necessary and required service in behavioral health care settings. In response to those challenges, occupational therapists have worked to differentiate occupational therapy practice from that of other mental health providers, particularly from recreational therapy and to some extent from nursing, social work, and psychology (Allen, 1988). The efforts to establish a jurisdictional claim (Abbott, 1988) have evolved in various ways on the basis of the unique characteristics of the specific practice settings and the support for occupational therapy in those settings.

With regard to evaluation, then, various configurations have emerged that position occupational therapy differently in relation to other mental health providers. In some inpatient settings, occupational therapists have chosen to target particular client factors and performance skills, including cognitive disabilities (Allen, 1988; Allen, Earhart, & Blue, 1992), sensory processing patterns or disorders (Champagne, 2005, 2006; Champagne & Stromberg, 2004), or both. In those instances, the occupational therapy evaluation focuses on how the client factors and performance skills affect occupational engagement, support resilience and recovery, and stand as a unique, specialized component of the patient assessment process. Alternatively, using a transdisciplinary perspective (Paul & Peterson, 2001; Rushmer & Pallis, 2003), occupational therapists may collaborate with other psychiatric rehabilitation–activity therapy providers (i.e., recreational therapy, vocational rehabilitation) to develop a comprehensive psychiatric rehabilitation–activity assessment that any one of these providers is qualified to complete as a rehabilitation–activity therapy generalist. This approach is distinct from an interdisciplinary or multidisciplinary approach, in which each provider completes a discipline- or profession-specific assessment and then team members collaborate on the development of the treatment plan (Paul & Peterson, 2001). In addition, although not the most common configuration, in some community hospital inpatient psychiatric settings, occupational therapists may be the sole or lead psychiatric rehabilitation–activity therapy provider and as a result responsible for completing all evaluations (Mary Kay Wolfe, OTD, personal communication, September 25, 2007).

In community-based service models, occupational therapists have been equally committed to establishing their practice's proper relationship with other mental health providers. Although occupational therapy's presence in the U.S. community mental health service system is modest, internationally occupational therapists are typically represented on community mental health teams. Despite this representation, however, tension has arisen between the generalist (i.e., case manager) and specialist roles available to occupational therapists in those settings (Fossey, 2001; Harries & Gilhooly, 2003; Harrison, 2003; Parker, 2001). A particular aspect of this generalist versus specialist tension focuses on what the occupational therapy evaluation can contribute to the community mental health team's general understanding of the occupational needs of people with a psychiatric disability. Some occupational therapists have adopted an occupation-based perspective and have intentionally incorporated into their discourse the use of *occupation* over *activity* as a strategy to underscore their unique contribution. Moreover, those therapists have elected to practice explicitly from a particular frame of reference that foregrounds *occupation* and its role in facilitating resilience and recovery, for example, the Person–Environment–Occupation model (Creek, 2002) or the Model of Human Occupation (Haglund, Ekbladh, Thorell, & Hallberg, 2000). The Model of Human Occupation in particular has a richly developed set of evidence-based assessment tools that occupational therapists can use to demonstrate their specialty perspective in mental health practice settings (Kielhofner, 2008).

Micro-Level Influences

At the micro level, contextual influences that must be taken into account are the occupational therapist's individual characteristics and his or her unique biography (Meyer, 1957), including not only the therapist's developmental life experiences but also the educational and practice experiences that have helped to shape his or her occupational therapy values, knowledge, and skill sets. People are encouraged from the beginning of their education to continually reflect on the ways in which their own sensibilities shape what they see, how they interpret what they see, and how they prioritize what actions need to be taken.

Each configuration affords both opportunities and constraints as to how effectively the occupational therapy evaluation is situated as a component of the comprehensive understanding of a client's needs with regard to his or her resilience and recovery goals. It has been argued that transdisciplinary (also identified as post-disciplinary; Holmes, 2001) and generalist practice models are necessary given the complexity of the dilemmas that must be addressed in modern health care practices. Disciplines and professions have criticized this perspective, however, because they feel that it places the uniqueness of a given profession at serious risk. Discipline- and profession-specific approaches are preferred because they are more likely to avoid the blurring of boundaries associated with the transdisciplinary approach, and individual providers then have more confidence in their contribution to and visibility in the treatment process. Given the variations on occupational therapists' role in mental health, therapists must fully understand the practice landscape at all levels.

Evaluation as an Evidence-Based Practice

As noted in the previous section, occupational therapy, like other health care disciplines and professions, is responding to the call for EBP (Holm, 2000) and an emerging alternative referred to as *practice-based evidence* (McDonald & Viehbeck, 2007), including the need to use evaluation practices and assessment tools that are identified as best practices (Law, Baum, & Dunn, 2001). Law and Baum (2005) argued that many occupational therapists across practice settings "engage in 'standard practice,' which is employing more traditional, routine, and established ways of providing services" (p. 9). This call for EBP is intended to counter the use of standard practice to ensure that occupational therapists are continually updating their practices with the latest evidence. EBP has been criticized for a high reliance on randomized controlled trials as the best evidence. As a result, efforts to clarify that EBP "requires the integration of *current best evidence, practitioner expertise,* and *client preferences*" [italics added] (Cohen & Kearney, 2005, p. 264) are under way. What then counts for best practice in occupational therapy evaluation?

Eliciting the Client's Preferences

The second edition of the *Occupational Therapy Practice Framework* (American Occupational Therapy Association [AOTA], 2008) described two components of an occupational therapy evaluation: (1) the occupational profile and (2) the analysis of occupational performance. Each step in the occupational therapy evaluation process assists the therapist and the client in collaborating to develop interventions to facilitate occupational engagement in the service of building resilience and recovery. The occupational profile in particular is understood to be that part of the evaluation in which the client's perceptions of his or her occupational performance are elicited as well as his or her perception of the need for change and preferences for the nature of that change.

Hinojosa (2007) has argued that in some clinical situations, completing the occupational profile would be "of little use" (p. 631), suggesting that diagnostic-based procedural reasoning rather than narrative reasoning may be more appropriate as an initial first step in completing an occupational therapy evaluation. Some in the psychiatric community might agree, given the view that people with a psychiatric disability, particularly schizophrenia, are considered to have poor insight and awareness into the nature of their disability (Amador, 2007; Amador & Strauss, 1993). Supporting this viewpoint are studies that have determined that the use of self-report quality of life measures should be taken up with caution because they "are likely to contain biases due to cognition, periodic affective swings, and recent life events that may better reflect psychopathology and symptoms than actual life conditions or functions" (Atkinson, Zibin, & Chuang, 1997, p. 104)

That said, the occupational therapist practicing in the mental health context who does not begin with the thoughtful and skilled development of an occupational profile would be out of step with the demand from the mental health consumer–survivor–ex-patient movement for full participation in all aspects of the delivery of mental health services (Bassman, 2001; Chamberlin, 1979, 1997). In addition, alternative views regarding the insight and awareness of people with a psychiatric disability have been developed and provide meaningful guidance for making sense of what is considered insight (Davidson, 2003; Roe & Kravetz, 2003) and quality of life self-reports (Hasson-Ohayon, Kravetz, Roe, David, & Weiser, 2006; Voruganti, Heslegrave, Awad, & Seeman, 2000). These authors emphasized the importance of phenomenological–narrative interviewing approaches for eliciting people's lived experience of psychiatric disorder and disability, its impact on their life course, their understanding of the disorder's etiology, and their desire for change. Moreover, these perspectives argue that quality of life is a complex phenomenon that is best understood in light of people's personal illness–recovery narrative (Lysaker, Buck, Hammoud, Taylor, & Roe, 2006; Lysaker, Buck, Taylor, & Roe, 2008; Lysaker, Campbell, & Johannesen, 2005; Lysaker & Louria, 2007; Lysaker, Roe, & Yanos, 2007; Marin et al., 2005; Sells et al., 2005).

The use of narrative approaches has been documented in occupational science and occupational therapy as being meaningful for eliciting the client's lived experience of occupation and occupational disruptions (Clark, Larson, & Richardson, 1996; Frank, 1996; Kielhofner & Mallinson, 1995; Mallinson, Kielhofner, & Mattingly, 1996; Mattingly, 1991, 1998a, 1998b). Evidence-based occupational therapy assessment tools informed by specific theoretical models or frames of reference in keeping with the perspective discussed earlier are available and in wide use both nationally and internationally. Both the Canadian Occupational Performance Measure, informed by the Canadian Model of Occupational Performance (www.otworks. com; Law et al., 2005) and the Occupational Therapy Performance History Interview–II (Version 2.1), informed by the Model of Human Occupation (Kielhofner et al., 2004), have been demonstrated to be effective and have utility for use with people with a psychiatric disability (Cresswell & Rugg, 2003; Ennals & Fossey, 2007; Pan, Chung, & Hsin-Hwei, 2003; Warren, 2002).

Drawing on the Therapist's Expertise

Although therapist expertise is identified as a component of EBP, research evidence or technical rationality (i.e., application of scientific theory and technique; Polkinghorne, 2004; Schon, 1983) has obtained a privileged position in health care, including mental health and behavioral health care. Because EBP has become established as a framework for all health care practice, efforts to place therapist expertise on equal footing with research evidence have grown (Polkinghorne, 2004; Tanenbaum, 1994, 1999, 2003, 2005). These perspectives emphasize that practical knowledge is essential because it "allows for the complexity of [therapist] experience and for the immediacy and individuality of [patients, clients, or persons served]" (Tanenbaum, 1999, p. 757).

The expertise that the occupational therapist in mental health develops over time to successfully conduct an evaluation includes first—and perhaps most important—an understanding of the nature of occupational engagement, particularly the generative influence of occupational engagement on optimizing a person's mental health status as well as it protective influence on minimizing his or her mental health risk from adverse psychosocial circumstances. Additionally, the mental health occupational therapist builds a practical knowledge of the phenomena that may disrupt occupational engagement. Psychiatric disorder or disability, trauma, exposure to occupationally deprived environments, and other contextual barriers may disrupt occupational engagement in characteristic ways. Although each person has a unique illness experience, specific psychiatric disorders do affect occupational engagement in particular ways. For example, people with schizophrenia commonly experience cognitive (van den Bosch, Rombouts, & van Asma, 1993), self (Parnas & Handest, 2003), and sensory (Brown, Cromwell, Filion, Dunn, & Tollefson, 2002) disruptions (Davidson, 2003). Although the entry-level occupational therapist will initially have learned this in his or her coursework, interacting and working with people with schizophrenia, and then reflecting on those interactions, will provide knowledge-in-action of how occupational engagement can be disrupted. Finally, as the occupational therapist engages in the process of selecting, administering, and interpreting assessments and using particular assessment approaches, he or she builds knowledge-in-action of specific assessment tools.

Knowing the Meaningful Current Best Evidence

Resources and guidance on how to find and make sense of the current best evidence have been developed within health care at large, within mental health or behavioral health care specifically, and for occupational therapy interventions delivered in a variety of health care and social service contexts. AOTA's EBP and research resources (available through its Web site, www.aota.org) include evidence briefs, critically appraised topics, and critically appraised papers that target mental health populations. A common strategy to facilitate access to the current best evidence, as well as to engage in the development of practice-based evidence, is for individual therapists and or agencies to develop partnerships with academic occupational therapy, psychiatric rehabilitation, or other mental health professional faculty. What, then, counts as meaningful current best evidence needed to effectively conduct meaningful occupational therapy evaluations?

Evidence Regarding Occupational Engagement for People at Risk for or With a Psychiatric Disability

Occupational therapists must in particular target literature that investigates the protective and generative influences of engagement for promoting optimum mental health and well-being (Yerxa, 1998) and facilitating recovery and resilience for people at risk for or with a psychiatric disability (Borg et al., 2005; Eklund & Bäckström, 2005; Eklund et al., 2004; Iannelli & Wilding, 2007; Kennedy-Jones et al., 2005; Krupa, 2004; Laliberte-Rudman, 2002; Lloyd & Waghorn, 2007; Mee & Sumsion, 2001; Mee et al., 2004; Mezzina et al., 2006; Wilding, May, & Muir-Cochrane, 2005). Occupational science research—as well as psychology, sociology, anthropology, geography, public health, and leisure studies, for example—are critical sources for this area of knowledge. This literature should also be considered for deepening therapists' understanding of the very real barriers to occupational participation for people with a psychiatric disability (Brekke, Prindle, Bae, & Long, 2001; Rebeiro, 1999). Moreover, it can facilitate critical thinking regarding the experience of occupational justice (Townsend, 2003), structural violence (Kelly, 2005), and the more controversial occupational apartheid (Kronenberg, Algado, & Pollard, 2004; Kronenberg & Pollard, 2006).

Evidence Regarding Phenomena That Disrupt Satisfying and Successful Occupational Engagement for People at Risk for or With a Psychiatric Disability

Occupational therapists should consider the literature that addresses the subjective and functional aspects of psychiatric disorders and disability (Chugg & Craik, 2002; Laliberte-Rudman et al., 2000; Leufstadius & Eklund, 2008; Nagle, Cook, & Polatajko, 2002), in particular sensory modulation (Brown et al., 2002) and cognitive impairments (Green, 1996; van den Bosch et al., 1993). Additional areas that need to be investigated and understood include trauma (Mueser, Rosenberg, Goodman, & Trumbetta, 2002), exposure to occupationally deprived environments, and other contextual factors such as stigma (Link, Struening, Neese-Todd, Asmussen, & Phelan, 2001; Perlick et al., 2001), poverty (Wilton, 2004), and the structure and design of the mental health service system itself (Bryant, Craik, & McKay, 2004; Rebeiro, 1999).

Evidence Regarding the Effectiveness of Rehabilitation and Biomedical Interventions That Have Been Designed to Support Recovery and Resilience

SAMHSA (n.d.) has identified a core set of interventions that are or have been adopted by state and local mental health authorities with which occupational therapists practicing in mental health services should be familiar. The interventions include illness management and recovery (Mueser et al., 2004, 2006), assertive community treatment (Bond, Drake, Mueser, & Latimer, 2001; Phillips et al., 2001), family psychoeducation (Dixon et al., 2001), supported employment (Bond, Drake, & Becker, 2008; Bond, McHugo, Becker, Rapp, & Whitley, 2008), and integrated dual treatment for co-occurring disorders (Minkoff, 2001). Additional approaches have also been documented and are being implemented, including supported housing (Chilvers, Macdonald, & Hayes, 2006; Fakhoury, Murray, Shepherd, & Priebe, 2002; Humberstone, 2002) and supported education (Collins, Mowbray, & Bybee, 2000). Evidence-based mental health interventions for children (Hoagwood, Burns, Kiser, Ringeisen, & Schoenwald, 2001; Ramchandani, Joughin, & Zwi, 2001), including the role of occupational therapy (Lougher, 2001), and for older adults (Bartels et al., 2004; Clark et al., 1997; Ludwig, 1997) have also been documented.

Evidence Regarding the Effectiveness of Specific Assessment Tools and Approaches for Developing the Occupational Profile and Completing an Analysis of Occupational Performance

Advanced practice therapists have developed their knowledge and skill sets for the meaningful and effective selection, administration, and interpretation of specific assessments that are well suited to their specific meso- and micro-level practice contexts. Guidance regarding how to meaningfully critique assessments has been documented elsewhere and should be reviewed (Bass-Haugen, 2005; Cohen, Hinojosa, & Kramer, 2005; Crist, 2005; Polgar, 2009).

Narrative–phenomenological assessment approaches and tools, as noted earlier, have been identified and documented as effective for completing the occupational profile in mental health settings. Regarding assessment approaches and tools for the analysis of occupational performance, recent efforts by psychiatric researchers to understand the relationship of cognitive capacity to real-world functioning through the development of performance-based ecologically valid assessments has been documented (Mausbach, Harvey, Goldman, Jeste, & Patterson, 2007; McKibbin, Brekke, Sires, Jeste, & Patterson, 2004; Patterson, Goldman, McKibbin, Hughs, & Jeste, 2001; Worrall, McCooey, Davidson, Larkins, & Hickson, 2002). Hamera, Rempfer, and Brown (2005) challenged these researchers regarding their failure to thoroughly investigate the research on assessments developed by or in collaboration with occupational therapy researchers (Hamera et al., 2005; McKibbin, Patterson, Brekke, & Jeste, 2005)—for example, the Test of Grocery Shopping Skills (Hamera & Brown, 2000). Beyond the need for performance-based, ecologically valid assessments is the need to develop and use assessments that are effective for use in the natural environment, such as work (MacDonald-Wilson, Rogers, & Anthony, 2001; McGuire, Bond, Evans, Lysaker, & Kim, 2007), school (Coster, 1998), and engagement in instrumental activities of daily living (Rempfer, Hamera, Brown, & Cromwell, 2003).

As noted earlier, EBP "requires the integration of current best evidence, practitioner expertise, and client preferences" (Cohen & Kearney, 2005, p. 264). How does this integration process occur? "Down on the ground" health care practices have been described as improvisations (Mattingly & Fleming, 1994; Schon, 1983), which may be a useful frame for addressing the integration that is expected with EBP. Various perspectives on improvisation can be found in the social science and humanities literature (Becker, 2000a, 2000b; Cash, 2000; Montuori, 1997) and in literature on the performing arts, particularly dance (Clark-Rapley, 1999; Schwartz, 2000; Sheets-Johnston, 2000), theater, and jazz (Day, 2000; Kodat, 2003; Sawyer, 2000a, 2000b). The next sections consider some of the dimensions of improvisation that may be useful in this context.

Improvisation Involves Interaction and Collaboration. In the dance literature, this process is described as "leading and following"; that is, any dancer at a particular time during the improvisation could be leading or following. This process is described as a democratic one in which all participants have equal power to move the dance forward (Schwartz, 2000; Sheets-Johnston, 2000). This leading and following process requires a "mindful" (Langer, 1990) attentive stance on the part of each participant. Improvisation, it is argued, cannot go just anywhere—it is not chaotic, it has an implicit structure. Improvisation has boundaries. In jazz improvisation, the boundaries are set by the original piece of music on which the improvisation is made (Sawyer, 2000b). In theater, the boundaries are set by the first person to begin the improvisation; within a few exchanges, the "plot" is established, and the improvisers must work within that plot or disrupt the improvisation. To be able to have such "conversations," improvisers must be able to understand each other; they must have what social scientists call *shared cultural knowledge*. This shared cultural knowledge provides the actors with "ready-mades" used to create novel performances (Sawyer, 2000a, 2000b).

Each Improvisation Is Unique—A One-Time Performance. What makes a performance improvisational is that each improvisation is a new or novel performance that emerges out of the transactions among players. Given its emergent properties, improvisation always develops within the situation or context as presented, which is why advanced practice therapists have been found to be more effective improvisers than novice therapists.

When considered in light of evidence-based assessment, each element of improvisation provides the occupational therapist with the practice space to respond to the unique and immediate context of a particular care encounter. The therapist is, of course, required to be familiar with the established protocol but must also be mindful of others with whom he or she is interacting and of the immediate context when conducting an evaluation.

Evaluation as a Political Practice

Although most therapists would acknowledge that the settings in which they work have political dimensions, they are less likely to acknowledge or frame their own practice or care encounters as political, so to suggest that the occupational therapy evaluation is a political practice may seem overstated. However, if we think of therapeutic relationships as having elements of power and authority (Foucault, 1982), despite the move to a health care ethic that promotes partnership and collaboration (Cole & McLean, 2003; Peloquin, 1990, 1993; Taylor, 2008), is it not reasonable to consider professional acts, like evaluation, as political or at least as having political dimensions? Pollard, Sakellariou, and Kronenberg (2009) described political activities of daily living, arguing for "political literacy and engagement with occupational therapy" (p. 3). They clarified that *politics* "refers to a politics that is not determined by party ideologies but by local conditions, the intricacies of accountability, interprofessional relationships, user and carer needs and individual motivations, issues that are often managerial concerns" (p. 3).

The sociologist Foucault, whose work many philosophers of professional practices have used to frame these practices as political, argued that professional care relationships are inherently about "power", that is "the way the everyday practices of individuals and groups are coordinated so as to produce, perpetuate, and delimit what people can think, do and be" (Dreyfus, 1996, p. 2). This perspective positions professional acts, especially communicative acts such as the written documentation of an evaluation or the oral reporting of evaluation results to key stakeholders, as being representative of particular "discourses." According to Mackey (2007), "[o]ccupational therapy discourses consist of languages and practices that enable occupational therapists to be distinguishable and visible and through which the dominant knowledges about the occupational therapy world come into play" (p. 97). Occupational therapists practicing in mental health are encouraged to consider the political, particularly the rhetorical, power of language inherent in the process of interpreting, documenting, and communicating the findings of the evaluations that they conduct.

Making sense of what one has come to know about the person with a psychiatric disability as a result of the evaluation process is certainly informed by the theoretical perspective that informs the assessment tool, as well as the philosophical perspective of the specific work environment. With regard to philosophical and theoretical perspectives on recovery, tensions have arisen between what are defined as scientific and consumer (Bellack, 2006) or clinical and social models (Secker et al., 2002). Roughly, these divergent models parallel arguments regarding the ongoing tension in occupational therapy between a reductionist biomedical perspective and an occupational perspective (Mattingly & Fleming, 1994) as well as the move from a deficits perspective to a strengths perspective for people with a psychiatric disability in particular (Rapp & Goscha, 2006).

Work settings that adopt or practice from the scientific or clinical models of recovery will interpret the findings of an assessment differently from those informed by the consumer or social models. The determination of the need, or perceived need, for intervention may be significantly different between the two perspectives. What is understood from the consumer or social model perspective as an adaptive or natural human response to life's challenges (Deegan, 1988) may be seen from the scientific and clinical models as symptomatic. Although these perspectives have been argued to be complementary (Bellack, 2006), others have taken a critical psychiatry perspective and challenged the psychiatric community to radically reframe how it makes sense of what is labeled *mental illness* (Thomas & Bracken, 2004).

Given the tensions attendant in the differences between the models and the unequal power balance common to care relationships, the understanding to which the therapist comes about the client's occupational engagement and disruptions as a result of the occupational therapy evaluation becomes a political act. As a result, therapists must be aware of and acknowledge the frame or lens through which they are interpreting what they have come to know and adopt an ethical stance that acknowledges that frame and its unique risks.

The form and content of documentation of the occupational therapy evaluation can also be understood as having political force, especially because it is thoughtfully crafted to represent a particular account of the client's experiences and needs and is used as the rationale for the client's need for a particular type of intervention (i.e., medical necessity). In addition, it is a means by which occupational therapists demonstrate their expertise and position themselves in relation to other mental health professionals.

Conclusion

In considering the advanced practice nature of the occupational therapy evaluation in mental health, this chapter has focused on its contextualized, evidence-based, and political dimensions. For each dimension, it highlights influences, perspectives, and tensions that affect occupational therapists as they complete the occupational profile and analysis of occupational performance. First, it identifies the contextual influences specific to mental health practice at the macro, meso, and micro levels. Next, it uses the assertion that EBP represents an integration of the client's perspective, the therapist's expertise, and the best evidence to frame issues important to evaluation as an EBP in mental health practice settings. Finally, it describes evaluation as a political practice in which interpretation and documentation of the findings of an occupational therapy evaluation have rhetorical power.

References

Abbott, A. (1988). *The system of professions: An essay on the division of expert labor.* Chicago: University of Chicago Press.

Allen, C. K. (1988). Occupational therapy: Functional assessment of the severity of mental disorders. *Hospital and Community Psychiatry, 39*(2), 140–142.

Allen, C. K., Earhart, C. A., & Blue, T. (1992). *Occupational therapy treatment goals for the physically and cognitively disabled.* Bethesda, MD: American Occupational Therapy Association.

Allen, M., & Smith, V. F. (2001). Opening Pandora's box: The practical and legal dangers of involuntary outpatient commitment. *Psychiatric Services, 52*(3), 342–346.

Amador, X. F. (2007). *I am not sick, I don't need help.* Peconic, NY: Vida Press.

Amador, X. F., & Strauss, D. H. (1993). Poor insight in schizophrenia. *Psychiatric Quarterly, 64*(4), 305–318.

American Occupational Therapy Association. (2008). Occupational therapy practice framework: Domain and process (2nd ed.). *American Journal of Occupational Therapy, 62,* 625–683.

Anthony, W. A. (1993). Recovery from mental illness: The guiding vision of the mental health service system in the 1990s. *Psychosocial Rehabilitation Journal, 16,* 11–23.

Anthony, W., Rogers, E. S., & Farkas, M. (2003). Research on evidence-based practices: Future directions in an era of recovery. *Community Mental Health Journal, 39*(2), 101–113. doi: 10.1023/A:1022601619482

Atkinson, M., Zibin, S., & Chuang, H. (1997). Characterizing quality of life among patients with chronic mental illness: A critical examination of the self-report methodology. *American Journal of Psychiatry, 154*(1), 99–105.

Bartels, S. J., Dums, A. R., Oxman, T. E., Schneider, L. S., Arean, P. A., Alexopoulos, G. S., et al. (2004). Evidence-based practices in geriatric mental health care. *Focus, 2*(2), 268–281.

Bass-Haugen, J. (2005). Assessment identification and selection. In J. Hinojosa, P. Kramer, & P. Crist (Eds.), *Evaluation: Obtaining and interpreting data* (2nd ed., pp. 37–50). Bethesda, MD: AOTA Press.

Bassman, R. (2001). Whose reality is it anyway? Consumers/survivors/ex-patients can speak for themselves. *Journal of Humanistic Psychology, 41*(4), 11–35.

Becker, H. S. (2000a). The etiquette of improvisation. *Mind, Culture and Activity, 7*(3), 171–176.

Becker, H. S. (2000b). Examples and generalizations. *Mind, Culture and Activity, 7*(3), 197–200.

Bejerholm, U., & Eklund, M. (2004). Time use and occupational performance among persons with schizophrenia. *Occupational Therapy in Mental Health, 20*, 27–47.

Bellack, A. S. (2006). Scientific and consumer models of recovery in schizophrenia: Concordance, contrasts, and implications. *Schizophrenia Bulletin, 32*, 432–442. doi: 10.1093/schbul/sbj044

Bond, G., Drake, R., & Becker, D. (2008). An update on randomized controlled trials of evidence-based supported employment. *Psychiatric Rehabilitation Journal, 31*(4), 280.

Bond, G., Drake, R., Mueser, K., & Latimer, E. (2001). Assertive community treatment for people with severe mental illness: Critical ingredients and impact on patients. *Disease Management and Health Outcomes, 9*(3), 141–159.

Bond, G., McHugo, G., Becker, D., Rapp, C., & Whitley, R. (2008). Fidelity of supported employment: Lessons learned from the National Evidence-Based Practice Project. *Psychiatric Rehabilitation Journal, 31*(4), 300.

Borg, M., Sells, D., Topor, A., Mezzina, R., Marin, I., & Davidson, L. (2005). What makes a house a home: The role of material resources in recovery from severe mental illness. *American Journal of Psychiatric Rehabilitation, 8*, 243–256.

Brekke, J. S., Prindle, C., Bae, S. W., & Long, J. D. (2001). Risks for individuals with schizophrenia who are living in the community. *Psychiatric Services, 52*(10), 1358–1366.

Brown, C., Cromwell, R. L., Filion, D., Dunn, W., & Tollefson, N. (2002). Sensory processing in schizophrenia: Missing and avoiding information. *Schizophrenia Research, 55*(1–2), 187–195.

Bryant, W., Craik, C., & McKay, E. (2004). Living in a glasshouse: Exploring occupational alienation. *Canadian Journal of Occupational Therapy, 71*(5), 282–289.

Campbell, J. (1997). How consumers/survivors are evaluating the quality of psychiatric care. *Evaluation Review, 21*(3), 357–363.

Cash, D. (2000). Response to Becker's "The etiquette of improvisation." *Mind, Culture and Activity, 7*(3), 177–179.

Chaffey, L., & Fossey, E. (2004). Caring and daily life: Occupational experiences of women living with sons diagnosed with schizophrenia. *Australian Occupational Therapy Journal, 51*(4), 199–207.

Chamberlin, J. (1979). *On our own: Patient-controlled alternatives to the mental health system.* New York: McGraw-Hill.

Chamberlin, J. (1997). The ex-patients' movement: Where we've been and where we're going. In L. Spaniol, C. Gagne, & M. Koehler (Eds.), *Psychological and social aspects of psychiatric disability* (pp. 541–551). Boston: Center for Psychiatric Rehabilitation.

Champagne, T. (2005). Expanding the role of sensory approaches for acute inpatient psychiatry. *Mental Health Special Interest Section Quarterly, 28*(1), 1–4.

Champagne, T. (2006). Creating sensory rooms: Environmental enhancements for acute inpatient mental health settings. *Mental Health Special Interest Section Quarterly, 29*(4), 1–4.

Champagne, T., & Stromberg, N. (2004). Sensory approaches in inpatient psychiatric settings: Innovative alternatives to seclusion and restraint. *Journal of Psychosocial Nursing, 42*(9), 35–44.

Chilvers, R., Macdonald, G., & Hayes, A. (2006). Supported housing for people with severe mental disorders. *Cochrane Database of Systematic Reviews, 3*, Article CD000453. doi: 10.1002/14651858.CD000453.pub2

Chugg, A., & Craik, C. (2002). Some factors influencing engagement for people with schizophrenia living in the community occupational. *British Journal of Occupational Therapy, 65*, 67–74.

Clark, F., Azen, S. P., Zemke, R., Jackson, J., Carlson, M., Mandel, D., et al. (1997). Occupational therapy for independent-living older adults. A randomized controlled trial. *JAMA, 278*(16), 1321–1326.

Clark, F., Larson, B., & Richardson, P. (1996). A grounded theory of the techniques for occupational story telling and occupational story making. In R. Z. F. Clark (Ed.), *Occupational science: The evolving discipline* (pp. 373–393). Philadelphia: F. A. Davis.

Clark-Rapley, C. (1999). Dancing bodies: Moving beyond Marxian views of human activity, relations, and consciousness. *Journal for the Theory of Social Behavior, 29*(2), 89–107.

Cohen, M., Hinojosa, J., & Kramer, P. (2005). Administration of evaluation and assessments. In J. Hinojosa, P. Kramer, & P. Crist (Eds.), *Evaluation: Obtaining and interpreting data* (2nd ed., pp. 81–100). Bethesda, MD: AOTA Press.

Cohen, M. E., & Kearney, P. J. (2005). Use of evaluation data to support evidence-based practice. In J. Hinojosa, P. Kramer, & P. Crist (Eds.), *Evaluation: Obtaining and interpreting data* (2nd ed., pp. 263–282). Bethesda, MD: AOTA Press.

Cole, M. B., & McLean, V. (2003). Therapeutic relationships re-defined. *Occupational Therapy in Mental Health, 19*(2), 33–56.

Collins, M. E., Mowbray, C. T., & Bybee, D. (2000). Characteristics predicting successful outcomes of participants with severe mental illness in supported education. *Psychiatric Services, 51*(6), 774–780.

Cooper, B. (2003). Evidence-based mental health policy: A critical appraisal. *British Journal of Psychiatry, 183*(2), 105–113.

Corrigan, P. W., Giffort, D., Rashid, F., Leary, M., & Okeke, I. (1999). Recovery as a psychological construct. *Community Mental Health Journal, 35*(3), 231–239.

Coster, W. (1998). Occupation-centered assessment of children. *American Journal of Occupational Therapy, 52*(5), 337–344.

Creek, J. (2002). *Occupational therapy and mental health* (3rd ed.). New York: Churchill Livingston.

Cresswell, M. K., & Rugg, S. A. (2003). The Canadian Occupational Performance Measure: Its use with clients with schizophrenia. *International Journal of Therapy and Rehabilitation, 10*(1), 544–553.

Crist, P. (2005). Scoring and interpretation of results. In J. Hinojosa, P. Kramer, & P. Crist (Eds.), *Evaluation: Obtaining and interpreting data* (2nd ed., pp. 147–174). Bethesda, MD: AOTA Press.

Davidson, L. (2003). *Living outside mental illness: Qualitative studies of recovery in schizophrenia.* New York: New York University Press.

Davidson, L., Borg, M., Marin, I., Topor, A., Mezzina, R., & Sells, D. (2005). Processes of recovery in serious mental illness: Findings from a multinational study. *American Journal of Psychiatric Rehabilitation, 8*(3), 177–201.

Davidson, L., O'Connell, M., Tondora, J., Styron, T., & Kangas, K. (2006). The top ten concerns about recovery encountered in mental health system transformation. *Psychiatric Services, 57*(5), 640–645.

Day, W. (2000). Knowing as instancing: Jazz improvisation and moral perfectionism. *Journal of Aesthetics and Art Criticism, 58*(2), 100–111.

Deane, F. P., Crowe, T. P., King, R., Kavanagh, D. J., & Oades, L. G. (2006). Challenges in implementing evidence-based practice into mental health services. *Australian Health Review, 30*(3), 305–309. Retrieved from www.aushealthreview.com.au/publications/articles/issues/ahr_30_3_0806/ahr_30_3_305.html

Deegan, P. (1988). Recovery: The lived experience of rehabilitation. *Psychosocial Rehabilitation Journal, 11,* 11–19.

Dixon, L., McFarlane, W. R., Lefley, H., Lucksted, A., Cohen, M., Falloon, I., et al. (2001). Evidence-based practices for services to families of people with psychiatric disabilities. *Psychiatric Services, 52*(7), 903–910.

Dreyfus, H. (1996). Being and power: Heidegger and Foucault. *International Journal of Philosophical Studies, 4*(1), 1–16.

Eklund, M. (2001). Psychiatric patients' occupational roles: Changes over time and associations with self-rated quality of life. *Scandinavian Journal of Occupational Therapy, 8*(3), 125–130.

Eklund, M., & Bäckström, M. (2005). A model of subjective quality of life for outpatients with schizophrenia and other psychoses. *Quality of Life Research, 14*(4), 1157–1168.

Eklund, M., Hansson, L., & Ahlqvist, C. (2004). The importance of work as compared to other forms of daily occupations for wellbeing and functioning among persons with long-term mental illness. *Community Mental Health Journal, 40*(5), 465–477.

Ennals, P., & Fossey, E. (2007). The Occupational Performance History Interview in community mental health case management: Consumer and occupational therapist perspectives. *Australian Occupational Therapy Journal, 54*(1), 11–21.

Fakhoury, W. K. H., Murray, A., Shepherd, G., & Priebe, S. (2002). Research in supported housing. *Social Psychiatry and Psychiatric Epidemiology, 37,* 301–315.

Farkas, M., Gagne, C., Anthony, W., & Chamberlin, J. (2005). Implementing recovery oriented evidence-based programs: Identifying the critical dimensions. *Community Mental Health Journal, 41*(2), 141–158.

Fidler, G. (1991). The challenge of change to occupational therapy practice. *Occupational Therapy in Mental Health, 11*(1), 1–11.

Fossey, E. (2001). Effective interdisciplinary teamwork: An occupational therapy perspective. *Australasian Psychiatry, 9*(3), 232–235.

Foucault, M. (1982). The subject and power. *Critical Inquiry, 8*(4), 777–795.

Frank, G. (1996). Life histories in occupational therapy clinical practice. *American Journal of Occupational Therapy, 50*(4), 251–264.

Frese, F., Stanley, J., Kress, K., & Vogel-Scibilia, S. (2001). Integrating evidence-based practices and the Recovery Model. *Psychiatric Services, 52*(11), 1462–1468. Retrieved from http://psychservices.psychiatryonline.org/cgi/content/full/52/11/1462

Ganju, V. (2003). Implementation of evidence-based practices in state mental health systems: Implications for research and effectiveness studies. *Schizophrenia Bulletin, 29*(1), 125–131.

Goldman, H. H., Ganju, V., Drake, R. E., Gorman, P., Hogan, M., Hyde, P. S., et al. (2001). Policy implications for implementing evidence-based practices. *Psychiatric Services, 52*(12), 1591–1597. Retrieved from http://psychservices.psychiatryonline.org/cgi/reprint/52/12/1591.pdf

Green, M. F. (1996). What are the functional consequences of neurocognitive deficits in schizophrenia? *American Journal of Psychiatry, 153*(3), 321–330.

Haglund, L., Ekbladh, E., Thorell, L.-H. K., & Hallberg, I. R. (2000). Practice models in Swedish psychiatric occupational therapy. *Scandinavian Journal of Occupational Therapy, 7*(3), 107–113.

Hamera, E., & Brown, C. E. (2000). Developing a context-based performance measure for persons with schizophrenia: The test of grocery shopping skills. *American Journal of Occupational Therapy, 54*(1), 20–25.

Hamera, E., Rempfer, M., & Brown, C. (2005). Performance in the "real world": Update on Test of Grocery Shopping Skills (TOGSS). *Schizophrenia Research, 78*(1), 111–112.

Harries, P. A., & Gilhooly, K. (2003). Generic and specialist occupational therapy casework in community mental health teams. *British Journal of Occupational Therapy, 66,* 101–109.

Harrison, D. (2003). The case for generic working in mental health occupational therapy. *British Journal of Occupational Therapy, 66,* 110–112.

Hasson-Ohayon, I., Kravetz, S., Roe, D., David, A. S., & Weiser, M. (2006). Insight into psychosis and quality of life. *Comprehensive Psychiatry, 47*(4), 265–269.

Hinojosa, J. (2007). Becoming innovators in an era of hyperchange. *American Journal of Occupational Therapy, 61*(6), 629–637.

Hoagwood, K., Burns, B. J., Kiser, L., Ringeisen, H., & Schoenwald, S. K. (2001). Evidence-based practice in child and adolescent mental health services. *Psychiatric Services, 52*(9), 1179–1189.

Holm, M. B. (2000). Our mandate for the new millennium: Evidence-based practice. *American Journal of Occupational Therapy, 54*(6), 575–585.

Holmes, C. A. (2001). Postdisciplinarity in mental health-care: An Australian viewpoint. *Nursing Inquiry, 8*(4), 230–239.

Honey, A. (1999). Empowerment versus power: Consumer participation in mental health services. *Occupational Therapy International, 6*(4), 257–276.

Humberstone, V. (2002). The experiences of people with schizophrenia living in supported accommodation: A qualitative study using ground theory methodology. *Australian and New Zealand Journal of Psychiatry, 36,* 367–372.

Iannelli, S., & Wilding, C. (2007). Health-enhancing effects of engaging in productive occupation: Experiences of young people with mental illness. *Australian Occupational Therapy Journal, 54*(4), 285–293.

Isett, K. R., Burnam, M. A., Coleman-Beattie, B., Hyde, P. S., Morrissey, J. P., Magnabosco, J., et al. (2007). The state policy context of implementation issues for evidence-based practices in mental health. *Psychiatric Services, 58*(7), 914–921.

Jackson, G. A. (1984). Short-term psychiatric treatment: How will occupational therapy adapt? *Occupational Therapy in Mental Health, 4*(3), 11–17.

Jacobson, N., & Curtis, L. (2000). Recovery as policy in mental health services: Strategies emerging from the states. *Psychiatric Rehabilitation Journal, 23*(4), 333–342.

Jacobson, N., & Greenley, D. (2001). What is recovery? A conceptual model and explication. *Psychiatric Services, 52*(4), 482–485.

Kelly, B. D. (2005). Structural violence and schizophrenia. *Social Science and Medicine, 61*(3), 721–730.

Kennedy-Jones, M., Cooper, J., & Fossey, E. (2005). Developing a worker role: Stories of four people with mental illness. *Australian Occupational Therapy Journal, 52*(2), 116–126.

Kielhofner, G. (Ed.). (2008). *Model of Human Occupation: Theory and application* (4th ed.). Baltimore: Lippincott Williams & Wilkins.

Kielhofner, G., & Burke, J. (1977). Occupational therapy after 60 years: An account of changing identity and knowledge. *American Journal of Occupational Therapy, 31*(10), 675–689.

Kielhofner, G., & Mallinson, T. (1995). Gathering narrative data through interviews: Empirical observations and suggested guidelines. *Scandinavian Journal of Occupational Therapy, 2*(2), 63–68.

Kielhofner, G., Mallinson, K., Crawford, C., Nowak, M., Rigby, M., Henry, A., et al. (2004). *Occupational Performance History Interview–II* (Version 2.1). Chicago: Model of Human Occupation Clearinghouse, Department of Occupational Therapy, College of Applied Health Sciences, University of Illinois at Chicago.

Kodat, C. (2003). Conversing with ourselves: Canon, freedom, jazz. *American Quarterly, 55*(1), 1–28.

Kronenberg, F., Algado, S. S., & Pollard, N. (2004). *Occupational therapy without borders: Learning from the spirit of survivors.* Oxford, England: Churchill Livingstone.

Kronenberg, F., & Pollard, N. (2006). Political dimensions of occupation and the roles of occupational therapy. *American Journal of Occupational Therapy, 60*(6), 617–625.

Krupa, T. (2004). Employment, recovery, and schizophrenia: Integrating health and disorder at work. *Psychiatric Rehabilitation Journal, 28*(1), 8–15.

Laliberte-Rudman, D. (2002). Linking occupation and identity: Lessons learned through qualitative exploration. *Journal of Occupational Science, 9*(1), 12–19.

Laliberte-Rudman, D., Yu, B., Scott, E., & Pajouhandeh, P. (2000). Exploration of the perspectives of persons with schizophrenia regarding quality of life. *American Journal of Occupational Therapy, 54*(2), 137–147.

Lamberti, J. S., Weisman, R. L., Schwarzkopf, S. B., Price, N., Ashton, R. M., & Trompeter, J. (2001). The mentally ill in jails and prisons: Towards an integrated model of prevention. *Psychiatric Quarterly, 72*(1), 63–77.

Langer, E. (1990). *Mindfulness.* Reading, MA: Addison-Wesley.

Law, M., Baptiste, S., Carswell, A., McColl, M. A., Polatajko, H., & Pollock, N. (2005). *Canadian Occupational Performance Measure* (4th ed.). Ottawa, Ontario, Canada: CAOT Publications.

Law, M., & Baum, C. (2005). Measurement in occupational therapy. In M. Law, C. Baum, & W. Dunn (Eds.), *Measuring occupational performance: Supporting best practice in occupational therapy* (pp. 3–20). Thorofare, NJ: Slack.

Law, M., Baum, C., & Dunn, W., (Eds.). (2001). *Measuring occupational performance: Supporting best practice in occupational therapy.* Thorofare, NJ: Slack.

Leufstadius, C., & Eklund, M. (2008). Time use among individuals with persistent mental illness: Identifying risk factors for imbalance in daily activities. *Scandinavian Journal of Occupational Therapy, 15*(1), 23–33.

Liberman, R. P., Kopelowicz, A., Ventura, J., & Gutkind, D. (2002). Operational criteria and factors related to recovery from schizophrenia. *International Review of Psychiatry, 14*(4), 0954–0261. Retrieved from www.jhsph.edu/mental_health_initiatives/Events/2007_Symposium/Articles/Liberman_2002_Operational_Criteria_Factors_Related_to_Recovery_from_Schizophrenia.pdf

Link, B. G., Struening, E. L., Neese-Todd, S., Asmussen, S., & Phelan, J. C. (2001). Stigma as a barrier to recovery: The consequences of stigma for the self-esteem of people with mental illnesses. *Psychiatric Services, 52*(12), 1621–1626.

Lloyd, C., & Waghorn, G. (2007). The importance of vocation in recovery for young people with psychiatric disabilities. *British Journal of Occupational Therapy, 70*, 50–59.

Lougher, L. (Ed.). (2001). *Occupational therapy for child and adolescent mental health*. London: Churchill Livingstone.

Ludwig, F. (1997). How routine facilitates wellbeing in older women. *Occupational Therapy International, 4*(3), 215–230.

Lysaker, P., Buck, K., Hammoud, K., Taylor, A., & Roe, D. (2006). Associations of symptoms, psychosocial function, and hope with qualities of self-experience in schizophrenia: Comparisons of objective and subjective indicators of health. *Schizophrenia Research, 82*(2–3), 241–249.

Lysaker, P., Buck, K., Taylor, A., & Roe, D. (2008). Associations of metacognition and internalized stigma with quantitative assessments of self-experience in narratives of schizophrenia. *Psychiatry Research, 157*(1–3), 31–38.

Lysaker, P., Campbell, K., & Johannesen, J. (2005). Hope, awareness of illness, and coping in schizophrenia spectrum disorders: Evidence of an interaction. *Journal of Nervous and Mental Disease, 193*(5), 287–292.

Lysaker, P., & Louria, S. (2007). Insight and quality of life in schizophrenia spectrum disorders. In M. S. Ritsner & A. G. Awad (Eds.), *Quality of life impairment in schizophrenia, mood, and anxiety disorders* (pp. 227–240). Dordrecht, the Netherlands: Springer.

Lysaker, P., Roe, D., & Yanos, P. (2007). Toward understanding the insight paradox: Internalized stigma moderates the association between insight and social functioning, hope, and self-esteem among people with schizophrenia spectrum disorders. *Schizophrenia Bulletin, 33*(1), 192–199.

MacDonald-Wilson, K., Rogers, E. S., & Anthony, W. A. (2001). Unique issues in assessing work function among individuals with psychiatric disabilities. *Journal of Occupational Rehabilitation, 11*(3), 217–232.

Mackey, H. (2007). "Do not ask me to remain the same": Foucault and the professional identities of occupational therapists. *Australian Occupational Therapy Journal, 54*, 95–102.

Mallinson, T., Kielhofner, G., & Mattingly, C. (1996). Metaphor and meaning in a clinical interview. *American Journal of Occupational Therapy, 50*(5), 338–346.

Marin, I., Mezzina, R., Borg, M., Topor, A., Staecheli Lawless, M., Sells, D., et al. (2005). The person's role in recovery. *American Journal of Psychiatric Rehabilitation, 8*, 223–242.

Mattingly, C. (1991). The narrative use of clinical reasoning. *American Journal of Occupational Therapy, 45*, 998–1005.

Mattingly, C. (1998a). *Healing dramas and clinical plots: The narrative structure of experience*. Cambridge, England: Cambridge University Press.

Mattingly, C. (1998b). In search of the good: Narrative reasoning in clinical practice. *Medical Anthropology Quarterly, 12*(3), 273–297.

Mattingly, C., & Fleming, M. (1994). *Clinical reasoning: Forms of inquiry in a therapeutic practice*. Philadelphia: F. A. Davis.

Mausbach, B. T., Harvey, P. D., Goldman, S. R., Jeste, D. V., & Patterson, T. L. (2007). Development of a brief scale of everyday functioning in persons with serious mental illness. *Schizophrenia Bulletin, 33*(6), 1364–1372.

McDonald, P. W., & Viehbeck, S. (2007). From evidence-based practice making to practice-based evidence making: Creating communities of (research) and practice. *Health Promotion Practices, 8*(2), 140–144.

McGuire, A., Bond, G., Evans, J., Lysaker, P., & Kim, H. (2007). Situational assessment in psychiatric rehabilitation: A reappraisal. *Journal of Vocational Rehabilitation, 27*(1), 49–55.

McKibbin, C., Brekke, J., Sires, D., Jeste, D., & Patterson, T. (2004). Direct assessment of functional abilities: Relevance to persons with schizophrenia. *Schizophrenia Research, 72*(1), 53–67.

McKibbin, C., Patterson, T., Brekke, J., & Jeste, D. (2005). Response to letter entitled "Performance in the 'real world': Update on test of grocery shopping skills (TOGSS)." *Schizophrenia Research, 78*(1), 113–114.

Mee, J., & Sumsion, T. (2001). Mental health clients confirm the motivating power of occupation. *British Journal of Occupational Therapy, 64*(3), 121–128.

Mee, J., Sumsion, T., & Craik, C. (2004). Mental health clients confirm the value of occupation in building competence and self-identity. *British Journal of Occupational Therapy, 67*(5), 225–233.

Merryman, B., & Riegel, S. K. (2007). The recovery process and people with serious mental illness living in the community: An occupational therapy perspective. *Occupational Therapy in Mental Health, 23*(2), 51–73.

Meyer, A. (1922). The philosophy of occupation therapy. *Archives of Occupational Therapy,* *1*(1), 1–10.

Meyer, A. (1957). *Psychobiology: A science of man.* Springfield, IL: Charles C Thomas.

Mezzina, R., Borg, M., Marin, I., Sells, D., Topor, A., & Davidson, L. (2006). From participation to citizenship: How to regain a role, a status, and a life in the process of recovery. *American Journal of Psychiatric Rehabilitation, 9,* 39–61.

Minkoff, K. (2001). Best practices: Developing standards of care for individuals with co-occurring psychiatric and substance use disorders. *Psychiatric Services, 52*(5), 597–599.

Montuori, A. (1997). Social creativity, academic discourse, and the improvisation of inquiry. *ReVision, 20*(1), 34–38.

Mowbray, C., Moxley, D., & Collins, M. (1998). Consumers as mental health providers: First-person accounts of benefits and limitations. *Journal of Behavioral Health Services and Research, 25*(4), 397–411.

Mueser, K. T., Corrigan, P. W., Hilton, D. W., Tanzman, B., Schaub, A., Gingerich, S., et al. (2004). Illness management and recovery: A review of the research. *Focus, 2*(1), 34–47.

Mueser, K. T., Meyer, P. S., Penn, D. L., Clancy, R., Clancy, D. M., & Salyers, M. P. (2006). The Illness Management and Recovery Program: Rationale, development, and preliminary findings. *Schizophrenia Bulletin, 32*(Suppl. 1), S32–S43.

Mueser, K. T., Rosenberg, S. D., Goodman, L. A., & Trumbetta, S. L. (2002). Trauma, PTSD, and the course of severe mental illness: An interactive model. *Schizophrenia Research, 53*(1–2), 123–143.

Nagle, S., Cook, J. V., & Polatajko, H. J. (2002). I'm doing as much as I can: Occupational choice of persons with a severe and persistent mental illness. *Journal of Occupational Science, 9*(2), 72–81.

Pan, A.-W., Chung, L., & Hsin-Hwei, H. (2003). Reliability and validity of the Canadian Occupational Performance Measure for clients with psychiatric disorders in Taiwan. *Occupational Therapy International, 10*(4), 269–277.

Parker, H. (2001). The role of occupational therapists in community mental health teams: Generic or specialist? *British Journal of Occupational Therapy, 64,* 609–610.

Parnas, J., & Handest, P. (2003). Phenomenology of anomalous self-experience in early schizophrenia. *Comprehensive Psychiatry, 44*(2), 121–134.

Patterson, T. L., Goldman, S., McKibbin, C. L., Hughs, T., & Jeste, D. V. (2001). UCSD performance-based skills assessment: Development of a new measure of everyday functioning for severely mentally ill adults. *Schizophrenia Bulletin, 27*(2), 235–245.

Paul, S., & Peterson, C. Q. (2001). Interprofessional collaboration: Issues for practice and research. *Occupational Therapy in Health Care, 15*(3/4), 1–12.

Peloquin, S. (1990). The patient–therapist relationship in occupational therapy: Understanding visions and images. *American Journal of Occupational Therapy, 44*(1), 13–21.

Peloquin, S. (1993). The patient–therapist relationship: Beliefs that shape care. *American Journal of Occupational Therapy, 47*(10), 935–942.

Perlick, D. A., Rosenheck, R. A., Clarkin, J. F., Sirey, J. A., Salahi, J., Struening, E. L., et al. (2001). Stigma as a barrier to recovery: Adverse effects of perceived stigma on social adaptation of persons diagnosed with bipolar affective disorder. *Psychiatric Services, 52*(12), 1627–1632.

Phillips, S. D., Burns, B. J., Edgar, E. R., Mueser, K. T., Linkins, K. W., Rosenheck, R. A., et al. (2001). Moving assertive community treatment into standard practice. *Psychiatric Services, 52*(6), 771–779.

Polgar, J. (2009). Critiquing assessments. In E. Crepeau, E. Cohn, & B. Boyt Schell (Eds.), *Willard and Spackman's occupational therapy* (11th ed.). Philadelphia: Lippincott Williams & Wilkins.

Polkinghorne, D. (2004). *Practice and the human sciences: The case for a judgement-based practice of care.* Albany: State University of New York Press.

Pollard, N., Sakellariou, D., & Kronenberg, F. (Eds.). (2009). *A political practice of occupational therapy.* Philadelphia: Churchill Livingstone.

President's New Freedom Commission on Mental Health. (2003). *Achieving the promise: Transforming mental health care in America* (Final Report, DHHS Pub. No. SMA–03–3832). Rockville, MD: Author.

Ralph, R. O. (2000). *Review of recovery literature: A synthesis of a sample of recovery literature 2000.* Alexandria, VA: National Technical Assistance Center for Mental Health Planning, National Association for State Mental Health Program Directors.

Ralph, R. O., Lambert, D., & Kidder, K. A. (2002). *The recovery perspective and evidence-based practice for people with serious mental illness: A guideline developed for the Behavioral Health Recovery Management Project.* Portland: University of Southern Maine, Edmund S. Muskie School of Public Service, Institute for Health Policy.

Ramchandani, P., Joughin, C., & Zwi, M. (2001). Evidence-based child and adolescent mental health services: Oxymoron or brave new dawn? *Child and Adolescent Mental Health, 6*(2), 59–64.

Rapp, C., & Goscha, R. (2006). *The Strengths Model: Case management with people with psychiatric disabilities.* Oxford, England: Oxford University Press.

Rebeiro, K. (1999). The labyrinth of community mental health: In search of meaningful occupation. *Psychiatric Rehabilitation Journal, 23*(2), 143–152.

Rebeiro-Gruhl, K. L. (2005). Reflection on . . . The recovery paradigm: Should occupational therapists be interested in recovery? *Canadian Journal of Occupational Therapy, 72*(2), 99–101.

Rempfer, M. V., Hamera, E. K., Brown, C. E., & Cromwell, R. L. (2003). The relations between cognition and the independent living skill of shopping in people with schizophrenia. *Psychiatry Research, 117*(2), 103–112.

Roe, D., & Kravetz, S. (2003). Different ways of being aware of a psychiatric disability: A multifunctional narrative approach to insight in to mental disorder. *Journal of Nervous and Mental Disease, 191*(7), 417–424.

Rushmer, R., & Pallis, G. (2003). Inter-professional working: The wisdom of integrated working and the disaster of blurred boundaries. *Public Money and Management, 23*(1), 59–66.

Salzer, M. S. (1997). Consumer empowerment in mental health organizations: Concept, benefits, and impediments. *Administration and Policy in Mental Health and Mental Health Services Research, 24*(5), 425–434.

Sawyer, R. K. (2000a). Improvisation and the creative process: Dewey, Collingwood, and the aesthetics of spontaneity. *Journal of Aesthetics and Art Criticism, 58*(2), 149–151.

Sawyer, R. K. (2000b). Improvisational cultures: Collaborative emergence and creativity in improvisation. *Mind, Culture and Activity, 7*(3), 180–185.

Schon, D. (1983). *The reflective practitioner: How professionals think in action.* New York: Basic Books.

Schultz-Krohn, W., & Cara, E. (2000). Occupational therapy in early intervention: Applying concepts from infant mental health. *American Journal of Occupational Therapy, 54*(4), 550–554.

Schwartz, P. (2000). Action research: Dance improvisation as a dance technique. *JOPERD, 71*(5), 42–46.

Secker, J., Membrey, H., Grove, B., & Sebolm, P. (2002). Recovering from illness or recovering your life? Implications of clinical versus social models of recovery from mental health problems for employment support services. *Disability and Society, 17*(4), 403–418. doi: 10.1080/09687590220140340

Sells, D., Andres-Hyman, R., Lawless, M. S., Borg, M., Topor, A., Mezzina, R., et al. (2005). Contexts and narratives of recovery. *American Journal of Psychiatric Rehabilitation, 8*(3), 203–221.

Sheets-Johnston, M. (2000). Dance improvisation: A paradigm of thinking in movement. *Thinking: The Journal of Philosophy for Children, 15*(3), 2–8.

Shore, A. (2001). Effects of a secure attachment relationship on right brain development, affect regulation, and infant mental health. *Infant Mental Health Journal, 22*(1–2), 7–66.

Substance Abuse and Mental Health Services Administration. (n.d.). *SAMHSA's national outcome measures.* Retrieved May 29, 2008, from www.nationaloutcomemeasures.samhsa.gov/

Substance Abuse and Mental Health Services Administration. (2005). *Transforming mental health care in America—the federal action agenda: First steps.* Rockville, MD: Author.

Swartz, M. S., & Swanson, J. W. (2004). Involuntary outpatient commitment, community treatment orders, and assisted outpatient treatment: What's in the data? *Canadian Journal of Psychiatry, 49*(9), 585–591.

Tanenbaum, S. (1994). Knowing and acting in medical practice: The epistemological politics of outcomes research. *Journal of Health Politics Policy and Law, 19*(1), 27–44.

Tanenbaum, S. (1999). Evidence and expertise: The challenge of the outcomes movement to medical professionalism. *Academic Medicine, 74*(7), 757–763.

Tanenbaum, S. (2003). Evidence-based practice in mental health: Practical weaknesses meet political strengths. *Journal of Evaluation in Clinical Practice, 9*(2), 287–301. doi: 10.1046/j.1365-2753.2003.00409.x

Tanenbaum, S. (2005). Evidence-based practice as mental health policy: Three controversies and a caveat. *Health Affairs, 24*(1), 163–173.

Taylor, R. (2008). *The intentional relationship: Occupational therapy and use of self.* Philadelphia: F. A. Davis.

Thomas, P., & Bracken, P. (2004). Critical psychiatry in practice. *Advances in Psychiatric Treatment, 10*(5), 361–370.

Torrey, W. C., Drake, R. E., Dixon, L., Burns, B. J., Flynn, L., Rush, A. J., et al. (2001). Implementing evidence-based practices for persons with severe mental illness. *Psychiatric Services, 51*(1), 45–50. Retrieved from http://psychservices.psychiatryonline.org/cgi/reprint/52/1/45.pdf

Townsend, E. (2003). Reflections on power and justice in enabling occupation. *Canadian Journal of Occupational Therapy, 70*(2), 74–87.

U.S. Department of Health and Human Services. (1999). *Mental health: A report of the Surgeon General.* Rockville, MD: U.S. Department of Health and Human Services, Substance Abuse and Mental Health Services Administration, Center for Mental Health Services & National Institute of Mental Health. Retrieved November 17, 2009, from www.surgeongeneral.gov/library/mentalhealth/home.html

van den Bosch, R. J., Rombouts, R., & van Asma, M. J. O. (1993). Subjective cognitive dysfunction in schizophrenic and depressed patients. *Comprehensive Psychiatry, 34*(2), 130–136.

Voruganti, L., Heslegrave, R., Awad, A. G., & Seeman, M. V. (2000). Quality of life measurement in schizophrenia: Reconciling the quest for subjectivity with the question of reliability. *Psychological Medicine, 28*(1), 165–172.

Warren, A. (2002). An evaluation of the Canadian Model of Occupational Performance and the Canadian Occupational Performance Measure in mental health practice. *British Journal of Occupational Therapy, 65,* 515–521.

Wilding, C., May, E., & Muir-Cochrane, E. (2005). Experience of spirituality, mental illness and occupation: A life-sustaining phenomenon. *Australian Occupational Therapy Journal, 52*(1), 2–9.

Wilton, R. (2004). Putting policy into practice? Poverty and people with serious mental illness. *Social Science and Medicine, 58*(1), 25–39.

Worrall, L., McCooey, R., Davidson, B., Larkins, B., & Hickson, L. (2002). The validity of functional assessments of communication and the activity/participation components of the ICIDH–2: Do they reflect what really happens in real-life? *Journal of Communication Disorders, 35*(2), 107–137.

Yerxa, E. (1998). Health and the human spirit for occupation. *American Journal of Occupational Therapy, 52,* 412–418.

Young, S. L., & Ensing, D. S. (1999). Exploring recovery from the perspective of people with psychiatric disabilities. *Psychiatric Rehabilitation Journal, 22*(3), 219–232.

CHAPTER 9

Occupational Therapy Intervention for Children and Youth With Mental Illness

Sarah Nielsen, MMGT, OTR/L, and
Renee Watling, PhD, OTR/L

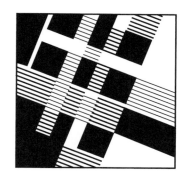

Learning Objectives

After reading this material and completing the examination, readers will be able to

- Identify assessments used in the treatment of children and youth with mental illness;

- Identify appropriate assessment tools on the basis of client cases;

- Identify assessment challenges and general evaluation strategies to be used with children and youth with mental illness that increase the success of the evaluation process;

- Delineate occupation-based and impairment-based models used in the treatment of children and youth with mental illness;

- Recognize the unique role and involvement of the family in interventions for children and youth with mental illness; and

- Identify occupational therapists' possible roles in transition planning for children and youth with mental illness.

Children and youth with mental illness frequently experience challenges in adapting to change, achieving a sense of mastery, and developing a healthy identity (American Occupational Therapy Association [AOTA], 2008). This chapter addresses occupational therapy practice for these young people. It focuses on evaluation practices to provide readers with a better understanding of the factors that interrupt a child's occupational performance and the intervention methods that support development of social and emotional competence and success in childhood occupations and roles.

Evaluation

Occupational therapy evaluation for children and youth with emotional and behavioral difficulties should be comprehensive in nature to gain a complete understanding of the factors affecting the child's functional performance. The evaluation's focus should be guided by the domain of occupational therapy, the concerns for which the child was referred, and the treatment philosophy of the facility in which the child receives services. For children and youth with mental illness, evaluation frequently includes performance of activities of daily living; motor skills; cognitive skills; sensory–perceptual skills; emotional regulation; and participation in education, play, leisure, and social activities. Information can be gathered from performance-based measures and clinical or structured observations of the child and an interview with the child and parent.

The process of evaluation can be particularly challenging with children and youth who have emotional and behavioral difficulties because of the complexity of factors affecting their performance and because of difficulties the child may experience while participating in the evaluation process (Davidson, 2005). The occupational therapist should make every attempt to gather pertinent information from past records, caregivers, teachers, and other service providers who are familiar with the child. Gathering information in advance will limit the performance demands placed on the child and provide the therapist with insights from the people who interact with the child in natural environments. Next, the therapist should gather data directly from the child, allowing comparison of the child's and other people's perceptions of occupational performance. A variety of assessment tools available from within and outside of occupational therapy yield important information in understanding a child's capacity for occupational performance. Selected measures relevant to occupational therapy in the area of pediatric mental health are listed in Table 9.1.

The next section uses case examples to illustrate the selection and use of assessment tools and methods with children and youth with mental illness; it is not intended to be a comprehensive guide, however, because more assessment tools are available than can be covered here.

Case Example: Tara

Tara, age 17, was recently admitted to a day treatment program with the diagnoses of anxiety disorder and depressive disorder. She was referred from the inpatient psychiatric unit to which she was admitted after threatening to kill herself because of feeling overwhelmed and anxious. Inpatient staff reported she had difficulty making her own decisions and contributing to her treatment. Chart review and a brief interview with her parents revealed the following presenting problems: Tara is having significant anxiety, possibly related to preparing to leave her parents' home, fear her parents might die, fear of being in large crowds, and fear of driving on gravel roads. She has a history of significant sleep difficulties, has always been difficult to soothe, and struggles with a variety of food textures. Tara is a senior in high school and performs well academically. She is the youngest of three children and the only one left at home. She also volunteers at the Humane Society.

The therapist began the evaluation with the Canadian Occupational Performance Measure (COPM; Law et al., 2005) to give Tara a voice in describing her struggles. The interview process used in the COPM enabled the therapist to gain more insight into factors surrounding Tara's problems. Tara's history of problems with sleep, feeding, and self-soothing suggests that she may have sensory processing

Table 9.1. Selected Assessment Tools Used With Children and Youth With Mental Illness

Measure	Purpose, Population, and Administration
Adaptive Behavior Assessment System–Second Edition (Harrison & Oakland, 2003)	*Purpose:* Provides a complete assessment of adaptive skills functioning, including conceptual, practical, and social skills. *Population:* Ages 0–89 *Administration:* Parent and teacher form available. Administration time is 15–20 min.
Behavioral Assessment System for Children, Second Edition (Reynolds & Kamphaus, 2002)	*Purpose:* Provides an understanding of a child's or adolescent's adaptive and problem behaviors. *Population:* Ages 2–21 *Administration:* Rating scales for teacher and parent and self-report. Administration time is 10–20 min.
Bruininks–Oseretsky Test of Motor Proficiency (Bruininks & Bruininks, 2006)	*Purpose:* Motor proficiency test measuring fine manual control, manual coordination, body coordination, and strength and ability. *Population:* Ages 4–21 *Administration:* 53 performance-based tasks taking 45–60 min to administer.
Canadian Occupational Performance Measure (Law et al., 2005)	*Purpose:* Assesses client perception of occupational performance over time and assists in client-centered goal setting. *Population:* Children to adults with a variety of disabilities *Administration:* Semistructured interview of child, parent, or both with five steps: problem definitions, problem weighting, scoring, reassessment, and follow-up. (20–40 min)
Child Occupational Self-Assessment (Keller, Kafkes, Basu, Federico, & Kielhofner, 2005)	*Purpose:* Assesses competence and value of occupations including self-care, play, and school-based activities. Communication and interaction skills, motor skills, and process skills are addressed. *Population:* Ages 8–17 for a variety of settings and diagnoses *Administration:* 25 self-rated items via paper and pencil or card sort. Follow-up interview.
Children's Assessment of Participation and Enjoyment (CAPE) and Preferences for Activities With Children (PAC; King et al., 2004)	*Purpose:* The CAPE investigates child's participation in activity across five dimensions: diversity and intensity, with whom, where, and leisure and recreation outside of school. The PAC quantifies preference for activity. *Population:* Ages 6–21 with or without disabilities *Administration:* Self-administered or interviewer-administered using activity cards and visual response (55 items)
KidCOTE (Kunz & Brayman, 1999)	*Purpose:* Provides a comprehensive overview of patient behaviors and development by looking at general behaviors, sensory–motor performance, cognitive behaviors, and psychosocial behaviors. *Population:* Children and young adolescents *Administration:* Observation rating of behaviors on a 4-point scale, based on intensity and frequency of occurrence. Admit and discharge rating are given.
Occupational Therapy Psychosocial Assessment of Learning (Townsend et al., 1999)	*Purpose:* Measures the psychosocial aspects of student performance within the classroom for making choices, habits and routines, and roles and environment. Facilitates optimal student–environment fit. *Population:* Ages 6–12 demonstrating difficulty meeting functional expectations and roles in the classroom *Administration:* Classroom observation and teacher, student, and parent interviews. Scoring consists of a rating scale ranging from 1 to 4.
Piers–Harris Children's Self-Concept Scale, Second Edition (Piers, Harris, & Herzberg, 2002)	*Purpose:* Measures psychological health in children, specifically identifying areas of conflict, typical coping and defense mechanisms, and appropriate intervention techniques. *Population:* Ages 7–18 *Administration:* 60-item self-report form taking 10–15 min to administer. Scores given for six subscales.
Sensory Processing Measure Home/School (Parham, Ecker, Miller-Kuhaneck, Henry, & Glennon, 2007)	*Purpose:* Assesses sensory processing, praxis, and social participation to provide information about sensory facilitators of and barriers to successful functional performance. *Population:* Ages 5–12 *Administration:* Home Form—caregiver completes 75 items. Main Classroom Form—teacher completes 62 items. School Environment Form—10–15 items per environment. Yields eight standard scores of *typical*, *some problems*, or *definite dysfunction*.

(Continued)

Table 9.1. Selected Assessment Tools Used With Children and Youth With Mental Illness (*cont.*)

Measure	Purpose, Population, and Administration
Sensory Profile (Dunn, 1999) and Adolescent/Adult Sensory Profile (Brown & Dunn, 2002)	*Purpose:* Sensory Profile assesses the frequency with which the child responds to sensory experiences and addresses sensory processing, modulation, and behavioral and emotional responses. Adolescent/Adult version gathers information about a person's sensory processing and links sensory processing to everyday experiences. *Population:* Sensory Profile, ages 5–10; Adolescent/Adult Sensory Profile, 11–65+ *Administration:* The Sensory Profile is a 125-item caregiver questionnaire providing scores for nine factor groupings. The Adolescent/Adult Sensory Profile is a 60-item self-report measure with items rated on a 5-point scale for four factor groupings.
Social Skills Rating System (Gresham & Elliot, 1990)	*Purpose:* Provides a picture of social skills and problem behaviors that guide intervention. *Population:* Ages 3–18 *Administration:* Teacher, parent, and self-report forms available. 10–25 min to administer. Provides standard scores for social skills, problem behaviors, and academic competence.
Test of Visual–Motor Skills–Revised (Gardner, 1995)	*Purpose:* Standardized measure of visual–motor functioning. Used to identify neurosensory integration dysfunction. *Population:* 3 years–13 years, 11 months *Administration:* Child copies 25 designs. Administration 3–6 min. Scoring 15–20 min.
Test of Visual–Perceptual Skills (Nonmotor), Third Edition (Martin, 2006)	*Purpose:* Standardized measure to determine a child's visual–perceptual strengths and weaknesses. *Population:* Ages 4–13 years, 11 months *Administration:* Seven untimed subtests taking 30–40 min. Scoring 5 min.
Vineland Adaptive Behavior Scales, Second Edition (Sparrow, Balla, & Cicchetti, 1984)	*Purpose:* Assess personal and social skills through the following components: Daily Living Skills, Communication, Socialization, and Motor Skills. *Population:* Birth–18 years, 11 months *Administration:* Semistructured interview and questionnaire. 60- to 90-min administration.

difficulties. The therapist used the Adolescent/Adult Sensory Profile (Brown & Dunn, 2002) to evaluate behaviors related to sensory processing and provide recommendations to address sensory processing difficulties that may be causing anxiety. The psychologist will evaluate personality and underlying thought processes that are contributing to Tara's anxiety and make recommendations to the therapist for occupational therapy intervention from the cognitive–behavioral standpoint.

Case Example: Corey

Corey, age 12, was recently admitted to the inpatient psychiatric unit after physically attacking his mother while arguing about his chores. The unit physician diagnosed him with oppositional defiant disorder and attention deficit hyperactivity disorder (ADHD), combined type, and considered a diagnosis of bipolar disorder. During the interview, Corey's mother was tearful as she reported that she is a single parent, has two other children, and does not know how to control her children. Corey had trouble with fighting at school and was doing okay academically until recently. Corey's mom says he likes to play basketball but recently has not been playing. He becomes angry and argumentative about everything at home. At times, he says he is not good at anything.

On the basis of Corey's comments indicating poor self-concept and inability to cope, along with the descriptions of oppositional behavior, the therapist selected the Piers–Harris Children's Self-Concept Scale, Second Edition (Piers, Harris, & Herzberg, 2002), to better understand how Corey perceives himself and his current struggles.

The therapist also used the Child Occupational Self-Assessment (COSA; Keller, Kafkes, Basu, Federico, & Kielhofner, 2005) to better understand Corey's competency in and value of occupations. Although Corey stated that he is not good at anything, he has a history of doing well in several areas. This assessment will provide insight into whether Corey has competency issues or whether he has lost value in certain occupations.

Case Example: Sue

Sue is an 8-year-old third grader who transferred a few weeks ago and attends class in the self-contained classroom for children with severe emotional disturbance. She lives with her mother and father and an older half-sibling. Mrs. Olson, Sue's classroom teacher, reported that Sue is having difficulty adjusting to the classroom; she is struggling with attention during academics and is easily distracted by auditory and visual stimuli. Sue often interrupts the class with talk about bugs and the pain of childbirth. Mrs. Olson said that Sue picks at her skin and becomes tearful if the teacher raises her voice. During free time, Sue often argues with the other students. Mrs. Olson also reported that Sue handles the classroom hamster roughly. Her diagnoses are Asperger's disorder and ADHD, combined type.

The occupational therapist chose the Occupational Therapy Psychosocial Assessment of Learning (OT PAL; Townsend et al., 1999) to evaluate Sue's adjustment to the classroom. The OT PAL is designed to evaluate performance in the classroom context and facilitate optimal student–environment fit. Sue's school records did not indicate a past sensory processing evaluation. Given her difficulties with visual and auditory stimuli, fixation on the perception of pain, picking, and history of ADHD and Asperger syndrome, the therapist also chose the Sensory Processing Measure Home/School (SPM; Parham, Ecker, Miller-Kuhaneck, Henry, & Glennon, 2007). The combined results of the OT PAL and the SPM will help the therapist develop the optimal student–environment fit.

Challenges to Evaluation

The cases illustrate the process of gathering data from chart review, parents, guardians, client interview, and assessment tools. Sometimes gathering assessment data can be difficult. Families may be reluctant to trust the helping professional because of past negative experiences or fear of having their child removed from the home. Forming a partnership involves taking time to visit with parents about their needs for support and specifically what they want the child to be able to do at discharge. The therapist should not assume that parents can read and should always offer to read the assessment tools to parents, for example, by simply stating that the parent can choose to either answer the questions through interview or by reading and checking the assessment form. The therapist should also be sure to explain the results of assessments in language parents can understand.

Sometimes gaining a child's compliance with assessments can be a challenge. In such cases, behavioral principles can be applied to facilitate completion of the evaluation. For example, an arrangement can be made in which the child agrees to complete portions of the evaluation in exchange for a privilege such as playing a game or doing a physical activity. In addition, engaging children in follow-up discussion, such as in the COSA, can also be difficult. Engaging the child in an activity of his or her choice while talking can be a useful strategy. Using behavioral principles and activity and breaking assessments into short periods of time can increase compliance, which in turn results in more accurate assessment results. Other strategies are offering to read the assessment questions to the child and letting him or her mark the appropriate response on the questionnaire form or providing visual scales, such as the Adolescent/Adult Sensory Profile rating scale, to the child.

Intervention

Contemporary occupational therapy practice is guided by three overarching principles: client-centered practice, occupation-centered practice, and evidence-based practice (Crepeau, Cohn, & Boyt Schell, 2004), which should be reflected in both the theoretical models and the specific intervention strategies used in pediatric psychosocial occupational therapy. However, Haglund, Ekbladh, Thorell, and Hallberg (2000) reported that 75% of therapists surveyed used interdisciplinary impairment-based models (e.g., cognitive, behavioral) that are not reflective of client-centered or occupation-based practice. Using only impairment-based models can lead occupational therapists to feel a lack of professional identity and other professionals to be unaware of occupational therapy's unique contributions. The use of occupation-based and client-centered treatment in intervention is a distinguishing professional feature.

Model of Human Occupation

Therapists using the Model of Human Occupation (MOHO) have reported that its client-centered focus helps them to structure thinking around occupation-based treatment and enhance their professional identity and competence (Lee, Taylor, Kielhofner, & Fisher, 2008). MOHO challenges a therapist to look beyond impairment and focus on the client's perspective and lifestyle (Lee et al., 2008) The model is not prescriptive in nature but can be combined with other conceptual practice models in guiding treatment. In psychosocial occupational therapy practice, group and individual interventions using MOHO independently or with other conceptual models focus on the constructs of volition, roles and habits, performance, and environment. Refer to the MOHO text (Kielhofner, 2008) for a detailed description of the principles for therapeutic intervention.

Consider MOHO applied to the case of Corey. The COSA identified Corey as having "a big problem" with four occupations that were most important to him: (1) getting chores done, (2) getting enough sleep, (3) doing things with friends, and (4) calming down when upset. In the follow-up interview, Corey reported that he forgets his chores and does not do them well enough. He was unable to describe a bedtime routine, stating that he goes to bed at 1:00 a.m. or 2:00 a.m. Corey said that he often fights with peers and has difficulty calming down when he is upset with his friends and family. On the basis of this evaluation, Corey indicated that he feels he lacks skills in those areas. Corey's results on the Piers-Harris Children's Self-Concept Scale, Second Edition, suggest that he has serious doubts about his self-worth, feels negatively about his behaviors, and feels he often causes trouble. He also acknowledges a dysphoric mood. Intervention will teach him skills and structure his environment to facilitate success and increase self-worth.

Group intervention focused on supporting Corey in working cooperatively with peers. The first group session began with setting up a safe environment by sharing and discussing the group rules: Stay an arm's length away from peers, take turns talking, and use good sportsmanship. Next, relaxation exercises were used as a warm-up, with the three group participants selecting one to use if they became frustrated. The group then set to the task of making a spider web with yarn and then untangling it. Supportive prompts for using the relaxation strategies, taking turns talking, and being respectful were provided. The group then discussed the activity, reflecting on what skills they used to cooperate, what they might like to do better, and what activity they would do in the next group session.

Before discharge, the occupational therapist met with Corey and his mother to discuss Corey's concern about chores. Corey and his mother agreed on a chore that was of value to Corey, clearing the supper table. Corey and his mother both reported that he does not stay focused to get the job done. The performance skills of attention and sequencing were addressed by having Corey and his mom work together to write a step-by-step process to clear the table. Environmental modification included having only Corey and his mother in the room to limit distractions. Corey's mom was instructed in providing calm, step-by-step feedback to Corey. This plan was also communicated to the therapist at the day treatment program where Corey would be starting the following week.

Occupational Adaptation

The Occupational Adaptation Model (Schkade & Schultz, 1992) focuses on the client's internal adaptation, which is achieved through occupation. The occupational therapist serves as the facilitator and the client as the agent of change. A key feature of this approach is that the child evaluates his or her own progress by self-assessing relative mastery (Jackson & Schkade, 2001). The model supports compensatory techniques if needed. An example of applying the Occupational Adaptation model when preparing youth for transition in a residential center is to place children in "in vivo" (i.e., within the residential center) worker roles to focus on work and community social participation (Stelter & Whisner, 2007). Schultz (2003) developed a program for students with emotional and behavioral disorders that emphasizes therapeutic use of self as the tool to facilitate adaptation through occupation. Rather than teaching skills or role-playing, therapy occurs within the context of the child's roles.

Consider the Occupational Adaptation Model applied to the case of Sue. Sue's OT PAL results revealed that during free time Sue and five other students attempted to play games together. They would argue about which game to play and rules, at which point the teacher would intervene to resolve the conflict, hindering the students' learning of appropriate adaptive responses. Sometimes, instead of facilitating a cooperative activity, the teacher directed the students to play on their own. The occupational therapist used an Occupational Adaptation approach to facilitate improvement in the student's adaptive responses in cooperative play. Intervention began with environmental modification, including using two small groups and providing two game choices. The therapist applied therapeutic use of self by providing supportive prompts and modeling to encourage appropriate decision making and sportsmanship. Prompts consisted of facilitating exploratory processes. For example, when peers said that someone was not following the rules, the therapist responded, "It doesn't seem like things are working. This seems similar to yesterday; why don't you think about what you did then?" When the students sought reassurance, the therapist said, "How do you it think it worked?" As the group demonstrated relative mastery through their actions and comments, the therapist added choices and increased the number of students in the group. Sue became more confident in play with peers and was able to carry over the adaptive responses for cooperative play into the community.

Canadian Model of Occupational Performance and Engagement

The Canadian Model of Occupational Performance and Engagement (CMOP–E; Townsend & Polatajko, 2007) is an emerging client-centered model of practice based on occupational performance that focuses on the dynamic relationships among person, environment, occupation, and engagement. The model's focus on occupational performance addresses a person's ability to choose, organize, and perform meaningful occupations in his or her environment. Finally, the CMOP–E addresses engagement in occupation and more specifically the concept of enablement.

The CMOP–E explains the nature and process of client-centered practice (Kielhofner, 2004) without prescribing specific intervention processes; therefore, it can be helpful to therapists who are seeking to integrate client-centered and occupation-based interventions into their interdisciplinary models. The seven steps of the CMOP–E's occupational performance process (Fearing, Law, & Clark, 1997) are outlined in Table 9.2, illustrating the CMOP–E intervention with Tara.

Sensory Integration

Children and youth diagnosed with mental illness often experience difficulties in processing and integrating sensory information (Dunn, 2007; Schilling, Washington, Billingsley, & Deitz, 2003; Watling, Bodison, Henry, & Miller-Kuhaneck, 2006). Using the sensory integration frame of reference in mental health practice helps occupational therapists, clients, and family members to understand and address situations in which inadequate integration of sensory information compounds psychosocial functioning.

Intervention is a holistic approach that focuses on increasing self-awareness of sensory response patterns, modifying environments, and implementing sensory-based strategies to facilitate coping and improved adaptive responses to stimuli (Champagne, 2005; Champagne & Stromberg, 2004; Costa, Morra, Solomon, Sabino, & Call, 2006). Williams and Shellenberger's (1994) Alert Program, which assists in teaching self-regulation strategies, is a common approach used in intervention with children with emotional and behavioral difficulties (Barnes, Schoenfeld, Garza, Johnson, & Tobias, 2005; Nielsen & Zimmerman, 2008; Salls & Bucey, 2003). Sensory strategies such as seating devices (Schilling et al., 2003), weighted vests (Vandenberg, 2001), and sensory diets (Champagne, 2005) are also common in practice.

Consider Sue's case using the sensory integration approach to intervention. Sue's therapist had the classroom teacher complete the SPM. Results revealed that Sue had definite dysfunction in the areas of sensory processing related to vision, hearing, and touch and that she had behaviors related to sensory processing that

Table 9.2. Canadian Model of Occupational Performance and Engagement: Application to Tara

Step	Description
1. Identify occupational performance issues.	During Canadian Occupational Performance Measure interview, Tara identified many of the same concerns as her parents, stating that noise and congestion in crowded places caused panic. She identified wanting to work on socializing with her friends. She reported wanting to be able to hold a job but was anxious about interviewing and worried that she could not handle people. She wanted to be able to sleep better, saying sounds made it difficult for her to sleep and that she worried about things, such as lights in her room starting a fire at night.
2. Select potential intervention models.	Sensory integration and cognitive–behavioral therapy (CBT).
3. Identify occupational performance components and environmental conditions.	The assessments used to identify components and environmental conditions include the Adolescent/Adult Sensory Profile and psychological testing (see the Sensory Integration and CBT sections for a discussion of these results).
4. Identify strengths and resources.	*Strengths:* volunteering, academic ability. *Resources:* parents, grandparents, counselor.
5. Identify target outcomes and action plans.	Tara identified three target outcomes: (1) I will be able to go to the mall with my friends for 1 hr; (2) I will have completed one job interview; and (3) I will develop and use a sleep habit schedule. *Action plan:* Participate in the partial hospitalization program for 4–6 weeks, engaging in group, individual, and family therapy for 4 hr per day and school for 3 hr per day and completing daily homework assignments relating to treatment goals.
6. Implementing plans through occupation.	Tara selected the following occupations to practice and apply the skills and strategies she is learning: engaging in board games and free time with peers in treatment; community outings, including going to the mall and eating out with the treatment group, family, and friends; role-playing and a real-life interview; and developing a sleep habit schedule in group and applying this schedule daily at home.
7. Evaluating occupational performance outcomes.	Tara reported that she was able to meet her target outcomes and now wanted to focus on maintaining a job and using supports she identified to assist her in dealing with anxieties.

were affecting her performance in social interactions, body awareness, and planning and ideas. The occupational therapist worked with Sue and the classroom teacher to create environmental modifications and a sensory diet for Sue. Classroom modifications included moving Sue's desk to the front corner of the room near the teacher's desk, providing her with a removable study carrel for use when visually distracted, and creating a cozy corner in the classroom for Sue to use when she feels overwhelmed or frustrated. The sensory diet included classroom calisthenics at the beginning of the school day, a 2-minute isometric exercise routine for the entire class to perform before seat work, and an agreement that recess would not be withdrawn from Sue as a consequence for inappropriate behavior. In addition, Sue was enrolled in a weekly social skills group led by the occupational therapist and school counselor.

Behavioral Modification

Although entry-level occupational therapists are typically not trained in applied behavioral analysis, those strategies may be beneficial when working with children with disabilities (Watling & Schwartz, 2004). *Applied behavioral analysis* is an approach to changing behavior based on the principles of Skinner's work with antecedents, behaviors, and consequences (Lutzker & Whitaker, 2005). Behavioral approaches use strategic manipulation of factors that influence behavior rather than allowing natural environmental occurrences to influence the child's learning, which in effect places a significant amount of control in the hands of the therapist using the behavioral strategies (Schultz, 2003). Behavioral intervention principles commonly referenced in the literature include consequences (positive or negative reinforcement and punishment) and antecedent strategies.

Of the behavioral principles, punishment is considered the least desirable approach because although it reduces the behavior, it does not teach a new positive behavior (Bruce & Borg, 2002). In addition, behavior stopped through punishment is likely to reoccur and create negative feelings in the therapeutic relationship (Bruce & Borg). Clinicians are cautioned to carefully consider the downfalls of this method before selecting punishment as an intervention strategy and before instructing families to use punishment.

A better alternative is use of consequential strategies. Of the consequential strategies, positive reinforcement is the most widely used in the educational and clinical setting (Watling & Schwartz, 2004). Using naturally occurring reinforcers is a more desirable intervention strategy because of the likelihood that spontaneous performance of the desired behavior will be reinforced in generalized contexts (Rhode, Jenson, & Reavis, 1996). For example, a child who complies with the classroom schedule throughout the day may earn the privilege of caring for a classroom pet at school, and a child who cooperates with completing homework before dinner may earn 15 minutes of video game time at home. Visiting with each child to determine his or her preferred reinforcing items is crucial because using items or activities not desired by the child will not be effective. In addition, the timing of reinforcement is critical. Reinforcement should occur immediately after the target behaviors so that the reinforcer is associated with the behavior. A lag between the behavior and the reinforcer will decrease the reinforcer's power to effect behavior change. The schedule of reinforcement is another important principle of applied behavioral analysis. Continuous reinforcement is used when a new behavior or skill is being learned, and intermittent reinforcement is applied until the behavior or skill is firmly established.

In contrast to reinforcing a behavior after it has occurred, therapists can use antecedent strategies to set the stage for appropriate behavior to occur (Rhode et al., 1996). Antecedents can be environmental conditions, a sequence of events, a preferred person, or other conditions that support the child in executing a desired behavior. For example, the therapist can use encouraging statements and structuring incentives at the beginning of a group session, such as saying, "Everyone who is in their seat when the group starts can pick their favorite sensory tool to use this morning." Antecedent control approaches have been found to decrease aggression and agitation in separation anxiety and reduce the need for physical restraint (Luiselli, 2000; Luiselli, Kane, Treml, & Young, 2000).

Although they are not necessarily labeled as antecedent strategies, occupational therapists already use this approach through activity analysis. When preparing for a group, the activity and the client are analyzed for the best fit, and needed supports are identified. For example, the therapist may place supplies where children cannot see them until it is time to start, eliminating an opportunity for distraction and off-task behavior. Using the same group routine in each session can provide structure, which decreases behavioral difficulties for children with anxieties and pervasive developmental delays. The sensory strategies previously discussed, such as those used with Sue and Tara, are also examples of antecedent approaches that occupational therapists frequently use.

A behavioral modification program is unlikely to be the only theoretical framework an occupational therapist uses with a child; however, those strategies may be useful in increasing the success of other therapeutic approaches. For example, Corey was asked to use his relaxation exercise in the context of group. Reinforcing him for using the strategies would likely increase his follow-through. Occupational therapists may also teach parents about behavioral management strategies, including antecedents and reinforcers. Reinforcement programs frequently used in the home are chore charts, where the child earns preferred activities, such as computer time, on completion of the chores. Parents also can be taught to use antecedent approaches, such as adding structure and predictable schedules to decrease the likelihood of behavioral difficulties.

Oppositional children can resist behavior modification programs, in which case a behavioral contract, which allows the child to have more control, may be appropriate. For example, the unit nurse reported that Corey will not go to bed at night and Corey's COSA identified getting enough sleep as an occupation of value to him with which he was having difficulty at this time. The therapist addressed developing a sleep habit as the group topic of the day; as a part of this group, Corey developed the behavioral contract shown in Figure 9.1.

Because inpatient stays are short and Corey's mom indicated that she was unable to control her children, the therapist and mother agreed she should take part in a community-based program addressing parenting. The 14-week series used the Strengthening Families Program, which addresses parenting skills, child skills, and family skills. Parenting skills sessions teach strategies for increasing desired behaviors in children through attention and rewards, clear communication, effective discipline, substance use education, problem solving, and limit setting (Substance Abuse and Mental Health Services Administration, 2007).

Each day Corey follows his bedtime routine, he will earn 30 minutes of extra gym time to be used the next day.

Bedtime Routine

8:30	Snack
8:45	Shower, teeth, pajamas
9:00	In bed reading
9:30	Lights out, stay in bed, and do my mental imagery and relaxation exercises

Corey's Signature _____ Therapist Signature _____

Figure 9.1. Corey's behavioral modification contract.

Cognitive–Behavioral Therapy

Cognitive–behavioral therapy (CBT) is based on the belief that four symptom clusters emerge in psychologically meaningful environments (Beck, 1985). The four symptom clusters are (1) physiological changes, (2) behavioral changes, (3) emotional changes, and (4) cognitive changes. Symptoms in the four clusters are triggered by stressful events, such as divorce, death, or moving. CBT directs intervention toward cognitive–behavioral symptoms as a way to change physiological and affective stress. Identifying stressors and experimenting with new ways of thinking and doing help youth gain new ways of coping (Friedberg, Friedberg, & Friedberg, 2001). This approach uses homework as an essential component of treatment. CBT is often used with people with depression, whose thinking patterns are skewed; the resultant behaviors are the focus of intervention. Types of skewed thought patterns include all-or-nothing thinking and "fortune telling," such as believing that everything in the future will be the same as it is in the present.

The Program for Innovative Self-Management (Wexler, 1991) and the EQUIP Program (Gibbs, Potter, & Goldstein, 1995) are two programs developed for adolescents that use cognitive–behavioral approaches. Therapeutic Exercises for Children (Friedberg et al., 2001), which is based on the Preventing Anxiety and Depression in Youth Program, was developed for children ages 8 to 11. All three programs are excellent for applying CBT in practice. The programs often include worksheet-based exercises that engage youth in reflection and changing thinking patterns. Whether teaching the concepts related to CBT or working with other mental health professionals, occupational therapists can facilitate transferring those skills into occupation.

Tara's psychologist recommended a CBT approach on the basis of results of psychological testing revealing that Tara was having excessive anxiety fueled by feelings of inadequacy and a belief that she could not change her situation. Intervention began with Tara's participating in a group that helped her to identify faulty self-talk (cognitive distortions) and then apply approaches to correct the self-talk. The therapist helped Tara understand that what she thinks controls how she feels and acts. Moving skill into occupation is the next step. A simple brain-teaser was used in the group process as a way of showing this concept. The brain-teaser was started, and breaks were taken to record faulty self-talk. The remainder of the group time focused on analyzing the negative self-talk and then changing it. As a homework assignment, Tara was asked to log self-talk each day, increasing her generalization and application. She set goals related to changing self-talk on weekly community outings and was encouraged to use her sensory strategies along with progressive muscle relaxation and mental imagery to assist in handling the anxiety that occurred.

Working With Families

Although the cases in this chapter provide examples of how occupational therapists work with families, it is important to highlight some key points. When children and youth enter treatment, the client is actually the family system (Haiman, Lambert, & Rodrigues, 2005). Principles of family-centered care include families and practitioners working together in the child's best interests. Respect, trust, open communication, negotiation, and mutual decision making are all tenets of family-centered care (Maternal and Child Health Bureau, 2005).

Family-centered care should be reflected throughout the entire occupational therapy process. During evaluation, the family system is addressed by identifying the family structure, strengths and resources, and stressors in the family unit. Intervention may include referring the family to support services, such as homeless coalitions, parenting groups, food pantries, and social services. The therapist and youth teach the parents the skills the youth is learning to facilitate the skill's generalization. Parents also are taught skills to handle their own stress. Modeling and teaching in the context of family groups can help in situations in which the family and child have difficulty interacting, such as in family recreation and play activities.

Therapists are encouraged to focus on family strengths, honor family traditions, and celebrate success throughout the occupational therapy process. Focusing on using community and natural supports and developing family-friendly practice are key to family-centered care (Maternal and Child Health Bureau, 2005). Finally, occupational therapists can support families by providing (1) information about the nature, course, and treatment of their child's disability; (2) skills to cope with their child's disability; and (3) support for themselves (Abelenda & Helfrich, 2003).

Transition Services

Children and youth with emotional and behavioral disabilities have traditionally had poorer outcomes than other students with disabilities (Maag & Katsiyannis, 1998). In fact, in one study the academic functioning of young adults with emotional and behavioral disabilities was equal to or higher than that students with learning disabilities or mental retardation, but they still had more difficulty adjusting to young adulthood (Frank, Sittlington, & Carson, 1995). Despite having the skills and proximity to address transition planning, only 16% of occupational therapists surveyed reported providing transition services for youth ages 13 to 21 (AOTA, 2000). However, occupational therapists working in community mental health have identified supporting independent living as one primary goal (Auerbach & Jeong, 2005).

Whether working in a school system, residential treatment, or community mental health, occupational therapists are challenged to address transition in adolescents. Spencer and Emery (2006) highlighted the following four priorities for transition planning: (1) Engage in assistive technology consultation and task modification; (2) develop work skills, such as job performance skills, job assessment, and postsecondary skills; (3) provide independent living transition services, such as in problem-solving skills, decision-making skills, and self-advocacy skills; and (4) provide community and residential exploration. Occupational therapy models, such as Occupational Adaptation and MOHO, can guide transition planning services. Behavioral interventions are commonly also used to teach skills required in vocational training (Lieberman, Fujitsubo, & Murray, 1997; Maag & Katsiyannis, 1998). Each youth with behavioral and emotional disabilities will require individualized transition services. We use Tara's case here as an example of transition services.

Tara had identified participating in a job interview as a goal. She also had significant anxiety about transitioning to adulthood. In the context of partial hospitalization, her treatment focused on developing the skills necessary for job interviewing, including communication skills and coping skills to handle her anxiety. She searched for jobs and, with the therapist, analyzed jobs for best fit. Tara and her parents also participated in developing a 5-year plan regarding her goals. The plan included paying for college, arranging housing, and outlining the supports that would be provided by her parents. This plan appeared to alleviate Tara's anxiety because she no longer believed she would be on her own immediately after high school graduation.

Outcomes

The process of occupational therapy intervention concludes with measurement of outcomes. "Supporting health and participation in life through engagement in occupation is the broad, overarching outcome of the occupational therapy intervention process" (AOTA, 2008, p. 660). Measurable outcomes include occupational performance, adaptation, health and wellness, participation, prevention, self-advocacy, quality of life, and occupational justice (AOTA, 2008). The cases presented in this chapter include those outcomes as they are exemplified in the occupations of children and youth. We should note that outcome evaluation includes the client and his or her perception of change. Outcome data may be gathered by readministering standardized or nonstandardized measures used at admission, assessing client perceptions through satisfaction scales, or discussing goals and revisiting the occupational profile with the client.

References

Abelenda, J., & Helfrich, C. A. (2003). Family resilience and mental illness: The role of occupational therapy. *Occupational Therapy in Mental Health, 19*(1), 25–39.

American Occupational Therapy Association. (2000). *AOTA 2000 member compensation survey*. Bethesda, MD: Author.

American Occupational Therapy Association. (2008). Occupational therapy practice framework: Domain and process (2nd ed.). *American Journal of Occupational Therapy, 62,* 625–683.

Auerbach, E. S., & Jeong, G. (2005). Vocational programming. In E. Cara & A. MacRae (Eds.), *Psychosocial occupational therapy: A clinical practice* (pp. 591–619). Clifton Park, NY: Thomson Delmar Learning.

Barnes, K., Schoenfeld, H., Garza, L., Johnson, D., & Tobias, L. (2005). Preliminary: Alert Program for boys with emotional disturbances in the school setting. *School System Special Interest Section Quarterly, 12*(2), 1–4.

Beck, A.T. (1985). Cognitive therapy, behavior therapy, psychoanalysis, and pharmacotherapy: A cognitive continuum. In M. J. Mahoney & A. Freeman (Eds.), *Cognition and psychotherapy* (pp. 325–347). New York: Plenum.

Brown, C., & Dunn, W. (2002). *Adolescent/Adult Sensory Profile user's manual*. San Antonio, TX: Psychological Corporation.

Bruce, M. A., & Borg, B. A. (2002). Model of Human Occupation: Systems perspective of occupational performance. In M. A. Giroux Bruce & B. Borg (Eds.), *Psychosocial frames of reference: Core for occupation-based practice* (3rd ed., pp. 209–240). Thorofare, NJ: Slack.

Bruininks, R., & Bruininks, B. (2006). *Bruininks–Oseretsky Test of Motor Proficiency* (2nd ed.). Bloomington, MN: Pearson.

Champagne, T. (2005). Expanding the role of sensory approaches in acute psychiatric settings. *Mental Health Special Interest Section Quarterly, 28*(1), 1–4.

Champagne, T., & Stromberg, N. (2004). Sensory approaches in inpatient psychiatric settings: Innovative alternatives to seclusion and restraint. *Journal of Psychosocial Nursing, 42*(9), 1–8.

Costa, D., Morra, J., Solomon, D., Sabino, M., & Call, K. (2006, March 6). Snoezelen and sensory-based treatment for adults with psychiatric disorders. *OT Practice, 11,* 19–23.

Crepeau, E. B., Cohn, E. S., & Boyt Schell, B. A. (2004). Occupational therapy practice. In E. B. Crepeau, E. S. Cohn, & B. B. Schell (Eds.), *Willard and Spackman's occupational therapy* (10th ed., pp. 27–45). Philadelphia: Lippincott Williams & Wilkins.

Davidson, D. (2005). Psychosocial issues affecting social participation. In J. Case-Smith (Ed.),*Occupational therapy for children* (pp. 449–480). St. Louis, MO: Mosby.

Dunn, W. (1999). *Sensory Profile user's manual.* San Antonio, TX: Psychological Corporation.

Dunn, W. (2007). Supporting children to participate successfully in every life by using sensory processing knowledge. *Infants and Young Children, 20*(2), 84–101.

Fearing, V. G., Law, M., & Clark, J. (1997). An Occupational Performance Process Model: Fostering client and therapist alliances. *Canadian Journal of Occupational Therapy, 64*(1), 7–15.

Frank, A. R., Sittlington, P. L., & Carson, R. R. (1995). Transition of adolescents with behavioral disorders. Is it successful? *Behavioral Disorders, 16,* 180–191.

Friedberg, R., Friedberg, B., & Friedberg, R. (2001). *Therapeutic exercises for children: Guided self-discovery using cognitive–behavioral techniques.* Sarasota, FL: Professional Resource Press.

Gardner, M. F. (1995). *Test of Visual Perceptual Skills* (Rev.). Noveto, CA: Academic Therapy.

Gibbs, J. C., Potter, G. B., & Goldstein, A. P. (1995). *The EQUIP program: Teaching youth to think and act responsibly through a peer-helping approach.* Champaign, IL: Research Press.

Gresham, F. M., & Elliott, S. N. (1990). *Social Skills Rating System.* Circle Pines, MN: American Guidance Service.

Haglund, L., Ekbladh, E., Thorell, L. H., & Hallberg, I. R. (2000). Practice models in Swedish psychiatric occupational therapy. *Scandinavian Journal of Occupational Therapy, 7,* 107–113.

Haiman, S., Lambert, W. L., & Rodrigues, B. J. (2005). Mental health of adolescents. In E. Cara & A. MacRae (Eds.), *Psychosocial occupational therapy: A clinical practice* (pp. 299–333). Clifton Park, NY: Thomson Delmar Learning.

Harrison, P., & Oakland, T. (2003). *Adaptive Behavior Assessment System* (2nd ed.). San Diego, CA: Elsevier.

Jackson, J. P., & Schkade, J. K. (2001). Occupational adaptation model versus biomechanical-rehabilitation model in the treatment of patients with hip fractures. *American Journal of Occupational Therapy, 55,* 531–537.

Keller, J., Kafkes, A., Basu, S., Federico, J., & Kielhofner, G. (2005). *The Child Occupational Self-Assessment* (Version 2.1). Chicago: Model of Human Occupation Clearinghouse, Department of Occupational Therapy, College of Applied Health Sciences, University of Illinois at Chicago.

Kielhofner, G. (2004). The Canadian Model of Occupational Performance. In G. Kielhofner (Ed.), *Conceptual foundations of occupational therapy* (3rd ed., pp. 94–109). Philadelphia: F. A. Davis.

Kielhofner, G. (2008). *Model of Human Occupation: Theory and application* (4th ed.). Baltimore: Lippincott Williams & Wilkins.

King, G., Law, M., King, S., Hurley, P., Hanna, S., Kertoy, M., et al. (2004). *Children's Assessment of Participation and Enjoyment (CAPE) and Preferences for Activities of Children (PAC).* San Antonio, TX: Harcourt Assessment.

Kunz, K. R., & Brayman, S. J. (1999.) The Comprehensive Occupational Therapy Evaluation. In B. Hemphill-Pearson (Ed.), *Assessments in occupational therapy mental health: An integrative approach* (pp. 259–274). Thorofare, NJ: Slack.

Law, M., Baptiste, S., Carswell, A., McColl, M., Polatajko, H., & Pollock, N. (2005). *Canadian Occupational Performance Measure* (4th ed.). Ottawa, Ontario: CAOT Publications.

Lee, S. W., Taylor, R., Kielhofner, G., & Fisher, G. (2008). Theory use in practice: A national survey of therapists who use the Model of Human Occupation. *American Journal of Occupational Therapy, 62,* 106–117.

Lieberman, R., Fujitsubo, L., & Murray, P. D. (1997). A prevocational training project for emotionally disturbed adolescents. *Behavioral Interventions, 12*(1), 41–54.

Luiselli, J. K. (2000). Case demonstration of a fading procedure to promote school attendance of a child with Asperger's disorder. *Journal of Positive Behavior Interventions, 2,* 47–52.

Luiselli, J. K., Kane, A., Treml, T., & Young, N. (2000). Behavioral intervention to reduce physical restraint of adolescents with developmental disabilities. *Behavioral Interventions, 15,* 317–330.

Lutzker, J. R., & Whitaker, D. J. (2005). The expanding role of behavior analysis and support: Current status and future directions. *Behavior Modification, 29*(3), 575–594.

Maag, J. W., & Katsiyannis, A. (1998). Challenges facing successful transition for youth with E/BD. *Behavioral Disorders, 23*(4), 209–221.

Martin, N. (2006). *Test of Visual–Perceptual Skills (Non-Motor)* (3rd ed.). Novato, CA: Academic Therapy.

Maternal and Child Health Bureau. (2005). *Definition of family-centered care.* Retrieved November 2, 2009, from www.medicalhomeinfo.org/health/Downloads/rollout%20 letter%202%20(2).rtf

Nielsen, S., & Zimmerman, S. (2008, April). *Occupational therapy in an interdisciplinary program for children with behavioral and emotional problems.* Short course presented at the AOTA Annual Conference & Expo, Long Beach, CA.

Parham, L. D., Ecker, C., Miller-Kuhaneck, H., Henry, D. A., & Glennon, T. J. (2007). *Sensory Processing Measure manual.* Los Angeles: Western Psychological Services.

Piers, E. V., Harris, D., & Herzberg, D. S. (2002). *Manual for the Piers–Harris Children's Self-Concept Scale 2.* Los Angeles: Western Psychological Services.

Reynolds, C. R., & Kamphaus, R. W. (2002). *A clinician's guide to the BASC.* New York: Guilford.

Rhode, G., Jenson, W. R., & Reavis, H. K. (1996). *The tough kid book: Practical classroom management strategies.* Longmont, CO: Sopris West.

Salls, J., & Bucey, J. C. (2003, March 10). Self-regulation strategies for middle school students. *OT Practice, 8,* 11–16.

Schilling, D. L., Washington, K., Billingsley, F. F., & Deitz, J. (2003). Classroom seating for children with attention deficit hyperactivity disorder: Therapy balls versus chairs. *American Journal of Occupational Therapy, 57,* 534–541.

Schkade, J. K., & Schultz, S. (1992). Occupational adaptation: Toward a holistic approach for contemporary practice, Part 1. *American Journal of Occupational Therapy, 46,* 829–837.

Schultz, S. (2003, September 8). Psychosocial occupational therapy in schools. *OT Practice, 8*(16), CE-1–CE-8.

Sparrow, S., Balla, D., & Cicchetti, D. (1984). *Vineland Adaptive Behavior Scales manual.* Circle Pines, MN: American Guidance Service.

Spencer, J. E., & Emery, L. J. (2006). Priority transition services for adolescents with communication and behavioral disorders. *Developmental Disabilities Special Interest Section Quarterly, 29*(2), 1–4.

Stelter, L., & Whisner, S. M. (2007). Building responsibility for self through meaningful roles: Occupational Adaptation Theory applied in forensic psychiatry. *Occupational Therapy in Mental Health, 23*(1), 69–84.

Substance Abuse and Mental Health Services Administration. (2007). *Strengthening Families Program.* Retrieved August 7, 2008, from http://nrepp.samhsa.gov/programfulldetails. asp?PROGRAM_ID=211

Townsend, S., Cary, P. D., Hollins, N. L., Helfrich, C., Blondis, M., Hoffman, A., et al. (1999). *Occupational Therapy Psychosocial Assessment of Learning (OT PAL)* (Version 2.0). Chicago: Model of Human Occupation Clearinghouse, Department of Occupational Therapy, College of Applied Health Sciences, University of Illinois at Chicago.

Townsend, E., & Polatajko, H. (2007). *Enabling occupation II: Occupational therapy perspective and occupational therapy guidelines for client-centred practice.* Ottawa, Ontario, Canada: CAOT Publications.

Vandenberg, N. (2001). The use of a weighted vest to increase on-task behavior in children with attention difficulties. *American Journal of Occupational Therapy, 55,* 621–628.

Watling, R., Bodison, S., Henry, D. A., & Miller-Kuhaneck, H. (2006). Sensory integration: It's not just for children. *Sensory Integration Special Interest Section Quarterly, 29*(4), 1–4.

Watling, R., & Schwartz, I. S. (2004) Understanding and implementing positive reinforcement as an intervention strategy for children with disabilities. *American Journal of Occupational Therapy, 58,* 113–116.

Wexler, D. B. (1991). *The PRISM workbook: A program for innovative self-management.* New York: W. W. Norton.

Williams, M. S., & Shellenberger, S. (1994). *"How does your engine run?" A leader's guide to the alert program for self-regulation.* Albuquerque, NM: Therapy Works.

CHAPTER 10

Occupational Therapy Intervention for Adults With Mental Illness

Marian Kavanaugh Scheinholtz, MS, OT/L, and Linda T. Learnard, OTR/L

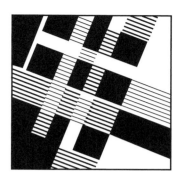

Learning Objectives

After reading this material and completing the examination, readers will be able to

- Differentiate a recovery paradigm from traditional rehabilitation intervention and models;

- Identify components and characteristics of the recovery paradigm as they apply to the therapeutic intervention;

- Identify the five cornerstones of the partnership between the occupational therapist and the consumer;

- Recognize the circularity of the process of planning, evaluation, and intervention in advanced mental health occupational therapy;

- Identify the implication of the nonlinear aspect of recovery for the occupational therapy process; and

- Recognize the meaning of the concept of circles of support and how it affects successful occupational therapy intervention with adults with mental illness.

This chapter addresses occupational therapy practice for adults diagnosed with a mental illness (termed *consumers*). Most of the education and training received by occupational therapists in mental health is in intervention for adults with mental illness. Adults with mental illness have also been the predominant population for which occupational therapy services in mental health have historically been delivered. This training, however, has not consistently incorporated the most current principles of psychiatric rehabilitation, particularly those related to the concept of recovery. Chapter 5 presented the "what" of these principles for the practice of occupational therapy for adults with mental illness (i.e., evidence-based practices supporting adults' occupational functioning in employment, education, and daily living skills). This chapter presents the "how"—that is, how occupational therapists can deliver appropriate interventions using knowledge of the "what" combined with a biopsychosocial understanding of the person and environments in which occupational behaviors are enacted.

Medical Model Replaced by Recovery Paradigm

Medical diagnosis is typically the start of care or intervention planning and implementation for many mental health professionals. In the practice of psychiatric rehabilitation, Anthony, Cohen, Farkas, and Gagne (2002) recommended the use of functional diagnosis for people diagnosed with mental illness. This approach is also appropriate for occupational therapists because medical labels or diagnoses are often secondary to the consumer's functional limitations and barriers, which create impediments to their desired occupational performance. Occupational therapy advanced practice in mental health is grounded in a transformed system of care that creates a new recovery-oriented paradigm for mental health care. In this paradigm, the Recovery Model (Ralph & Corrigan, 2005) is the frame of reference. Consumers work as partners with their care providers in directing their own care. The prevention of illness, both mental and physical, is as important as the treatment of illness, and evidence-based practice is the norm. The services and supports consumers need are readily available, accessible, and coordinated across multiple systems (Power, 2007).

In a recovery paradigm, mental illness does not impede consumers' life goals; hope is real, and psychological and physical well-being are possible despite the presence of symptoms and disability (Ralph & Corrigan, 2005). The recovery paradigm encompasses an environment of care for occupational therapy that is consumer driven—that is, based on consumers' personal choice. This paradigm provides for support during therapeutic intervention to empower consumers through jointly determined intervention plans and shared decision making (Deegan, Rapp, Holter, & Riefer, 2008; Schauer, Everett, del Vecchio, & Anderson, 2007) and through models of self-directed care (Cook, Russell, Grey, & Jonikas, 2008). The structure for providing services is to match the consumer's functional requirements with circles of support, which are described later. In this paradigm, the outcomes sought are wellness and hopefulness.

In a recovery paradigm, the rehabilitation process for adults is consumer driven (or directed) rather than consumer centered (or involved). A consumer-driven approach is essential to empower the consumer with control over his or her life. Having control over one's life is an essential part of the "flow" experience, about which Csikszentmihalyi (1990) wrote, "The effort to achieve self-control is one of the oldest goals of human psychology" (p. 243). The consumer is a partner in the process of service provision, and if care is to be consumer driven, this theme must be woven into its every aspect.

The shared decision-making process must begin with the occupational therapist's complete acceptance of the consumer's current level of functioning; by establishing a supportive relationship, the therapist and consumer together explore occupational goals, desires, and outcomes. To be consumer driven, the process must occur at the consumer's level and pace, and an intervention is successful only when the therapist creates an environment that allows the consumer to initiate the action. Ralph and Corrigan (2005) described positive and negative external influences in the environment of a person who is in recovery. Providing the consumer with information, support, and encouragement is a positive external influence that enables him or her to adapt to environmental demands or change his or her desired occupational goals. The consumer is not acted on; rather, the consumer acts as an integral part of the process by influencing its direction and the tools and techniques to be used. This occurs only when the therapist and consumer first establish a relationship and build a partnership, which is critical to the process of achieving effective outcomes.

This chapter focuses on the consumer–therapist partnership. It describes the five cornerstones of this partnership and the circular process of planning, evaluation, and intervention to deliver mental health occupational therapy services. It discusses the nonlinear aspect of recovery as it is seen in the rehabilitation process. The concept of circles of support to enable occupational performance is defined. The chapter concludes with an example that depicts the concepts it describes.

Consumer–Therapist Partnership

In a recovery paradigm, mental health occupational therapy is a rehabilitation process of working in partnership with consumers to enable them to function and access environments that allow and facilitate the use of their skills. It is essential to understand that the therapist and the consumer are equal citizens in this partnership; each should be valued, respected, and treasured for what they bring to the process.

Cornerstones of Partnership

The consumer–therapist partnership process has five cornerstones:

1. The consumer and the therapist have a mutual understanding of how the consumer is functioning.
2. The consumer and the therapist identify and understand the skills and functional requirements needed to achieve the desired tasks that are part of a specific occupation.
3. The consumer and the therapist develop strategies or methods for skill building that match the consumer's functional requirements.
4. The consumer and the therapist work to shape or adapt the environment to support and assist the consumer in achieving his or her highest level of functioning at any given time.
5. The therapist's and consumer's partnership teaches the consumer the skills to use the contextual or environmental supports provided when the consumer's skills are weak or absent.

In many cases, the consumer's level of functioning can change from day to day or even as the day progresses, so maintaining this understanding will be ongoing. When working in day-to-day programming (e.g., supported housing programs, supported employment, or peer-support drop-in centers), the therapist must be able to understand how the consumer is functioning in each encounter.

Case Example: Mr. Z

Mr. Z is a nonverbal consumer who wants to be employed but has had marginal success with past efforts at vocational rehabilitation. The occupational therapist is working with Mr. Z in a supported employment program and has determined that he is sensitive to external stimuli, which affects his ability to concentrate. One day, Mr. Z arrives at the job site moving in an all-or-none pattern of movement with rigid trunk movements. On the basis of their consumer–therapist partnership, the therapist understands Mr. Z's patterns of functioning and knows that this is a cue that he is at a high level of alertness and irritation. The therapist's goal is to enhance Mr. Z's level of functioning so that he can modulate his motor actions and focus on the identified work tasks. To do this, the therapist guides Mr. Z to the lower-sensory environment of the job site (e.g., stepping outside or into an uncluttered storage room or hallway). The therapist then provides calming sensory inputs until Mr. Z is ready to engage in the day's work tasks. On another day, Mr. Z's shoulders are drooping, he has low muscle tone, and his head is down. The therapist has learned that those cues indicate that Mr. Z has a low alertness level. That day, the rehabilitation process begins with the therapist patterning her movements after Mr. Z's and gradually increasing stimuli to bring him to a just-right level of alertness to begin his daily work tasks. For example, the therapist walks side by side with Mr. Z, gradually increasing their speed of walking, and goes to an area of the workplace with a slightly higher level of sensory stimulation, such as the employee kitchen.

Returning to our discussion of the five cornerstones, occupational therapists must know and understand each consumer's functional requirements to be able to shape the environment to support his or her function at an optimum level. In the consumer–therapist partnership, the occupational therapist's role is not only to learn the consumer's functional requirements but also to help the consumer to embrace and accept those traits as uniquely his or her own. Moreover, the occupational therapist's role is to coach the consumer to understand and feel that his or her level of functional requirements is not bad or good; rather, it is okay, a culture of his or her own.

The second critical cornerstone is to identify and understand the skills and functional requirements needed to achieve the desired tasks that are part of a specific occupation. The occupational therapist's role in the process is to work with the person to bring his or her functional requirements and the task's functional requirements into alignment; this process is described later in the evaluation and intervention sections of this chapter.

The third cornerstone is for the consumer and therapist to develop strategies or methods for skill building that match the consumer's functional requirements. For example, the psychosocial skills-building modules that are part of dialectical behavioral therapy (Linehan, 1993) can be used to build interpersonal and coping skills with people diagnosed with borderline personality disorder. This method breaks down performance into skill sets, presenting one concept at a time, with role playing for motor practice, repetition of skill-building activities, journal keeping for reinforcement, and visual review of actions by keeping a diary of daily activities, emotions, and drugs taken (prescribed and unprescribed), and so forth. The psychosocial skills program, as originally developed, is a match for consumers whose functional requirements enable them to learn from classroom-type teaching or coaching that they can generalize to other environments. However, this method is not a match for consumers whose functional requirement is that they must learn the skill set in the specific environment in which the skills are to occur.

The fourth cornerstone is that the consumer and therapist should work to shape or adapt the environment to support and assist the consumer in achieving his or her highest level of functioning at any given time.

The fifth and final cornerstone is that through the consumer–therapist partnership, the therapist teaches the consumer the skills to use the contextual or environmental supports provided when the consumer's skills are weak or absent. For example, providing a consumer with a homemaker service is not a support if the consumer is not able to let the homemaker know how he or she wants their apartment to be cleaned. Moreover, a consumer who is sensitive to strong smells and odors needs to be taught or enabled to let the homemaker know not to use such products in the cleaning process.

Nonlinearity of Recovery Process

Because consumers' recovery process may ebb and flow and occur at different times in their lifespan, the occupational therapist's role is to tailor the rehabilitation process to match where consumers are in their recovery. One of the characteristics of the Recovery Model is that recovery is nonlinear: "Recovery is not a step-by-step process but one based on continual growth, occasional setbacks, and learning from experience" (Substance Abuse and Mental Health Services Administration, 2005). Every occupational therapist must understand that his or her work with an individual, group, or system is just one step or stage in that process. To provide effective supports and interventions to consumers in the recovery process, the therapist must be able to envision the whole process. For example, if a therapist is working in an inpatient unit where a consumer first encounters mental health service provision, the desired outcome may be to expose the consumer to the recovery process. The goals of the occupational therapy process are to create a sense of hopefulness, improve the consumer's sense of his or her functional requirements, or provide the consumer simple success in performing a daily living task in the here and now. The therapist exposes the consumer to this type of support when they work together to identify the consumer's functional capacity and need for environmental supports, which should be the focus whether the consumer receives occupational therapy services for a short or long time. As consumers move through the recovery process, they will know they can come to the occupational therapist for that type of support and to experience success. They will understand that the occupational therapist is a specialist in facilitating their functioning and full participation as a member of the community.

Circles of Support

Circles of support are the types of assistance that surround a person in everyday life (e.g., family, friends, and community connections). The therapist needs to tailor intervention to all levels of consumers' circles of support. For example, providing training to assertive community support teams or residential staff to enable them to become better therapeutic agents is a way to empower consumers by making their support providers more skillful. An occupational therapist may also work as a consultant to a community program to improve the structure of its employment program, thereby improving the level of support the program is able to provide the consumer. Working with the state department of mental health to improve standards of practice and outcome guidelines is another method of building circles of support for consumers. The occupational therapist can be a meaningful and effective agent for consumers' recovery at any or all of these levels and must consider the impact of each level on consumers' personal recovery.

The partnership between the occupational therapist and the consumer is ongoing and lasts as long as the consumer chooses to be engaged in it. Members of the consumer's circles of support can be engaged in a supportive partnership with the therapist, even when the occupational therapist is not directly partnering with the consumer. For example, the consumer's legal guardian may receive training to improve his or her skills in advocating for the consumer. Another example is an occupational therapist's redesigning the environment or specific tasks in a supported housing program to match the functional requirements of the consumers living there.

Components of the Consumer–Therapist Partnership

The ongoing consumer–therapist partnership process is circular in nature. Components of this process are planning, evaluation, intervention, and evaluation, followed by a new or revised plan. Between each component is "thoughtful observation."

Planning: Shared Decision Making and Self-Direction

Planning is not a rigid process that begins at a specific point or must follow a specific protocol. Planning begins at whatever level at which the consumer is able to engage in the process. For example, a therapist was asked to evaluate Ms. A, who refused to work with any of the staff in the state hospital setting where she was living; she interacted and responded to staff in a limited manner. When the therapist first encountered Ms. A, she was sitting on a bench in the hallway of the hospital unit. The therapist sat down on the bench, so as to be at Ms. A's level. Ms. A looked at the therapist, who asked whether she could sit with her for 5 minutes. Ms. A nodded in agreement. This was the beginning of the planning stage of the partnership—sitting together.

Planning can be organized into three tiers—formal planning, environmental restructuring, and planning for skill and support building.

Formal Planning. Formal planning begins with big-picture thinking and future pursuits and involves discussing long-term goals, performance outcomes, and desired areas of occupation (American Occupational Therapy Association, 2008). Conducting an occupational therapy evaluation to develop a formal plan could be the reason for the therapist's referral to work with the consumer. The formal planning process is comparable to the conversations parents have with their high school–age children about their future life plans.

Formal planning is when occupational therapists need to clearly articulate to the consumer what they bring to the partnership. For example, when a therapist receives a referral from vocational rehabilitation to do a functional evaluation of a consumer to determine work capacity, he or she should first directly engage the consumer by asking, "What do you feel we are here to do?" The therapist can then let the consumer know that together they will go on a "treasure hunt" and explore how the consumer functions—the things the consumer can do well and the things that get in the way of functioning (their functional requirements) and for which adaptations need to be built into the job environment. Calling this process a treasure hunt is the therapist's way of letting the consumer know that the therapist thinks he or she is valuable and important. It implies that the consumer is respected and accepted for just who he or she is. It also frames the process as a journey the therapist and the consumer will take together rather than as something that will be done to the consumer. It presents the process as one of shared awareness and shared discovery.

Environmental Restructuring. Engaging in planning at the next level, environmental restructuring, involves finding out the types of environments the consumer will encounter (Learnard & Devereaux, 1992). Also, it is essential to identify the activity demands of the environment and cues, supports, and information-processing methods needed to allow the consumer to perform in the areas of occupation he or she chooses. Environmental restructuring can also be thought of as a means of providing access to specific environments where occupations occur for the consumer. For example, a consumer may identify at the start of the planning process that he or she wants to work but is slow to learn new things. The consumer and the therapist then agree to explore specific learning and information-processing requirements that will support the consumer to learn a new work task. In this situation, the therapist may identify the consumer's functional requirement as a need to demonstrate and immediately practice each skill step before being given more steps. This environmental restructuring will increase the consumer's ability to perform the job. The environmental restructuring involves modifying tasks, situations, patterns to be used, and strategies to be applied.

Skill and Support Building. The third tier of planning occurs at the level of skill and support building. This level of planning concerns three different skills the consumer needs to learn. First, the therapist determines the specific action steps the consumer will need to learn to achieve a desired outcome, based on an analysis of the tasks to be performed, an evaluation of the consumer's functional capacity, and a determination of environmental structuring, all of which will enable the consumer to perform the action steps. Once the therapist determines the action steps, the consumer needs to be taught the skills needed to access and use the identified environmental supports. A third skill that the consumer must be taught is to ask for the identified environmental supports needed to meet his or her functional requirements (Learnard & Devereaux, 1992). For example, Mr. B says he needs to have assigned work tasks written down so he will not forget to do them. In working at this level of planning, the therapist needs to determine how Mr. B should make this request and then teach him how to make it. However, before proceeding, the therapist needs to check with Mr. B to ascertain whether he agrees with this process. In this manner, Mr. B, the consumer, shares in the decision making regarding his care—a form of empowerment that contributes to his recovery.

Thoughtful Observation

Between each step in the planning process, the therapist always needs to engage in thoughtful observation of his or her interactions with the consumer, reflecting on the knowledge and insights he or she has gained. *Reflection* involves a review of the information gathered, prioritizing the consumer's response to the process (Henry, 2008). The therapist needs to thoughtfully process his or her observations and other information gathered to determine how to shape and adapt the environment to support the person at each step of the planning process. As an example of thoughtful observation during the evaluation process, at the initial contact with Ms. C, as the formal planning component began, the therapist noted that the Ms. C responded more quickly and accurately to simple, concrete questions. The therapist determined that when engaging in the formal assessment, simple, concrete questions would need to be used.

Consumer-Centered Evaluation

After the planning process and the development of an agreement with the consumer to proceed in a specific direction, the evaluation occurs. Evaluation can be a process that contributes to consumers' empowerment by providing them with valuable information about their functional requirements, that is, the functional capacity and environmental supports that enhance their ability to perform desired occupations, which enables them to meet their own needs by performing the tasks demanded by their environment to accomplish desired occupations.

Assessment tools and methods should be selected on the basis of the therapist's thoughtful observation of the cues provided by the consumer during the planning process. For example, during the planning process Mr. D identified a desire to move to a different housing situation with fewer supports and more freedom to access community activities in which he wanted to participate. The therapist needs to determine Mr. D's functional capacity and the environmental supports and structure he needs and then determine how his capacity and needs can be matched in the desired housing situation. During the planning process, Mr. D was able to describe this desire in some detail, and although he seems to have short-term memory problems, he appears to be able to verbally convey some of his wants and needs. On the basis of these facts, the therapist should initiate a detailed interview of Mr. D to gather information to provide a basic understanding of how he views himself, his skills, and his typical functioning.

Interview Skills

During this interview process, the therapist must be an attentive listener. Hemphill (1988) discussed how interviewing is an integral part of the occupational therapy evaluation process. She emphasized the importance of listening as a communication technique and outlined characteristics of effective listening skills with particular focus on attending. Effective attending involves the therapist's completely focusing on the consumer and the message being transmitted (Friedman, 1978). Gazada, Childers and Walters (1982) further described the characteristics of effective attending as including showing interest in the talker; increasing the talker's feelings of trust and self-worth; acting as a mark of respect for others; and having more impact on the talker than any other single communication skill. The therapist must use his or her listening skills to gather information in a nonjudgmental manner, which can be facilitated by effective attending. By listening to the consumer, the therapist develops a picture of the consumer's daily routine and his or her wants, skills, and needs for environmental supports—from the consumer's perspective (Henry, 2008).

Conducting the Evaluation

A semistructured interview is typically a good format for gaining understanding of a consumer's daily routine (Henry, 2008). In this type of interview, the evaluator listens to responses and asks probing questions to gather more information or to clarify information. The evaluator must compare and match this information with any information acquired through other formal assessments. Beginning the evaluation by listening to how the consumer's day unfolds can also help to build the assessment partnership. It provides the consumer with an opportunity to share what he or she knows of his or her own functioning. The therapist assessor has the opportunity to display interest in the person while attending to verbal and nonverbal cues regarding patterns of functioning.

Selection of Assessments

Returning to Mr. D's goal regarding residential placement, the therapist selects assessment tasks that will determine Mr. D's skill level and his needs for task adaptations and other environmental supports. To learn about Mr. D's functioning, the therapist uses the Allen Cognitive Level Screen (Allen, 1985; Allen, Kehrberg, & Burns, 1992) and completes the Routine Task Inventory (Allen, 1985; Allen et al., 1992) during the interview process. The therapist also asks Mr. D's care providers to complete the Routine Task Inventory. The information gathered by means of these tools provides an overview of Mr. D's functional capacity and environmental requirements in both new learning situations and routine daily living tasks. Using this information, the therapist then determines which of a variety of assessment tools for self-care and home management skills would be best to examine Mr. D's functional requirements for those skills. Mr. D's verbal skills and ability to concentrate on tasks independently (e.g., budgeting, check writing, community safety, and seeking needed supports and resources) indicate that he could complete some skills assessments in a paper-and-pencil format, such as the Kohlman Evaluation of Living Skills (KELS; Kohlman Thomson, 1992). For a consumer with fewer verbal skills—one who struggles with paper-and-pencil tasks—an assessment such as the Milwaukee Evaluation of Daily Living Skills (Leonardelli, 1988) would be appropriate; it also measures more instrumental activities of daily living than the KELS. However, paper-and-pencil assessments have limitations, and whenever possible the client should be observed performing a task in a real-life situation to verify his or her actual skills.

One characteristic of an advanced practitioner is keeping current with assessment tools and methods in a variety of areas of occupational performance skills, always having available tools that assess the different functional requirement levels of occupational performance, that is, verbal and nonverbal tasks, motor-based tasks, perceptual tasks, and simple, one-step tasks versus complex tasks. Compendiums of assessment tools for occupational therapy are available (Asher, 2007; Hemphill, 1988, Pitts, 2005). In addition, other evaluation techniques and tools specific to rehabilitation of consumers with mental illness are available (Anthony et al., 2002).

The selection of assessment tools must reflect the consumer's planning requests and functional requirements.

During the evaluation process, it is important for consumers to feel successful so they will be willing to engage in the intervention part of the rehabilitation process. Ensuring that tasks are simple and structured enables the consumer to establish a baseline of success. Therapists can also advise families or support staff to follow the "basic three Ss"—making tasks simple, structured, and successful. Using these baseline steps in each interaction will ensure the consumer's willingness to continue with the rehabilitation process.

Intervention

Intervention is a partnership with the consumer that provides encouragement, support, and information. Through the intervention, the consumer feels enabled to move forward to his or her desired goal and is able to initiate the process of "doing." Long, interesting discussions are not an intervention if the person leaves them feeling that the barriers to his or her "doing" are the same.

Part of the intervention process occurs during the evaluation. The therapist reports the findings of the evaluation to the consumer so that he or she can understand his or her own strengths and weaknesses. For example, during Mr. D's evaluation, the therapist determined that he needed demonstration or immediate practice for new learning to occur. The therapist recommended that Mr. D. ask others to show him what they want him to learn rather than verbally explaining it to him.

The therapist also made environmental recommendations for Mr. D's functional requirements. Using clear motor sequences and visual cues, support providers need to demonstrate new skills or tasks for Mr. D with immediate practice. The environmental recommendation for the system was that Mr. D's support providers learn and understand his functional requirements before providing services.

This example shows the importance of making recommendations not only to build the consumer's skills but also to build the supports and environments so that the consumer can perform those skills and ultimately perform his or her desired occupations. The therapist should always write recommendations for system requirements, environmental requirements, and the consumer's skills building.

Case Example: Mr. Y

Over the course of Mr. Y's 20 years of recovery, the occupational therapist had partnered with him at various stages of this process. Mr. Y was diagnosed with childhood schizophrenia at age 14. At age 21, he lived with his mother, stepfather, and half siblings. At that time, he was having increased periods of aggressive behavior toward family members, which culminated in a commitment to the state hospital for an extended period of time. On discharge, he was placed in an eight-person Housing and Urban Development–subsidized group home in the downtown area of a small city. The occupational therapist met Mr. Y for the first time when he was referred by the group home to the psychosocial rehabilitation agency where she worked as the clinical director for residential services.

Their working partnership began when the group home staff requested help from the occupational therapist in determining how to interact with Mr. Y to facilitate his functioning. To do this, the occupational therapist worked in partnership with Mr. Y to identify his strengths and areas in which he might need support. In addition, the occupational therapist and Mr. Y worked out a plan to solve issues that he felt were causing him difficulty. The occupational therapist used the information she gathered to address the priorities of the group home staff and Mr. Y and to train his care providers (circle of support) to adapt the context of Mr. Y's physical, social, and human environment.

The initial process occurred over several weeks as Mr. Y gradually felt more and more comfortable working in the partnership. Mr. Y and the therapist identified Mr. Y's specific functional requirements in terms of his sensory processing, information processing, working memory, and perceptual skills. He also had difficulties with emotional regulation and communication skills.

The occupational therapist worked to create a residential environment that would support Mr. Y in using his skills and feeling safe and comfortable. Mr. Y required a consistent, predictable daily routine in which the end of one activity or task was the cue to begin the next. Mr. Y needed staff support to maintain a consistent daily rhythm with routine patterns of action throughout the day, which would provide Mr. Y with strong cues and a sense of order. Mr. Y required a good sensory diet (Kinnealey, Oliver, & Wilbarger, 1995; Wilbarger & Wilbarger, 1991) in his daily routine to maintain comfort and mood stabilization. He needed support to develop and practice his daily routine until it became a habit for him. He also needed additional support to be precued to changes in his routine or changes in the group home's routine.

Routines were developed with Mr. Y, and he practiced them with staff working in parallel with him until he was doing the routine on his own. The residential staff were trained to observe and understand Mr. Y's sensory and processing issues. Staff were trained to observe slight changes in Mr. Y's functional performance signaling that he needed additional support to feel organized and regain his emotional stability. Staff also worked with Mr. Y to help him recognize the initial signs that he was becoming disregulated and to use certain tools and strategies to help himself or ask for the support he needed from others.

Ongoing support and training were provided to the staff to improve their skillfulness as therapeutic agents in providing Mr. Y support. Supervisory staff were trained to provide praise and encouragement to their staff for all attempts to maintain consistency and the environment that supported Mr. Y in functioning at his best.

After a period of time living in the residential program, Mr. Y stopped by the occupational therapist's office, saying that he wanted to talk with the women who worked in the local pharmacy (where he went daily to buy a soda), but he "didn't have the words to say." The occupational therapist worked with Mr. Y on developing social scripts for the various interactions in which he wished to engage. Residential staff were engaged to practice and role-play the social scripts with Mr. Y. Also, staff members were taught to work with Mr. Y to write social scripts in a format that was now familiar to him and in a way that he would understand. Mr. Y practiced using the social script and was able to ask staff for help when he needed to write new scripts or to adapt the one he had. In this way, he was enabled to interact and participate in community activities.

Several years later, the occupational therapist was managing a work program. Mr. Y was one of a group of consumers who were interested in working. The consumers had some specific functional requirements, such as a low sensory-stimulating environment, working in parallel with other workers, tasks broken down into one-step linear sequences, and tasks with repeated motor patterns. The occupational therapist decided to explore options to develop employment opportunities for the consumers through a special federal program that had set aside funds to create such opportunities for people with disabilities. The set-aside programs were federal contracts that required the company to employ a high percentage of people with disabilities. An important aspect of the jobs was that they paid federal rates, nearly twice the minimum wage. The federal set-aside that was available was to clean a federal building in town. A job for Mr. Y was developed so that he could work in the evening when the work environment had fewer sensory stimuli and more predictable routines. He was given an opportunity to work with the cleaning machines, which provided deep proprioceptive input. Mr. Y also worked in parallel with a peer on the work crew. He became skillful and had great pride in his job. The occupational therapist developed this work program so that it could become accredited as a supported employment model by the Commission on the Accreditation of Rehabilitation Facilities (CARF; www.carf.org). CARF is an organization similar to the Joint Commission. Although the Joint Commission primarily accredits hospitals, labs, and medical facilities, CARF accredits community rehabilitation programs and specialty rehabilitation units or hospitals. CARF accreditation enabled the program to receive funding from the state vocational rehabilitation department to pay for job coaches to assist Mr. Y and the other consumers on the work crew in sustaining their work careers.

Many years passed, and the occupational therapist and Mr. Y moved along different pathways. The state and local mental health service systems underwent changes, resulting in changes at the agency that provided support services to Mr. Y. He was placed in his own apartment and experienced significant change at his worksite that created an environment that was not supportive of Mr. Y's functional requirements. He became scared and panicked in response to living with less support in his housing and employment environments. He repeatedly went to the emergency room asking to be admitted to the state hospital. He reverted to his aggressive behaviors, which eventually resulted in admission to the state hospital after he assaulted a psychiatrist.

At the state hospital, many discharge plans were attempted with Mr. Y with unsuccessful results. With each attempt, Mr. Y became more resistive to leaving, and his functional performance decreased. His occupational performance deteriorated until he essentially became dependent on others for his total care and would only spend his days sitting by the nurse's station, which resulted in Mr. Y being placed under state guardianship.

By this time, the occupational therapist was working as a consultant to the state office of adult protective services. Mr. Y's care manager at the state hospital asked the occupational therapist to work with the hospital and community providers to develop a community placement that would support Mr. Y's functional requirements. As soon as the occupational therapist entered the unit, Mr. Y greeted her, saying, "Oh, good, you are here to help me have a safe place to live." His affective response improved almost immediately because he again had hope of gaining the future he desired. The occupational therapist worked with Mr. Y to describe the type of residential placement he needed. The occupational therapist collaborated with the social worker to describe Mr. Y's needs and emphasize his strengths to community service providers. The occupational therapist also worked with the activity therapy staff at the hospital to shape tasks and the environment to increase Mr. Y's willingness to participate. A community provider was found, and training was provided to its staff in Mr. Y's functional requirements. A daily routine was set up with Mr. Y for the new residence, along with a plan for him to become familiar with the new residential staff. A community volunteer job that used the skills Mr. Y already possessed was developed at a location familiar to him.

Mr. Y continues to be frightened when he leaves the group home, but he is adjusting to its routines and patterns. He is gradually building partnerships with the residential staff as his trust level increases and he feels more comfortable sharing his functional requirements. He has not begun working at his volunteer job in the community, but he is assisting with work tasks in the group home. Over 6 months, his personal care skills have improved, and he has not returned to the state hospital. The occupational therapist continues to partner with Mr. Y in the rehabilitation process.

Conclusion

This chapter describes the process of occupational therapy intervention with adult consumers according to current concepts of psychiatric rehabilitation within a paradigm of recovery. Much of the case-based information presented here is derived from Linda Learnard's private practice (which is also referenced in Chapter 2). Payment for services is primarily through contracts with state departments of mental health and vocational rehabilitation and adult protective services. An occupational therapist working in a mental health setting such as a hospital or outpatient program may be constrained by payment mechanisms. However, the concepts contained in this chapter can be applied to other mental health programs. The "how" of intervention is intended to be used with evidence-based or promising practices on the basis of the occupational therapist's clinical knowledge and experience. Advocating for funding and programs that enable this type of service is addressed in Chapter 20.

References

Allen, C. K. (1985). Assessment procedures. In C. K. Allen (Ed.), *Occupational therapy for psychiatric diseases: Measurement and management of cognitive disabilities* (pp. 105–129). Boston: Little, Brown & Co.

Allen, C. K., Kehrberg, K., & Burns, T. (1992). Evaluation instruments. In C. K. Allen, C. A. Earhart, & T. Blue (Eds.), *Occupational therapy treatment goals for the physically and cognitively disabled* (pp. 31–84). Rockville, MD: American Occupational Therapy Association.

American Occupational Therapy Association. (2008). Occupational therapy practice framework: Domain and process (2nd ed.). *American Journal of Occupational Therapy, 62,* 625–688.

Anthony, W., Cohen, M., Farkas, M., & Gagne, C. (2002). *Psychiatric rehabilitation* (2nd ed.). Boston: Center for Psychiatric Rehabilitation.

Asher, I. E. (2007). *Occupational therapy assessment tools: An annotated index* (3rd ed.). Bethesda, MD: AOTA Press.

Cook, J. A., Russell, C., Grey, D. D., & Jonikas, J. A. (2008). Economic grand rounds: A self-directed care model for mental health recovery. *Psychiatric Services, 59,* 600–602.

Csikszentmihalyi, M. (1990). *Flow: The psychology of optimal experience.* New York: HarperCollins.

Deegan, P. E., Rapp, C., Holter, M., & Riefer, M. (2008). Best practices: A program to support shared decision making in an outpatient psychiatric medication clinic. *Psychiatric Services, 59,* 603–605.

Friedman, P. (1978). *Listening process: Attention, understanding, evaluation.* Washington, DC: National Education Association.

Gazada, G., Childers, W., & Walters, R. (1982). *Interpersonal communication: A handbook for health professionals.* Rockville, MD: Aspen Systems.

Hemphill, B. J. (1988). Listening as an evaluative tool in the interviewing process. In B. J. Hemphill (Ed.), *Mental health assessment in occupational therapy: An integrative approach to the evaluation process* (pp. 23–33). Thorofare, NJ: Slack.

Henry, A. (2008). The interview process in occupational therapy. In E. Crepeau, E. Cohn, & B. A. Boyt Schell (Eds.), *Willard and Spackman's occupational therapy* (10th ed., pp. 285–297). Philadelphia: Lippincott Williams & Wilkins.

Kinnealey, M., Oliver, B., & Wilbarger, P. (1995). A phenomenological study of sensory defensiveness in adults. *American Journal of Occupational Therapy, 49*(5), 444–451.

Kohlman Thompson, L. (1992). *Kohlman Evaluation of Living Skills* (3rd ed.). Bethesda, MD: American Occupational Therapy Association.

Learnard, L. T., & Devereaux, E. (1992). A model for community practice. *Hospital and Community Psychiatry, 43*(9), 869–871.

Leonardelli, C. A. (1988). *The Milwaukee evaluation of daily living skills: Evaluation in long-term psychiatric care.* Thorofare, NJ: Slack.

Linehan, M. M. (1993). *Skills training manual for treating borderline personality disorders.* New York: Guilford Press.

Pitts, D. B. (2005) Evaluation and assessment. In E. Cara & A. MacRae (Eds.), *Psychosocial occupational therapy: A clinical practice* (2nd ed., pp. 477–507). Clifton Park, NY: Thomson Delmar Learning.

Power, A. K. (2007, July 23). *Putting consumers at the center of care.* Paper presented to Substance Abuse and Mental Health Services Administration National Advisory Council Subcommittee on Consumer/Survivor Issues, Rockville, MD.

Ralph, R. O., & Corrigan, P. W. (Eds.). (2005). *Recovery in mental Illness: Broadening our understanding of wellness.* Washington, DC: American Psychological Association.

Schauer, C., Everett, A., del Vecchio, P., & Anderson, L. (2007). Promoting the value and practice of shared decision-making in mental health care. *Psychiatric Rehabilitation Journal, 31,* 54–61.

Substance Abuse and Mental Health Services Administration. (2005). *National consensus statement on mental health recovery.* Rockville, MD: National Mental Health Information Center. Retrieved January 4, 2009, from http://mentalhealth.samhsa.gov/publications/allpubs/SMA05-4129/

Wilbarger, P., & Wilbarger, J. (1991). *Sensory defensiveness in children aged 2–12.* Denver, CO: Avanti Education Programs.

CHAPTER 11

Occupational Therapy Intervention for Older Adults With Mental Illness

Janie B. Scott, MA, OT/L, FAOTA

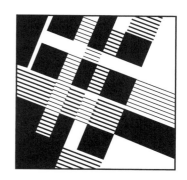

Learning Objectives

After reading this material and completing the examination, readers will be able to

- Identify contextual modifications of environments for traditional institutional and community-based settings as interventions for older adults with mental illness,

- Recognize how contexts can support occupational performance and participation of older adults,

- Identify how occupational therapists can use naturally occurring groups in the community as therapeutic interventions for older adults,

- Delineate the unique situations experienced by older adult veterans and identify intervention methods for mental illness and substance abuse for this group of people, and

- Identify occupation-based services that support older adults with mental illness or substance abuse and their caregivers.

This chapter addresses a range of occupational therapy interventions relevant to older adults with serious mental illness or substance abuse. Chapter 7 laid some of the groundwork for this chapter by identifying significant legislation and theories of occupational engagement for older adults with mental illness. This chapter applies that information to special aging-related topics—for example, Alzheimer's disease, substance abuse, and veterans—and also discusses occupational therapy interventions with caregivers. It places additional emphasis on specific interventions for this population and the variety of roles that occupational therapists may assume.

Risk factors that contribute to mental illness in older adults include isolation, poverty, and bereavement (Substance Abuse and Mental Health Services Administration [SAMHSA], 2004). Identification of risk factors can assist the advanced occupational therapist practicing in the area of mental health in creating effective interventions that prevent or reduce disability. Building interventions to address these risk factors also expands practice opportunities. Woven throughout this chapter are the therapists' roles in and options for delivering occupational therapy services to older adults with mental illness or substance abuse.

Special Aging-Related Topics

Alzheimer's Disease and Dementia

Alzheimer's disease and dementia are illnesses, not a typical part of aging. Mann et al. (2008) and Mahncke et al. (2006) have acknowledged cognitive declines for aging people. Depression is often a component of dementia or Alzheimer's disease; however, it can also be a reaction to a risk factor, such as the loss of a spouse or a significant other. The extra, related challenge for people with dementia and depression is that their short-term memory deficit may not allow for the accumulation of new memories or experiences; therefore, they are lost in memories involving the deceased. Moreover, a joyous moment with friends and family is good only in that moment and may not contribute to a greater sense of well-being. This fact does not suggest that introducing new and pleasurable activities into people's daily schedule is useless. Participation in arts and crafts activities, gardening, exercising, or listening to music may provide momentary pleasures and experiences that can be continued in the future. People should be encouraged to engage in meaningful occupations because occupational successes may help reduce depression.

Behavioral changes are often associated with Alzheimer's disease, and changes in behavior and memory impairments frequently challenge caregivers. Occupational therapists can teach coping strategies that will help both clients and caregivers. They can also teach family members and service providers that inability of people with dementia to remember, or their reaction to cognitive changes, is not necessarily within their control. For example, even though caregivers or therapists may ask people with dementia to write something down so that they can remember it, they may do so but forget where they put the note or be unable to understand the meaning of the words. Occupational therapists can identify devices (memory aids) that are appropriate for the client's specific needs and learning styles.

Therapists also need to consider whether challenging behaviors reflect the clients' or residents' sensory needs. They should assess the way in which people process sensory information and determine whether sensory diets, contextual adaptations, or incorporation of more sensory-based activities will positively change behavior and participation.

Sundowning

Mace and Rabins's (2006) work with people with dementia noted that behavior problems such as agitation appear to increase in the evening. Although the cause is unknown, the condition is often referred to as *sundowning* because symptoms often occur in the early evening, when the person may become more depressed, agitated, and suspicious. "Periods of restlessness or sleeplessness may be an unavoidable part of the brain injury" (Mace & Rabins, 2006, p. 132). Occupational therapists can help caregivers understand that those behaviors are not intentional.

Analyzing the client's daily activities and wake and sleep patterns will help the occupational therapist design a schedule that takes advantage of the times of day when the client's occupational performance is highest and reduce activity demands toward evening. The occupational therapist may also recommend using higher-wattage light bulbs and turning them on in the evening to reduce the impact of sundowning. If a caregiver cannot be with the person, particularly in the evening or overnight, the occupational therapist may suggest an emergency alert system so that the person can summon help in the event of an emergency. If the older adult stays awake late at night and sleeps the morning away, the primary care provider can be consulted to determine whether evening medications can be administered earlier to produce better sleep patterns. If agitation at night becomes problematic, the family may also want to request medications to be administered as needed. The occupational therapist may also suggest incorporating calming sensory stimuli into the client's afternoon and evening routine.

Substance Abuse

Substance abuse is a growing concern for elderly people and the providers who serve them. Between 15% and 20% of older adults intentionally or unintentionally abuse alcohol or medications (SAMHSA, 2005a). Alcohol use and abuse alone or in combination with over-the-counter or prescription medications create problems with mood, cognition, balance, and other daily activities (SAMHSA, 2005a, 2007).

> The elderly may be the group at highest risk for combined mood disorder and substance problems. . . . Episodes of mood disturbance generally increase in frequency with age. Older adults with concurrent mood and substance disorders tend to have more mood episodes as they get older, even when their substance use is controlled. (SAMHSA, 2005b, p. 375)

Some substance abuse is newly acquired; for other people, it has been a pattern of living. People who are substance abusers may age with more complex medical problems than their non–substance-abusing counterparts. The use of alcohol, prescription medications, and illegal drugs can have significant health consequences and is often overlooked by professionals serving the older population. "Because older adults are less likely to be diagnosed and receive the screening, assessment, and intervention they need, the whole community must help identify the problem" (SAMHSA, 2005a, p. 9). Occupational therapists who serve older adults, regardless of the environmental context, should be alert to the possibility of substance abuse and be knowledgeable about self-screenings or administered screenings that can be used. *Substance Abuse Among Older Adults: A Guide for Treatment Providers* (SAMHSA, 2005a) has screening tools and screening questions that may direct this form of inquiry. Identification and intervention with people who abuse alcohol or drugs may ultimately reduce falls, depression, and chronic health conditions. In some situations, if those issues are untreated, problems can arise with memory, cognition, mood, dementia, cirrhosis, sleep disturbances, and malnutrition (SAMHSA, 2005a).

Occupational therapists should investigate when their older clients have had car crashes, falls, bruises or fractures, changes in hygiene, agitation, or other behavior changes. A system of inquiry can provide an opportunity for occupational therapists to ask clients about their behavior patterns, leading to opportunities to screen for substance misuse or abuse. If treatment is warranted, many different levels of intervention exist, including informal counseling, inpatient or outpatient treatment, residential rehabilitation, and community-based services. Selection of treatment environments and modalities should be based on client needs and whether the treatment milieu is appropriate for an older adult. "Effective treatment for the older adult is more holistic, more supportive, and often a great deal more complicated than standard addiction treatment" (SAMHSA, 2005a, p. 25). For older people who are dependent on substances, effective treatment strategies to change the course of dependence are identified through a SAMHSA-funded project called Screening, Brief Intervention and Referral to Treatment (SAMHSA, n.d.).

Mood Disorders

Many factors can contribute to depression in elderly people, including heredity, environment, medication side effects, chronic illness, and the deaths of family and friends. Older people may have lived with a mood disorder for many years or may develop a mood disorder in older age. "Depressed elders do not typically report 'sadness.' . . . Instead they describe feelings of irritability, decreased pleasure, social withdrawal, physical symptoms (e.g., lack of appetite, decreased energy, insomnia), and hypochondriasis" (Mann et al., 2008, p. 10). Those feelings are often revealed through the occupational therapy evaluation. Developing an intervention plan to address these issues can promote recovery and enhance quality of life. One approach that complements occupational therapy philosophies is cognitive–behavioral therapy. This approach is client centered and educationally focused and helps the client set and achieve realistic goals to improve occupational performance. Occupational therapists may help clients identify step-by-step actions to return to their previous levels of participation. For example, a first step may be to create a list of phone numbers of friends whom they would like to see and designate a day and time to call one friend. The next step may be to identify previously pleasurable activities, contact a friend from the list, and invite the friend to participate in this activity.

Schizophrenia

Schizophrenia can affect cognition and performance skills. Occupational therapists play an important role in helping older clients identify what is important to them and what supports and resources may be available to stimulate their participation and facilitate their recovery process. The collaboration between client and therapist can direct goals and attention away from disability and toward self-satisfying occupational engagement. This collaborative model supports occupational therapy's emphasis on client-centered care. Basing interventions on improving performance patterns within the client's personal and environmental contexts will provide concrete learning opportunities through which to learn methods of adaptation.

Veterans

Older veterans with mental illness or substance abuse have special aging-related needs. This section briefly defines this population and explores issues related to veterans with mental illness or substance abuse, those who have posttraumatic stress disorder (PTSD) or brain injury, and those living in nursing homes.

The military is selective in its enlistment practices and therefore screens out people with preexisting mental illness or addiction. The incidence of mental illness or substance abuse in military service is essentially equivalent to the incidence of those conditions among college-age men and women (P. Eichmiller, personal communication, February 9, 2009).

This chapter focuses on adult veterans born before 1950. For this baby boom generation, social and cultural influences may have produced a greater tendency for substance abuse than in earlier periods. The psychological impact of war, or "shell shock," on veterans of all ages was described around World War I. The delayed onset of psychological symptoms after trauma became clearer with the Vietnam War. PTSD continues to have an impact on Vietnam War–era veterans and poses challenges to families and to the health care professionals responsible for veterans' treatment. The condition can persist for many years and requires psychiatric intervention. Interventions for older adult veterans with PTSD may be further complicated by co-occurring medical conditions and cognitive impairments (P. Eichmiller, personal communication, February 9, 2009). Occupational therapists can provide interventions geared toward reducing stress, improving organizational skills, and assessing vocational readiness.

The problem of substance abuse is likely to increase with baby boomers (both veterans and civilians) because they will live longer than past generations and their behavior patterns are perhaps more self-indulgent. This likelihood underscores the need for all health care practitioners to incorporate mental illness and substance abuse screening into their practice and to increase the availability of treatment programs.

Reid and Anderson (1997) investigated geriatric substance abuse. They reported evidence indicating that alcohol abuse among older veterans is a larger problem than previously recognized and that abuse of prescription medications in people older than 65 is more prevalent than previously observed. They also noted that alcohol and drug withdrawal among older adults is more prolonged and can be more complicated.

The Department of Veterans Affairs (VA) has a well-developed system of substance abuse treatment programs. Through the VA medical system, veterans may have substantially greater access to treatment than do nonveterans. Reid and Anderson (1997) also noted that older adults may respond to rehabilitation services in settings with peers as opposed to those delivered to multigenerational groups. The settings for service delivery may be outpatient clinics or inpatient facilities, including nursing homes.

"In 1990, nearly 25% of male veterans in nursing homes were *under* age 65. This compared to 19% of adult male civilians. The median age of male veterans in nursing homes was 73 compared to 80 for male civilians" (Klein & Stockford, 2001, p. 28). Veterans' military experiences and co-occurring conditions may complicate their clinical presentations. The rate of homelessness and nursing home admissions should alert occupational therapists in most practice areas of the likelihood that their client population will be composed in part of veterans. It is therefore imperative that occupational therapists understand the veteran experience and create interventions that will address their physical and psychosocial needs.

Although tabulating the rate of homelessness in any population is difficult, Klein and Stockford (2001) suggested that veterans have a high rate of homelessness. Whether their residential situation is related to their substance abuse or mental illness is not clearly understood. One advantage that veterans have is that their access to VA medical care includes specialized programming for veterans who are homeless or have mental illness or substance abuse.

Occupation-Based Interventions

Therapists may use a range of interventions with people with mental illness or substance abuse. Occupational therapists should become familiar with interventions that are used effectively in current occupational therapy practice and review other sources of gerontology research and literature, paying specific attention to occupational therapy's roles with caregivers. Awareness of these recent works provides a reference point for further independent investigation and application of evidence-based models that may be integrated into current practice. In this discussion of interventions, this chapter briefly reviews the Primary Care Research in Substance Abuse and Mental Health for the Elderly (PRISM–E) study, implications of the final report of the President's New Freedom Commission on Mental Health (2003), the use of assistive technologies, and Clark et al.'s (2001) study of community-dwelling older adults.

The PRISM–E study (SAMHSA, 2004, 2005a) indicated that older adults are more likely to use mental health or substance abuse services when they are integrated into a primary care services setting, which would suggest that occupational therapists specializing in mental health should inform primary care providers whose practice serves community-dwelling older adults about their services. This step would be the first in building a collaborative partnership that is onsite or in close proximity to services needed by seniors. Important but often neglected services for this population include transportation (or coordination of transportation); reminder phone calls, letters, or e-mails; and assistance with billing and reimbursement matters.

Consistent with the outcomes of the PRISM–E study, the 2004 SAMHSA publication *Community Integration for Older Adults With Mental Illnesses: Overcoming Barriers and Seizing Opportunities* concluded that many older adults would prefer to receive mental health care from their primary care providers; however, the majority of providers are not experienced in geriatrics or psychiatry. Mental health specialists, conversely, lack training and experience in geriatrics (SAMHSA, 2004). Occupational therapists can promote their services and skills to primary care providers to develop referral systems, in-clinic partnerships, and personnel training.

The President's New Freedom Commission on Mental Health (2003) final report reinforced the importance of emphasizing concepts of recovery and resilience in mental health intervention. This report helped bridge the outcomes of the PRISM–E studies by considering the environmental context, and it recommended use of the clubhouse or other models that offer supported housing to community-dwelling people with mental illness. Living options that include appropriate treatment and environmental details (e.g., safety features) enhance the opportunities for successful living (Mulligan, 2005).

Occupational therapists can facilitate individual environmental and contextual modifications by evaluating the institutional setting's fit with the clients it serves. On the basis of environmental evaluations, modifications may be made that incorporate color, art, and environmental adaptations (e.g., grab bars and other assistive technologies) to help inform and direct older adults and increase their safety. If an older client gets lost or confused in his or her living environment, the therapist should consider adding color to the hallway walls or flooring in a way that provides directional cues or signs, thereby helping clients move about with greater ease. For example, clients—by themselves or in collaboration with the therapist—can decorate the exterior door of their room. Decorations may include the client's name and photograph or a mailbox or plant that has meaning to the client and that he or she will recognize on returning to the room. Therapists may design rooms or areas to reduce sensory stimuli to promote relaxation and reduce agitation or stress.

Assistive Technology Interventions

Occupational therapists can be instrumental in recommending assistive technology (AT) and in training older adults and their caregivers in its proper use to ensure their safety and independence and support activities of daily living (ADLs) and instrumental ADLs within the home and community. Medication dispensing machines, motion detectors, wearable emergency alert systems, grab bars, and other technologies can be used to promote the safety and independence of both well older adults and those with disabilities. Digital technologies can help caregivers and health care providers monitor older adults' activities within the home. Research at the Massachusetts Institute of Technology's House_n Research Group, Microsoft HealthVault, and the Georgia Institute of Technology is leading to prototype development. The American Occupational Therapy Association's [AOTA's] Technology Special Interest Section, RESNA, the National Resource Center on Supportive Housing and Home Modifications, and similar organizations are also good resources for technology information (Bezaitis, 2008).

A study conducted by Mann et al. (2008) examined changes in impairment level, functional status, and the use of assistive devices by older people with depressive symptoms. They found that over a 3-year period, seniors had a reduction in their symptoms of depression even though their functional decline continued. "Older adults with depressive symptoms who are not prescribed or who do not use appropriate assistive devices to compensate for increasing disability as they age may be at risk for increased severity of depressive symptoms" (Mann et al., 2008, p. 15). Occupational therapists must be prepared to address the complex physical and psychosocial needs of clients and incorporate AT that may improve their quality of life.

Kaye, Yeager, and Reed (2008) reported on a survey of almost 2,000 clients of centers of independent living in California that focused on access to and use of AT. They stated that consumers may not reap the benefits of AT because they cannot obtain, afford, or understand AT's uses and benefits. Without AT for hearing, memory prompting, medication management, and mobility, physical and social isolation may result. Focusing specifically on older adults with mental illness who may have comorbidities, Kaye et al.'s (2008) study revealed that people with "mental health disabilities or with most types of cognitive impairment are less likely to use AT than others" (p. 198). According to this study, more than 75% of survey respondents with mental illness had another disability. Kaye et al. (2008) concluded that this population had a significantly reduced likelihood of continued AT use than other respondents with disabilities.

Occupational therapists may help address some of the issues that Kaye et al. (2008) identified by assisting clients, caregivers, and service providers with obtaining needed

Box 11.1. Case Example: Catherine

Catherine is 61 years old and lives in her own home with her partner of 17 years. She was diagnosed with bipolar disorder in her mid-30s. Because of her multiple hospitalizations, her employment history has not been consistent. Seven years ago, she was a passenger in a car that crashed, and she sustained a mild brain injury. Catherine's short-term memory became impaired, and she is having greater difficulty performing daily tasks like taking her medications, preparing meals, and keeping her home clean and organized. Catherine's psychiatrist referred her to an occupational therapist to help her with personal and home management.

The occupational therapist met with Catherine and her partner in their home. It was important to identify Catherine's and, to a lesser extent, her partner's primary concerns related to home management and personal safety. Catherine first identified a need for medication management, and they discussed what previous strategies had been tried and their outcomes. The occupational therapist researched medication-dispensing services and machines and found a machine; when it was delivered, she reviewed its operation with Catherine and her partner. The AT freed both Catherine and her partner from the concern that he needed to be around during medication times and reduced their anxiety. It provided Catherine with a greater sense of independence and control over her life, and she in turn found the courage to try things she had not done in quite a while, such as cooking her own meals and planning outings with her sister. This increased confidence and a sense of control also motivated Catherine to work with her occupational therapist to create systems to increase organization within the home and reduce years of clutter.

equipment and learning how to use AT devices and by following up to make sure clients continue to use AT (and address the causes if they are not). AT use, whether low tech or high tech, may help improve occupational engagement, maintain social participation, and potentially reduce secondary disabilities. Box 11.1 explores how the use of AT creates opportunities for greater independence within the home and community. Successful engagement in daily occupations reinforces self-concept and promotes health and participation.

Interventions for Aging Adults With Mental Illness and Dementia

Older adults with severe mental illness and dementia may want to spend more time reminiscing, engaging in self-stimulating activities, or seeking or avoiding contact with others. They may display a variety of behaviors, including resistance to bathing, showering, and changing clothes. Repeating the same questions over and over again may be an effort to fill a void, especially because it is increasingly difficult for older adults with mental illness or dementia to initiate and engage in conversations (Mace & Rabins, 2006, p. 163). Caregivers should avoid arguing or asking questions that the person can answer with a negative (e.g., "Do you want to take your shower now?" vs. "Do you want to take your shower now or before you go to bed?"). Occupational therapists can teach caregivers how to frame questions positively and redirect conversations to try to avoid tension. If decision making is stressful, the caregiver may want to state phrases in the affirmative or give the client a choice between two options.

Occupational therapists can introduce the use of prompts and step-by-step instructions to help older adult clients understand what is going to happen next; doing so may help reduce the anxiety associated with complex tasks (e.g., bathing, making the bed). The Picture Exchange Communication System (Bondy & Frost, 1985) is an option to help someone with limited language communicate and provide the caregiver with a pictorial way of breaking down and structuring everyday activities. Box 11.2 provides a case example of reducing mealtime conflicts with a client with dementia.

Clark et al. (2001) studied community-dwelling older adults and the impact of occupational therapy interventions. According to Clark et al.,

> [b]y considering each elder's personal concerns, values, and environmental resources and limitations, we intended to foster changes that were both intrinsically motivated and contextually feasible within the participant's life, factors jointly conducive to the potential for an enduring therapeutic effect. (p. 63)

This client-centeredness should be the focus of all occupational therapy interventions for older adults, especially those with mental illness. Clark et al. (2001) found that the impact of considering each person's values, concerns, and limitations and developing an individualized intervention plan made a significant difference in social engagement and reducing symptoms of depression.

Gitlin and Corcoran (2005) recommended direct clinical interventions for clients and caregivers. Although not all of their suggestions may be appropriate for every environment or client, they are listed in Box 11.3 to encourage the identification of client needs and environmental elements that may help increase occupational performance. Mahaffey (2007) provided additional guidance for occupational therapy interventions (Box 11.4), which may be geared to different populations and cultural contexts.

Older Adults and Their Caregivers

The education and support of caregivers is critical for older adults with mental illness and substance abuse. Occupational therapists can provide caregivers with

> **Box 11.2. Case Example: Margaret**
>
> Margaret, an 85-year-old widow with dementia and severe depression, was placed on a low-sodium diet after a recent diagnosis of congestive heart failure. An occupational therapist was engaged to help her in the home with activities of daily living and instrumental activities of daily living. Margaret had always enjoyed cooking, and according to her family, she was a great cook. The restriction of salt and other cooking ingredients was hard, especially because Margaret could not remember why she no longer had those ingredients in the house. Nothing tasted good to her, so eating balanced meals became a struggle.
>
> The caregiving team, led by the occupational therapist (and approved by the primary care provider), replaced the salt in the salt shakers with a salt substitute, which reduced some of the cooking conflicts. This strategy promoted Margaret's health (she was eating better), which in turn improved her energy level and, with the occupational therapist's encouragement, enabled her to increase her social engagement in the community. The client-centered approach to care led to solutions that benefited Margaret and promoted her well-being.

> **Box 11.3. Direct Clinical Interventions for Clients and Caregivers**
>
> Gitlin and Corcoran (2005) recommended direct clinical interventions for clients and caregivers. Not all of the suggestions may be appropriate for every environment or client, but they are listed here to encourage the identification of client needs and environmental elements that may help increase occupational performance.
>
> - Remove confusing and distracting elements from the environment. Do not have "objects around the toilet or commode, including washcloths, clothing, reading material, or telephone. These objects can confuse the care recipient about the intended purpose of the toilet or commode" (Gitlin & Corcoran, 2005, p. 244).
> - Create a safe environment, including proper lighting, glare-free work areas, low transitions between rooms, steps with edges highlighted or painted, and a house that is in good repair.
> - Use baby monitors to promote safety while providing the care recipient privacy.
> - Remove locks from interior doors.
> - Remove knobs from stoves or turn off the breaker for the oven when the care recipient is not supervised.
> - Place alarms on doors, cabinets with toxins, and windows.
> - Deciding what to wear can be stressful. Limit choices, purchase clothes that match each other, and remove old or last season's clothes from the closet.
> - Set the water heater at a temperature to prevent scalding.
> - "Avoid scolding, criticizing, or invading the care recipient's personal space, especially if there are signs of agitation" (Gitlin & Corcoran, 2005, p. 252).
> - Do not rush the person to eat; this causes stress and can lead to choking. Support social conversations during meals as long as they do not become stressful or too distracting.
> - Give simple, one-step directions. Use pictures, nonverbal communication, and the like to enhance understanding. Watch the pace of speech, and be patient in waiting for the person to respond. Frame comments, statements, and reactions positively. Watch for sarcasm and negativity in verbal and nonverbal communication.
> - To promote bathroom safety, install grab bars, tub seats, or benches.
> - "For a care recipient who likes to rummage, provide objects that are interesting to touch and manipulate. People with dementia who rummage through drawers and closets may be seeking tactile stimulation. The objects may be left out for easy access or placed all together in places where the care recipient typically rummages" (Gitlin & Corcoran, 2005, p. 272).
> - Help relieve stress and the need for wandering by taking walks, rocking in rocking chairs, using a stationary bike, swimming, or taking baths.
> - Establish predictable routines with consistent people available to provide support.
> - Be alert for signs of distress (e.g., changes in voice volume or tone, wringing of hands) and intervene quickly (Gitlin & Corcoran, 2005, p. 277).

Box 11.4. Additional Guidance for Occupational Therapy Interventions

The following suggestions based on Mahaffey (2007) may be geared to different populations and cultural contexts.

- Approach all clients from an occupational perspective; find out what gives their life purpose and provide treatment from that perspective. This information can be gathered during the initial interview or during completion of an occupational performance review. A cognitively intact older adult should be able to provide the interviewer with an occupational history and highlight occupations that brought the most satisfaction. Using those stories for future planning of employment or volunteer activities will help clarify future options.

  This approach is applicable to clients with cognitive impairment, depression, or other forms of mental illness. The therapist can ask questions about past occupational performance to the person with a cognitive impairment (e.g., ask for information about a position that they held during their youth that they enjoyed). The therapist might ask a person with a depressed mood to discuss a job, volunteer activities, or leisure activity in which he or she engaged that brought them satisfaction or pleasure. The goal is to limit the scope of the question to enable a response.

- Help clients find ways to feel a sense of control. Although many older adults may not have issues regarding control, people with cognitive impairment such as dementia may struggle with this issue because decision making may be difficult for them, leading to feelings of anxiety or not being in control. Provide clients with opportunities to choose the television program they wish to watch, add items to the grocery list, and so forth.

- Approach each person with true compassion: "What would it take in my life for me to act like this person?" Whether clients are typically aging or have disabilities, establishing empathy with them will increase therapists' understanding of their experiences and contribute to their ability to establish a therapeutic use of self.

the tools to manage their stress, prevent injuries, provide quality of care to older adults, and locate resources that promote independence and performance.

A 2007 study conducted by the Alzheimer's Association stated that almost 10 million caregivers are caring for someone with Alzheimer's disease or another form of dementia (Alzheimer's Association, 2009). "Clyburn et al. (2000) reported that the higher the number of problem behaviors, the more likely the family caregiver is to become depressed and that these behaviors are a more reliable predictor of caregiver burden than either cognitive or functional impairment" (Gitlin & Corcoran, 2005, p. 45).

Occupational therapists can help caregivers cope. Teaching stress management techniques to increase coping skills and recommending participation in support groups and programs that offer services to allow respite will promote caregivers' health and wellness. Families need to understand that taking good care of themselves will enable them to provide good care for their relative. Improved stress management also has a positive impact on the care recipient. Occupational therapists can also create opportunities to connect older adults and caregivers with formal support organizations and therapeutically designed groups. Organizations such as the National Alliance on Mental Illness, SAMHSA, Alzheimer's Association, Family Caregiver Alliance, National Family Caregivers Association, and National Coalition on Mental Health and Aging link families and providers to educational materials and information about support groups and services. Occupational therapists can lead such support groups.

Families and friends are naturally occurring caregiver groups that can support older adults with mental illness or substance abuse. Occupational therapists may identify ways for these groups to care for older adults while maintaining caregiver health and safety. After an evaluation of the client's self-management skills, the occupational therapist might outline the range of support the older adults needs, which will help caregivers identify tasks that can be delegated to others to reduce their burden. It is important for occupational therapists working with clients who have cognitive and psychosocial dysfunction to evaluate and alert caregivers to concerns regarding personal safety, security, and ability to respond in emergencies. Whichever caregiver system is identified, the occupational therapist can develop strategies with the client and caregivers to monitor the effectiveness of the care delivered and how to initiate any needed changes in service delivery.

Anticipating clients' and caregivers' needs is an opportunity for occupational therapy intervention. Clients' memory loss, confusion, and functional impairments can also make personal privacy difficult for caregivers. An older adult may have difficulty remembering where the caregiver is if he or she takes a shower, uses the bathroom, or goes on a quick trip to the store. The occupational therapist can provide strategies so that the client will feel safe while the caregiver obtains some relief. For example, the caregiver might leave a note in all the areas where the person might look, detailing where the caregiver is and when he or she will be available. Phone numbers can be added to the message if the client is able to dial the phone, so that she or he can call if worried. The caregiver will need to remember to remove the notes and destroy them on return.

> **Box 11.5. Case Example: Fred**
> Ninety-three-year-old Fred had paid companions with him throughout the day. Sometimes, when he became more depressed and agitated, he fired staff. The caregiving team developed procedures to deal with those situations, and the occupational therapist created a behavior checklist to help guide caregiver reactions. For example, the companion would go out of Fred's field of vision or house and see whether a few minutes apart would diminish the tension of the situation. Another option was to play calming music, and sometimes the caregiver would go home early (an option only if the client would not be in danger when left alone) or give Fred a medication to reduce his agitation.

Whether the client has paid or unpaid caregivers, he or she may occasionally not want the caregiver's assistance or presence. The occupational therapist can assess the client's safety and recommend strategies that may be useful under those circumstances. Strategy development should begin with identifying the antecedents to behaviors and what can be used to diffuse tense situations (e.g., music, relaxation techniques, or calming sensory stimuli). Caregivers can use these techniques whether clients are in their own home, assisted living, a skilled nursing facility, or an institution. Box 11.5 describes how behavior checklists can guide caregivers' responses to changes in their clients' moods or behaviors.

What Happens to Caregivers and Clients as They Age?

As clients and caregivers age, physical demands increase because of the caregiver's own aging process and the taxing demands of caring for another person who is not independent. Without access to and use of needed services and technologies, the physical, emotional, and financial burden rises. It becomes critical for the family to engage in life planning. Occupational therapists have the expertise to assist families in anticipating clients' needs and locating services before an emergency or change in resources occurs. The range of services available includes recreational services, day programs, financial planning, respite care, government assistance, and other support services. Consumers of mental health services are sometimes reluctant to use such services because of the stigma associated with receiving mental health services; however, the attitudes of caregivers, occupational therapists, and others in the support environment may have a positive impact on preconceived notions. Occupational therapists and occupational therapy assistants should teach caregivers transfer techniques, methods of energy conservation, signs of depression, and strategies for behavior management to promote the health and safety of both the caregiver and the client.

Helping families anticipate emergencies is another service appropriately delivered by occupational therapy. The occupational therapist or family member can complete an emergency contact card for the client living at home, which should be placed on the refrigerator and in the client's wallet. These cards are available through the Red Cross or MedsId.com; they contain the client's name, emergency contacts, doctors, primary medical conditions, allergies, and current medications. Occupational therapists can also encourage families and caregivers to have recent photos of the client just in case she or he goes missing. The photographs can be turned over to the police, who may help look for the client. Record a full description of the client on the back of each photograph.

Eklund (2007) reported that perceived control is an important indicator of well-being for people with severe mental illness and is thought to contribute to an improved quality of life, feelings of empowerment, and occupational performance. Eklund concluded that perceived control should be a factor in occupational therapists' clinical reasoning. If people have a sense of control, they feel empowered to make decisions about their life, their recovery, and their future goals. Assessing people's perception of control over their life should be a routine part of the interview and treatment implementation process. When clients establish personal outcomes and priorities, then the outcome of their achievements can be measured and mastery recognized (Eklund, 2007).

Consultation

Many therapeutic approaches to interventions address the needs of older adults with mental illness or substance abuse. In some situations, the occupational therapist can provide both direct and consultative services. For example, for many older adults, isolation and the loss of a spouse, close friend, or pet can contribute to both depression and a loss of independence. Support groups that use valued, age-appropriate, activity-based interventions can be led by occupational therapists or, in a consultative model, created and supervised by them.

Whether to offer direct or consultative services will be determined in part by the service delivery system, reimbursement streams, and human resources and frequently by policies and regulations that direct care. Consultation services are delivered to individuals, the community, or the agency. Occupational therapy consultants also have opportunities to collaborate with consumers to deliver peer counseling and support groups (Scott, 2008).

Consultation to Agencies

Occupational therapists often work with agencies to evaluate systems of care for institutionalized or community-dwelling older adults with mental illness or substance abuse. Efforts to keep clients integrated with their communities will help avoid segregation and promote use of least restrictive environments. Developing recommendations that caregivers can implement contributes to successful placement. Mental health agencies that provide care coordination will recognize that their elderly clients living in the community will only be able to age in place if home evaluations and modifications are considered. Occupational therapy consultants can provide the mental health agency and caregivers with direct services and in-service education about the aging processes and co-occurring conditions and assist with planning and improving services and aging-in-place opportunities.

Community-Based Consultation: Disaster Mental Health Services

One of the many ways in which occupational therapists can serve older adults with mental illness or substance abuse is through involvement with agencies in preparing for disasters and emergencies. "Older adults are classified in disaster mental health training literature as a special population or an 'at-risk' group" (Oriol, 2005, p. 3).

People with mental illness become more disorganized when their daily living schedule, environment, or access to support services is disrupted. Occupational therapists help to prepare people and systems to minimize disruptions. Local and state agencies will benefit from occupational therapists' guidance regarding how to identify at-risk groups in advance of a disaster and help them, nursing homes, assisted living facilities, day treatment programs, and so forth plan and rehearse evacuations. A familiar routine will make movement during emergencies easier. During times of disaster, occupational therapists can help survivors with practical functional activities that will meet their immediate needs. Activities may include helping people make a list of creditors and write to them to request an extension of payment deadlines. Helping evacuees locate food pantries so that meal planning and cooking can resume supports normalizing activities. The most important effort is to help people reestablish familiar routines. Occupational therapists' support of individual beliefs and customs will help them reintroduce activities and objects that offer comfort and provide feelings of normalcy. Therapists can also provide assistance in locating clergy and helping consumers resume their religious services and cultural connections. Professional contacts with suppliers of durable medical equipment may help facilitate donations of needed equipment and supplies.

Summary

Occupational therapists and occupational therapy assistants have many roles that they can assume with older adults with mental illness or substance abuse regardless of the environment in which they live. Occupational therapists serving older adults with mental illness or substance abuse have the latitude to define the environmental contexts in which they practice as clinicians, educators, researchers, advocates, and consultants. Occupational therapy practitioners will need to advocate for opportunities that can have a positive effect on consumers and ensure that funding exists to pay for them. The AOTA Web site (www.aota.org) provides connection to the Legislative Action Center and Resources through its Practitioners, Issues, and Advocacy tab. Occupational therapy practitioners should check this site regularly for important information that affects occupational therapy and mental health practice.

References

Alzheimer's Association. (2009). *Alzheimer's facts and figures. Alzheimer's and Dementia: Journal of the Alzheimer's Association, 5*(3), 234–271.

Bezaitis, A. G. (2008) New technologies for aging in place. *Aging Well, 1*(2), 26–30.

Bondy, A. S., & Frost, L. (1985). *Picture Exchange Communication System.* Newark, DE: Pyramid Educational Consultants.

Clark, F., Azen, S. P., Carlson, M., Mandel, D., LaBree, L., Hay, J., et al. (2001). Embedding health-promoting changes into the daily lives of independent-living older adults: Long-term follow-up of occupational therapy intervention. *Journal of Gerontology, Series B: Psychological Sciences, 56B*(1), 60–63.

Eklund, M. (2007) Perceived control: How is it related to daily occupation in patients with mental illness living in the community? *American Journal of Occupational Therapy, 61,* 535–542.

Gitlin, L. N., & Corcoran, M. A. (2005). *Occupational therapy and dementia care: The Home Environmental Skill-building Program for individuals and families.* Bethesda, MD: AOTA Press.

Kaye, H. S., Yeager, P., & Reed, M. (2008). Disparities in usage of assistive technology among people with disabilities. *Assistive Technology, 20,* 194–203.

Klein, R. E., & Stockford, D. D. (2001, May 31). *Data on the socioeconomic status of veterans and on VA program usage* [Slide presentation]. Retrieved February 2, 2009, from www1.va.gov/vetdata/docs/sesprogramnet5-31-01ppt

Mace, N. L., & Rabins, P. V. (2006). *The 36-hour day: A family guide to caring for people with Alzheimer disease, other dementias, and memory loss in later life* (4th ed.). Baltimore: Johns Hopkins University Press.

Mahaffey, L. (2007, October). *AOTA AudioInsight: Depression and the older adult—The role of occupational therapy.* Bethesda, MD: American Occupational Therapy Association.

Mahncke, H. W., Connor, B. B., Appelman, J., Ahsanuddin, O. N., Hardy, J. L., Wood, R. A., et al. (2006). Memory enhancement in healthy older adults using a brain plasticity-based training program: A randomized, controlled study. *Proceedings of the National Academy of Sciences, USA, 103,* 12523–12528.

Mann, W. C., Johnson, J. L., Lynch, L. G., Justiss, M. D., Tomita, M. D., & Wu, S. S. (2008). Changes in impairment level, functional status, and use of assistive devices by older people with depressive symptoms. *American Journal of Occupational Therapy, 62,* 9–17.

Mulligan, K. (2005). Recovery model seeks more than symptom relief. *Psychiatric News, 40,* 6. Retrieved February 25, 2008. from http://pn.psychiatryonline.org/cgi/content/full/40/18/6?maxtoshow=&HITS=10&hits=10&RESULTFORMAT=&fulltext=recovery+model&searchid=1&FIRSTINDEX=0&sortspec=relevance&resourcetype=HWCIT

Oriol, W. (2005). *Psychosocial issues for older adults in disasters* (DHHS Pub. No. SMA 99–3323). Rockville, MD: Center for Mental Health Services, Substance Abuse and Mental Health Services Administration.

President's New Freedom Commission on Mental Health. (2003). *Achieving the promise: Transforming mental health care in America* (Final Report, DHHS Pub. No. SMA 03–3832). Rockville, MD: Author.

Reid, M. C., & Anderson, P. A. (1997). Geriatric substance use disorders. *Medical Clinics of North America, 81,* 4.

Scott, J. B. (2008). Consultation. In E. B. Crepeau, E. S. Cohn, & B. A. Boyt Schell (Eds.), *Willard and Spackman's occupational therapy* (11th ed., pp. 964–972). Philadelphia: Lippincott Williams & Wilkins.

Substance Abuse and Mental Health Services Administration. (n.d.). *Screening, brief intervention, and referral to treatment.* Retrieved January 12, 2009, from http://sbirt.samhsa.gov/about.htm

Substance Abuse and Mental Health Services Administration. (2004). *Community integration for older adults with mental illnesses: Overcoming barriers and seizing opportunities* (DHHS Pub. No. SMA 05–4018). Rockville, MD: Author.

Substance Abuse and Mental Health Services Administration. (2005a). *Substance abuse among older adults: A guide for treatment providers* (DHHS Pub. No. SMA 05–4083). Rockville, MD: Author.

Substance Abuse and Mental Health Services Administration. (2005b). *Substance abuse treatment for persons with co-occurring disorders: A treatment improvement protocol TIP 42* (DHHS Pub. No. SMA 05–3992). Rockville, MD: Author.

Substance Abuse and Mental Health Services Administration. (2007). *SAMHSA action plan older adults fiscal years 2006–2007.* Retrieved October 2, 2007, from www.samhsa.gov/matrix/SAP_older.aspx

CHAPTER 12

Occupational Therapy in High-Risk and Special Situations

Tina Champagne, MEd, OTR/L, CCAP

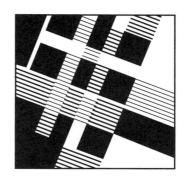

Learning Objectives

After reading this material and completing the examination, readers will be able to

- Identify populations at high risk;

- Differentiate risk and protective factors; and

- Recognize the value of traditional, evidence-based practices and nontraditional, recovery-focused, sensory supportive interventions when working with high-risk populations.

This chapter explores some of the ways in which advanced occupational therapists integrate the use of evidence-based and promising client-centered interventions when working with high-risk populations in mental health practice. Although many populations and situations may be identified as high risk, those that this chapter addresses include people with co-occurring disorders, people with complex trauma histories, and people who engage in self-injurious behavior (SIB). Note, however, that sensory supportive interventions are used for a broad range of purposes and not solely with high-risk populations.

In 2003, the President's New Freedom Commission on Mental Health was initiated for the purpose of increasing client-centered options in the areas of employment, education, assessment, treatment, and research, including assistive devices and universally designed technology, for people with mental illness. Paralleling the vision of the President's New Freedom Commission and the National Consensus Statement on Recovery (Substance Abuse and Mental Health Services Administration [SAMHSA], 2005), the National Association for State Mental Health Program Directors stated that for mental health systems of care to better support recovery, "trauma must be addressed on public policy, practice and educational levels" (Huckshorn, 2004, p. vii). The emerging science of trauma has revealed the high prevalence and pervasive impact of trauma on human development, functional performance, quality of life, health, and wellness (Felitti et al., 1998; Huckshorn, 2004; National Executive Training Institute [NETI], 2003; van der Kolk, 2005). Commonalities in populations at high risk often include having a trauma history, self-regulation and attachment issues, and engagement in SIB to a degree that negatively influences occupational performance. National mental health initiatives, therefore, include applications for populations at high risk, emphasizing resiliency and recovery as intrinsic abilities inherent in all human beings (SAMHSA, 2005; Ralph, 2000).

Growing evidence related to the impact of trauma symptoms and correlations to high-risk behaviors on individual and societal scales demonstrates the need for more sophisticated, comprehensive, and trauma-informed clinical assessment and intervention services (Boriskin, 2004). Without this knowledge, it can be difficult to work effectively with high-risk populations because of the greater probability of self-injurious habits, impulsivity, extreme emotional dysregulation, sensory processing challenges, violent behaviors, and fatality. Historically, difficulty working with high-risk populations has been evidenced in the high use of control-based measures with this group, such as seclusion and restraint (Brodsky, Cloitre, & Dulit, 1995; Linehan, 1993; NETI, 2006; Saxe, Chawla, & van der Kolk, 2002). Although people engage in violent and risky behaviors for many reasons, best practices and governmental initiatives have asserted the importance of assessing the level of risk, protective and risk factors, the function of the behaviors, and the provision of trauma-informed and recovery-focused interventions that do not further compound trauma experiences and symptoms (for clients and staff), such as seclusion and restraint (NETI, 2006).

Trauma-informed care is defined as mental health care that is grounded in and directed by a thorough understanding of the neurological, biological, psychological, and social effects of trauma; its prevalence among people who receive mental health services; and how it relates to each person's experiences and the therapeutic process (Jennings, 2004; NETI, 2006). When care is trauma informed, treatment providers become more empathetic and better able to offer therapeutic opportunities and environments of care that are specific to each person's needs. Hence, interventions weaving a blend of general mental health, trauma-informed, and recovery-focused services are considered best practices for high-risk populations (Drake, Mueser, Brunette, & McHugo, 2004; Gould, Greenberg, Velting, & Shaffer, 2003). The need for more humane and nurturing approaches, in addition to existing evidence-based practices, led (in part) to the introduction of sensory approaches (e.g., sensory modulation) for prevention and crisis intervention purposes, as well as maintenance, recovery, health, and wellness promotion (Champagne, 2003a, 2003b, 2006b, 2008b). Sensory modulation is considered a promising, emergent practice area within general mental health care services (Champagne & Stromberg, 2004; NETI, 2003). Occupational therapists have the knowledge base necessary to take a leadership role in this initiative to educate about and provide services in sensory approaches across client populations, as collaborative members of the transdisciplinary process.

Sensory Processing and Sensory Modulation

Sensory processing, according to Miller & Lane (2000), is

> an encompassing term that refers to the way in which the CNS and the pe-
> ripheral nervous system manage incoming sensory information from the
> seven peripheral sensory systems. The reception, modulation, integration,
> and organization of sensory stimuli, including the behavioral responses to
> sensory input, are all components of sensory processing. (p. 1)

Taken from the work of Ayres (1979) and similar to sensory processing, *sensory modulation* is part of the human condition across the lifespan and involves the ability to
adapt (accommodate), learn, and functionally participate in meaningful and purposeful activities (assimilate; Champagne, 2008b). Miller, Reisman, McIntosh, and
Simon (2001) referred to sensory modulation as

> the capacity to regulate and organize the degree, intensity and nature of re-
> sponses to sensory input in a graded and adaptive manner. This allows the
> individual to achieve and maintain an optimal range of performance and to
> adapt to challenges in daily life. (p. 57)

Difficulty with sensory modulation is evidenced by the emotional, behavioral, and
functional consequences that emerge (Dunn, 1997a, 1997b, 2001).

Research is being conducted to discern whether sensory modulation disorder
is a valid syndrome or part of other mental health diagnoses, addressing comorbidity and differentiation factors (Miller, Cermak, Lane, Anzalone, & Koomar,
2004). Although slight differences exist in the literature, it is generally proposed
that sensory modulation dysfunction (SMD) is regulatory in nature and includes
overresponsivity (hyperresponsivity), underresponsivity (hyporesponsivity), and
fluctuations or lability in the two (Lane, Miller, & Hanft, 2000). Sensory defensiveness, gravitational insecurity, aversive responses to movement, and low registration
are examples of atypical sensory modulation patterns (Dunn, 1997a, 1997b; Lane,
2002; Wilbarger & Wilbarger, 1991, 2002) and possible sensory discrimination
problems. Although many people are bothered by tags in clothes or loud noises,
SMD requires that the person show a patterned response to stimulation that may
be quantified in severity as mild, moderate, or severe, or fluctuate in degrees of
severity over time in a manner that creates barriers to occupational performance.
SMD may be a primary problem, may co-occur with other disorders, is not always
experienced as merely one extreme or the other, and is often evident among high-
risk populations. Research focused on neurophysiological indicators of SMD is limited (Zuckerman, 1994); however, it is growing and expanding to include mental
health indicators.

More recently, research on sensory modulation has expanded to include adults
with mental health symptoms, beyond the traditional realm of researching sensory
processing patterns among those with pervasive developmental disabilities, intellectual disabilities, and learning disabilities. Several studies have established initial links
to sensory processing patterns and adult mental health diagnoses, symptoms, and
treatment approaches, such as schizophrenia, bipolar disorder (Brown, Cromwell,
Filion, Dunn, & Tollefson, 2002; Brown & Dunn, 2002; Brown, Tollefson, Dunn,

Cromwell, & Filion, 2001), trauma, depression, anxiety, pain, and sensory defensiveness (Kinnealey & Fuiek, 1999; Kinnealey, Oliver, & Wilbarger, 1995; Moore & Henry, 2002; Mullen, Champagne, Krishnamurty, Dickson, & Gao, 2008; Pfeiffer & Kinnealey, 2003). Although more research is clearly needed to discern the validity of SMD as a syndrome, the efficacy of sensory modulation interventions with high-risk populations and the significance of sensory modulation as a construct applicable across mental health practice can no longer be disregarded or minimized.

High-Risk Habits and Habit Shaping

Trauma

Habits are created through learning across the lifespan and become one's consistent response in the face of stress or challenge or to what are perceived as adverse stimuli (Francis, 1998). For example, when stress or distress is prolonged or overwhelming, the habitual (whole-system) response self-organizes the whole being and may create stress-related disorders and decompensation (Chopra, 2004; Francis, 1998). Evidence has revealed that having a trauma history increases the likelihood of engagement in high-risk behaviors, such as suicidal acts, self-mutilation, substance abuse, and addiction, and addiction increases the probability of trauma-related disorders and SIB (Boriskin, 2004; Saxe et al., 2002). Through habit shaping, trauma experiences affect the whole system, increasing the likelihood of becoming involved in high-risk situations. (For more information on trauma and its potentially pervasive effects, refer to Chapter 14.) *Complex trauma* is used to describe traumatic experiences that are multiple and prolonged and that adversely influence the developmental process (van der Kolk, 2005). Additionally, developmental trauma disorder is being proposed for consideration in the fifth edition of the *Diagnostic and Statistical Manual of Mental Disorders* (van der Kolk, 2005). Although traumatic experiences occurring in adulthood are commonly understood to often have pervasive effects, significant evidence of a relationship between traumatic experiences in childhood and the onset of mental health symptoms (e.g., depression, anxiety), self-regulation and attachment issues, and SIB (e.g., suicide attempts, alcoholism, drug abuse, sexual promiscuity, and domestic violence) has been established (van der Kolk, 2006). Additionally, Atchinson (2007) identified the presence of SMD among children with complex trauma, supporting the need for the identification of related behaviors, occupational performance variables, and referrals to appropriate services.

Self-Injurious Behavior

Self-injury is often referred to as *self-harm, self-inflicted violence,* and SIB. Fatal self-injury includes SIB that is lethal (suicide). Suicide is a serious, complex, and preventable national public health problem, with no one identified cause (National Institute of Mental Health [NIMH], 2008b). Occupational therapists must be skilled, therefore, in the ability to comprehensively address suicidality and SIB. Most suicide attempts are ways of communicating extreme states of distress; common risk factors are outlined in Table 12.1.

Although debate is ongoing regarding what constitutes lethal versus nonlethal suicidal intent, *nonlethal SIB* refers to actions that lead to varied degrees of self-harm

Table 12.1. Risk Factors for Suicide

Biopsychosocial	Environmental	Sociocultural
More than 90% of people who die by suicide have the following risk factors: • Depression and other mental health issues or a substance abuse disorder (often in combination with a mental health disorder; Moscicki, 2001) • Hopelessness • Impulsive or aggressive tendencies • History of trauma or abuse • Some major physical illnesses • Previous suicide attempts • Family history of suicide, mental health, or substance abuse disorders.	• Job or financial loss • Easy access to lethal means • Firearms in the home (the method used primarily in male suicides; Miller, Azrael, Hepburn, Hemenway, & Lippmann, 2006) • Stressful life events occurring in combination with other risk factors, such as social or family loss (suicidal ideation and suicidal behavior are not typical responses to stress, and many people have these risk factors but do not commit suicide) • Incarceration • Local clusters of suicide events that have a contagious influence.	• Lack of social support and sense of isolation • Stigma associated with help-seeking behavior • Barriers to accessing health care, especially mental health and substance abuse treatment • Certain cultural and religious beliefs (e.g., the belief that suicide is a noble resolution of a personal dilemma) • Exposure to and influence of people who have died by suicide (including exposure through the media; Moscicki, 2001).

Sources. Suicide Prevention Resource Center (2001); U.S. Public Health Service (2001).

without the direct intent of suicide (e.g., self-mutilation, self-poisoning, substance abuse, starving one's self; Duberstein et al., 2000; Linehan, 1986; O'Carroll et al., 1996). Consequently, having a history of nonfatal self-harm often leads to SIB repetition and, sometimes, to suicide, whether suicide is intentional or not (Owens, Harrocks, & House, 2002). Repetitive engagement in SIB may also contribute to the development of other mental health disorders and some of the identified risk factors for child and adult nonfatal attempts (similar to those reported for fatal attempts), including depression, other mental health disorders, trauma history, substance abuse, disruptive behavior, low self-esteem, perfectionism, and parental separation or divorce (Kessler, Borges, & Walters, 1999; Petronis, Samuels, Moscicki, & Anthony, 1990). More recently, human suffering and poor ability to functionally self-regulate have been proposed as the primary source of most self-injurious acts (Khantzian, 2008).

Co-occurring Disorders

Co-occurring disorders include having both substance and other mental health disorders, also referred to as *comorbidity* or *dual diagnosis* (Center for Substance Abuse Treatment [CSAT], 2006b). Hodgson, Lloyd, and Schmid (2001) asserted that the recovery process from substance abuse includes "withdrawal and abstinence from a lifestyle as well as from chemicals" (p. 490), supporting the view that recovery from substance abuse requires a change in one's habits, roles, rituals, and routines, demonstrating the scope and magnitude of the recovery process. Roush (2008) asserted that feelings of loss typically accompany the attempt to change from one lifestyle to another. Co-occurring substance abuse and persistent mental health symptoms may also lead to occupational alienation (loss of intrinsic value), occupational deprivation (Stoffel & Moyers, 2005; Wilcock, 1998), and spiritual latency (Brockelman, 2002; Champagne, Ryan, Saccomando, & Lazzarini, 2007; Moyers, 1997). Khantzian

(2008) stated that "individuals self-medicate with addictive drugs because they provide short-term relief, or make more tolerable psychological pain or the distress associated with psychiatric disorders" (p. 16). Substances are often used (in part or entirely) for their self-regulating effects, which is related to sensory modulation. Although short-term relief may be achieved, SIB leads to long-term problems.

Self-Regulation and Sensory Modulation

The process of sensory modulation is regulatory in nature, and it has been well established that high-risk populations have difficulty with self-regulation, which is deeply interrelated with the complex autonomic nervous system and arousal responses. Wilbarger and Wilbarger (1997) developed a scale describing an "optimal arousal zone" and its relationship to sensory modulation. Siegel (1999) referred to the optimal zone as the "window of tolerance" where "various intensities of emotional and physiological arousal can be processed without disrupting the functioning of the system" (p. 253). At an optimal level of arousal clients are able to experience and integrate sensory–motor experiences and assimilate prior experiences with a greater degree of flexibility and without loss of emotion regulation or fragmentation of one's sense of self. Observations related to arousal and self-regulation must be part of the initial and ongoing assessment and intervention processes, particularly among populations at high-risk. Sensory supportive interventions (e.g., those that are related to sensory modulation) are used to provide a broad range of strategies to assist in the ability to adapt, to participate in meaningful roles and activities, and to increase quality of life. In this way, useful habits will be identified and enhanced through increased self-awareness. Over time, new habits will be learned (e.g., sensory diet), and dominating and impoverished habits will dissipate (e.g., SIBs).

Evidence-Based Practices and Populations at High Risk

Occupational therapy interventions are focused on the identification of and participation in meaningful and healthful roles and activities. Occupational therapists incorporate the use of evidence-based practices when working with people with complex trauma, SIB, and co-occurring disorders. Evidence-based interventions for high-risk populations include brief intervention (Barry, 1999), cognitive–behavioral therapy (CBT; Beck, Wright, Newman, & Liese, 1993; Brown et al., 2005), 12-step programs (Alcoholics Anonymous [AA], 2001), dialectical behavior therapy (Linehan, 1993), Seeking Safety (Najavits, 2002), harm reduction programs, and the community reinforcement approach (Meyers, Miller, Hill, & Tonigan, 1999). Advanced mental health practitioners also use promising sensory approaches to enhance evidence-based practices or as a primary intervention when warranted.

Sensory Modulation and the Occupational Therapy Process

Integrating sensory modulation interventions into practice involves much more than merely adding a few additional tools to one's tool kit. Occupational therapy intervention types include therapeutic use of self, therapeutic use of activities or occupations, education, advocacy, and consultation (American Occupational Therapy Association [AOTA], 2008). Occupational therapists therefore implement and promote the use of sensory modulation interventions in a variety of ways.

Therapeutic Use of Self

It has been well established that human experience and occupational performance can only be understood with respect to the dynamic interrelationship of person, context, and environment (Capra, 1999; Gleick, 1987). It is also well known that the key to successful therapeutic outcomes is the fostering of the therapeutic alliance (Hubble, Duncan & Miller, 1999), through client-centered care (AOTA, 2008) and relationship-centered (Suchman, 2006) principles. Moreover, it has been recognized that the skilled and responsible use of sensory modulation interventions fosters increased feelings of safety and security and the therapeutic relationship. Thus, the therapeutic use of self, one's most important sensory modulation tool, helps to facilitate the therapeutic alliance and build trust, ultimately cocreating, with the client, a "safe place." The way a therapist uses body positioning, tone of voice, speed of movement, energy level, intervention pace, and a host of other interpersonal strategies and interventions demonstrates how a sensory modulation lens is applied to help establish rapport and feelings of safety and security. Although a therapeutic alliance is necessary when working with all populations, it is critical and sometimes more difficult to establish with high-risk populations.

Hughes (2004, 2006, 2007) encouraged use of the PACE Model when working with children with trauma, self-regulation, and attachment issues. PACE promotes the therapeutic attitude of *p*layfulness, *a*cceptance, *c*uriosity, and *e*mpathy. Moreover, the PLACE model is encouraged for parents (*p*layfulness, *l*oving, *a*cceptance, *c*uriosity, and *e*mpathy). These models resonate with the profession's client-centered focus, and occupational therapists may use them when working with high-risk populations.

Readiness for change also has an impact on therapeutic outcomes. The transtheoretical model of the stages of change (Prochaska & DiClemente, 1982; Prochaska, Norcross, & DiClemente, 1994) and motivational interviewing (Miller & Rollnick, 1991) serve as frameworks for working with people at varied readiness-for-change phases. The stages of change (Prochaska & DiClemente, 1982) provide examples of interventions that may be particularly influential at each stage of change. Motivational interviewing (MI) draws on therapeutic strategies from client-centered counseling, CBT, systems theory, and the social psychology of persuasion (Miller & Rollnick, 1991); MI requires an empathetic approach and, similar to the stages of change, provides supportive suggestions for creating therapeutic interactions supporting the motivation to change.

Occupational Therapy Evaluation and Risk Assessment

Part of establishing a therapeutic alliance includes having a collaborative approach to initial evaluation while developing the occupational profile and engaging in the analysis of occupational performance (AOTA, 2008). Occupational therapists must integrate risk assessment into the evaluation process, recognizing that risk management begins with initial and ongoing screening and monitoring. Assessment of risk includes identification of ideation and intent related to harming self or others, risk and protective factors, and clinical observations based on the information obtained, severity, and physical, emotional, cognitive, and behavioral symptoms.

Risk and Protective Factors

Risk assessment and intervention planning require the collaborative assessment of the multiple factors involved and identification of the behavior's function to help identify the individualized interventions that will be most beneficial. Factors related to the likelihood of SIB are referred to as *risk and protective factors* (Suicide Prevention Resource Center [SPRC], 2001). Risk factors are variables that increase the likelihood of self-harm (e.g., death of a loved one, other traumatic events), whereas protective factors are preventive in nature, lowering the likelihood of fatal and nonfatal SIB (e.g., support system, access to health care; SPRC, 2001). Risk factors "vary with age, gender, or ethnic group and may occur in combination or change over time" (NIMH, 2008a, p. 1). People experiencing numerous risk factors are less likely to attempt suicide or self-injury if they are counteracted by protective factors (SPRC, 2001). Additionally, Linehan (1999) proposed the following initial steps for maintaining safety when suicidality is evident: (1) identifying the access to means of suicide, (2) limiting the access to means (e.g., firearms, drugs), (3) ensuring the person is not left alone, and (4) maintaining or increasing contact and support until the appropriate level of treatment is provided. Protective factors vary significantly from one person to the next but "enhance resilience and may serve to counterbalance" risk factors (U.S. Public Health Service, 2001, p. 1). One must understand the dynamic relationship between risk and protective factors and how to use this knowledge to affect SIB prevention (Moscicki, 1997). The SPRC (2001) and NIMH (2008a) provide examples of protective factors, outlined in Figure 12.1.

Self-Injurious Behavior and Evaluation

Skilled evaluation helps identify SIBs; related symptoms; the probable degree of risk; the function of the behaviors; and whether use, abuse, dependence, or addiction is evident. Formalized assessment tools contribute to the evaluation process by providing a systematic way to identify and gather clinical information in a consistent manner. Few standardized tools specifically assess trauma and SIB; two examples of tools focusing on SIB are the Self-Harm Inventory (Sansone, Weiderman, & Sansone, 1998) and the Self-Injurious Behavior Questionnaire (Schroeder, Rojahn, & Reese, 1997). Additionally, the Safety Tool questionnaire was developed to help identify trauma history, warning signs, triggers, and helpful strategies and is also meant to be used as an advance directive (MacLachlan & Stromberg, 2007; NETI, 2003). Occupational therapists assist in collaboratively creating and conducting these varied assessments and use the information during the intervention planning process.

Screening approaches used in substance abuse assessment include self-report (direct and indirect) and biological measures. Two common self-report screening tools used with adults include the CAGE Questionnaire and the Michigan Alcoholism Screening Test (Inaba & Cohen, 2007). Information obtained from biological screenings, typically conducted by nurses, include urinalysis and saliva, hair, and blood testing and provide information as to the accuracy of self-reported substance use and the degree of medical risk. Additional information on addiction-related interventions is available through CSAT (2006a).

- Easy access to a variety of clinical interventions and support for help seeking
- Effective clinical care for mental, physical, and substance use disorders
- Restricted access to highly lethal means of suicide
- Strong connections to family and community support
- Support through ongoing medical and mental health care relationships
- Skills in problem solving, conflict resolution, and nonviolent handling of disputes
- Cultural and religious beliefs that discourage suicide and support self-preservation
- Establishing a therapeutic alliance with the treatment providers
- Defining the thoughts and behaviors (vulnerability factors) that precede suicidal ideation and self-injurious behaviors for the purposes of increasing self-awareness and the ability to self-monitor
- Identifying and rehearsing steps and strategies to take to reduce self-injurious thoughts and behaviors (e.g., role play)
- Informing the person and his or her support network about how to access crisis care, including the existing treatment providers.

Sources. National Institute of Mental Health (2008a); Suicide Prevention Action Network (2001); Suicide Prevention Resource Center (2001).

Figure 12.1. Protective factors against suicide.

Sensory Processing and Assessment

The assessment of sensory processing patterns (e.g., sensory modulation tendencies) must be part of the occupational therapy evaluation process. In part, this assessment process helps collaboratively identify sensory processing–related facilitators and barriers as well as other sensory processing issues that may be in need of additional assessment. This process then helps the occupational therapist collaboratively establish goals and interventions specific to the client's sensory processing needs, as part of the risk management process. The formal and informal tools used or reviewed as part of the initial assessment of sensory processing patterns include standardized and nonstandardized sensory modulation screening tools, risk and trauma assessments, self-rating tools, clinical observation, narratives, art expression, and deescalation tools (Champagne, 2003b, 2008b; NETI, 2003). One example of standardized sensory modulation screening tools, with versions for different age ranges, is the Sensory Profile Series (Dunn, 1999).

Case Example: Abby

The case of Abby demonstrates why it is important to include sensory processing as part of the evaluation and risk management process. Abby was admitted to a long-term care unit because of extreme and ongoing self-mutilation and attempted overdoses. Once admitted to the unit, she appeared depressed; refused to get out of bed, eat, or shower; and would not go to groups or participate in the general milieu. Initially, staff assumed that because of her depression, what Abby needed was an increase in stimulation and activity. She was repeatedly and strongly encouraged by staff to get out of bed and go to groups, with subsequent deleterious effects. From a sensory modulation perspective, depression may be linked to low registration, for which activities affording increased, client-directed sensory modulation interventions may be beneficial. People with hypersensitivities, however, may withdraw from the milieu and activities of daily living because of overstimulation and subsequent distress.

Using the Adolescent/Adult Sensory Profile (Brown & Dunn, 2002), a standardized assessment tool, Abby scored much higher (++) than most people in her age range in both the sensory sensitivity and low registration categories, and her symptoms and demonstrated behaviors suggested difficulty with experiencing extreme sensory overload. Skilled assessment helped identify Abby's global sensory modulation patterns, indicated areas in need of further assessment, and enhanced the ability to collaboratively create a client-centered intervention plan specific to Abby's unique sensory processing and safety needs. Initial sensory modulation interventions included the collaborative identification of preparatory interventions that would help her to feel safe, reality oriented, and less anxious, which led to the increased ability to engage in self-care, leisure, social, and interdisciplinary treatment activities. Once Abby's hypersensitivities and anxiety were addressed, strategies targeting low registration patterns were initiated (Brown & Dunn, 2002).

Sensory Modulation Interventions

Sensory modulation interventions may be applied across any number of goal areas. Among high-risk populations, interventions are often initially introduced to increase self-awareness and to explore how to more skillfully self-regulate, adapt, engage in self-care activities, self-nurture, functionally communicate, and regulate emotions. Exploring how different interventions influence the person, when to use and when not to use each strategy, and intervention modifications typically follows. For example, a person who engages in self-mutilation for "grounding" purposes may use wrapping him- or herself tightly in a blanket, a cold cloth, or beanbag tapping followed by therapy ball exercises affording joint compressions as alternative ways to feel more centered, reality oriented, and bodily grounded. Similarly, the use of intense tastes or scented items may be used for distraction from negative thoughts and urges. Specific music selections identified by the client as calming may be organizing and used when feeling anxious or overwhelmed.

Sensory Diet Interventions

Occupational therapists promote the use of sensations to nourish the nervous system (Ayres, 1979), in recognition of the essential role of meaningful sensory experiences as enablers of occupational performance. Wilbarger (1984, 1995) coined the term *sensory diet*. Creating a sensory diet begins with the collaborative identification and organization of sensory modulation strategies to be strategically used at specific times throughout one's daily routine (Wilbarger & Wilbarger, 2002). For people at high risk, a sensory diet includes prevention and crisis interventions based on unique client factors, occupational performance skills, goals, values, and needs. Sensory-supportive strategies (e.g., sensory modulation interventions) are used as part of a sensory diet for a variety of purposes, such as fostering feelings of safety, improving the ability to engage in self-care tasks, promoting self-nurturance, and emotion regulation (Chiel & Beer, 1997). Moreover, a sensory diet may be used for health and wellness promotion and, therefore, is not solely used with high-risk populations. Sensory kits are often created to help identify and keep helpful strategies organized for use for prevention, maintenance, and crisis deescalation purposes (Champagne, 2003b).

In acute care settings, discharge planning must minimally include identifying and accessing community supports and plans for restricting access to means for suicide and other SIB as part of an individualized safety plan. Discharge and safety planning includes modifications to the person's sensory diet, a crisis deescalation plan, and collaboration with outpatient caregivers and providers to support follow-through. As part of relapse prevention, clients at high risk benefit from enhanced awareness of their own habits, rituals, and routines. This greater awareness supports the ability to create and use a sensory diet that mindfully promotes the specific lifestyle changes needed to support personal safety, wellness, and recovery.

Physical Environment Interventions

From a sensory modulation perspective, the physical environment is an essential therapeutic tool. Although many settings have created sensory modulation rooms and spaces (Champagne, 2003a, 2006a, 2007), the use of sensory carts and enhancements to the general physical environment is also advantageous. Different types of sensory rooms that occupational therapists often create and use include sensory modulation rooms, sensory integration (SI) rooms, and Snoezelen or what has been more recently classified as *multisensory environments* (Champagne, 2008a, 2008b). Although three general types of sensory rooms are listed for clarification purposes, note that sensory room types may also be combined if the setting has staff who are skilled in using the equipment and strategies applied therein. Sensory modulation rooms are most commonly used in general mental health settings because of their interdisciplinary applications and are often more homelike in nature or created around a specific theme. Sensory modulation rooms are created with input from consumers and staff, evolve over time, and are named according to their purpose (e.g., comfort room, serenity room, chill-ville, exploratorium, sanctuary room; Champagne, 2003b, 2006a, 2008b; Champagne & Caldwell, 2007a).

Operationalizing Sensory Modulation Approaches in Mental Health Care

Two examples of sensory modulation programs providing guidelines for operationalizing the use of sensory modulation approaches in mental health practice include the Alert Program for children ages 8 to 12 (Williams & Shellenburger, 1996) and the Sensory Modulation Program for adolescent through adult populations (Champagne, 2003b, 2006b, 2008b). Although developed for use with specific age ranges, both programs may be modified for use across varied age ranges, cultural groups, goals for use, and levels of care. The programs consist of screening tools, general goal areas, and a host of intervention suggestions. The aim of both programs is to help people at different ages learn to identify, change, monitor, and maintain appropriate levels of arousal and to advance strategies used for self-organization to promote occupational performance, recovery, and quality of life (Champagne, 2003b, 2006b, 2008b; Williams & Shellenberger, 1996). Parents, teachers, and interdisciplinary mental health professionals, under the direction of an occupational therapist, may be trained to implement the programs. Some of the key intervention areas include therapeutic use of self, group, and individual sensory–motor activities; sensory modalities; individual and programmatic recommendations; and enhancements and modifications to the physical environment.

Measuring Outcomes of Sensory Modulation Interventions

The quality and effectiveness of sensory modulation interventions may be evaluated in many ways. One acute care inpatient setting explored the effectiveness of providing 1 year of staff training (mandatory education and modeling) and the creation and implementation of a sensory modulation room using a quality improvement study at the end of the year. An assessment of the staff training and sensory room's effectiveness revealed that 89% of clients reported a positive effect, 10% had no change, and 1% had a negative effect, and the unit's restraint rates (episodes per 1,000 patient days) decreased by 54% (Champagne & Stromberg, 2004).

Sensory Modulation and the DESNOS Model

The Disorders of Extreme Stress Not Otherwise Specified (DESNOS) assessment and treatment models provide guidelines for working with people with complex trauma and disorders of extreme stress (Luxenberg, Spinazzola, Hidalgo, Hunt, & van der Kolk, 2001). Sensory-supportive interventions are promoted for use within the DESNOS model, which recognizes that "sensory input can automatically stimulate hormonal secretions and influence the activation of brain regions involved in attention and memory . . . which is particularly relevant for understanding and treating traumatized individuals" (van der Kolk, 2006, p. 1). The integration of the two approaches (sensory modulation and DESNOS) provides the comprehensive services necessary for high-risk populations.

The three phases of the DESNOS treatment model include (1) stabilization, (2) processing and grieving, and (3) transcendence (Luxenburg et al., 2001). When a person is in crisis or potentially headed toward crisis, therapeutic interventions must focus on the cultivation of stabilization, the first phase of the DESNOS model. The work at this phase is not focused on trauma (Luxenberg et al., 2001). Rather, interventions focus primarily on establishing feelings of safety and symptom reduction; enhancing somatic awareness, reality orientation, self-care, and a sense of containment; and fostering the therapeutic alliance. This intervention type is often categorized as *preparatory* in nature (AOTA, 2008). A person using a weighted shoulder wrap while rocking in a rocking chair is one example of a sensory modulation–related, preparatory intervention used for stabilization purposes. In this way, the client's state is recognized and validated, and client-directed, sensory modulation interventions are used to facilitate feeling more coherent, grounded bodily, and less vulnerable and to foster the increased ability to engage in meaningful life activities. The creation of an individualized sensory diet that affords the type and amount of stimulation needed throughout the day for stabilization purposes can be highly effective.

For some clients, the stabilization process may manifest quickly; for others, it may take a longer period of time. Consequently, it is important to use caution when shifting from stabilization-focused interventions to the other DESNOS phases. Although the client may sometimes seem or feel stabilized, this may be superficial (not a strong habitual pattern), and the client may, therefore, become easily destabilized.

The second DESNOS phase focuses on processing and grieving losses related to trauma experiences. Sensory modulation interventions are used in this phase to "help clients overcome traumatic imprints that dominate their lives, which are the sensations, emotions and actions that are not relevant to the demands of the present but are triggered by events that keep reactivating old trauma-based states of mind" (van der Kolk, 2002, p. 59). Therapists continue to use sensory modulation interventions when engaging in therapy sessions specifically addressing traumatic experiences to help clients cope with traumatic memories and related feelings and to prevent decompensation (Ogden, Minton, & Pain, 2006). Many of the traditional sensory modulation interventions that may be used during this phase include art expression, pet therapy, yoga, and the continued use of a sensory diet. Note that the sensory modulation strategies listed are not specific to any one phase of the DESNOS model.

Transcendence occurs when the person is able to move beyond the processing and grieving phase. According to Ogden et al. (2006), at this phase one's integrative capacity increases, one's window of tolerance widens, and "clients are now ready to expand their social connections, overcome their fears of daily life, evaluate and take appropriate risks, and explore change and intimacy" (p. 168). Thus, clients are more ready and able to expand their spiritual, social, leisure, educational, and vocational repertoires.

Case Example: Alex

Alex, age 16, was arrested and then committed to a juvenile justice program after being charged with robbery. He presented with symptoms of major depression and began drinking heavily and using substances at age 9. During the intake process, he reported having poor sleep, nightmares, and a history of witnessing extreme domestic violence and physical and emotional abuse. Initially, Alex demonstrated difficulty tolerating therapeutic groups and other activities requiring social participation. The Adolescent/Adult Sensory Profile was administered, and he scored much higher (++) than most people his age in the following areas: low registration, sensory sensitivity, and sensation avoiding.

After the occupational therapist explained the results, Alex was open to trying sensory modulation interventions to help increase his ability to sleep, engage in self-care tasks, feel less depressed, decrease emotional numbing, and feel more "alive." Alex began engagement in the Sensory Modulation Program in hopes of ultimately increasing his social participation, self-care, and ability to fully engage in therapeutic activities. One evidence-based strategy that helped him to rest more comfortably and sleep at night with fewer nightmares was the use of a weighted blanket (Mullen et al., 2008). Because of the positive impact of the use of the weighted blanket, he decided to test the use of a pressure vest during the daytime, having identified that the deep pressure helped him to feel more safe and centered. He was also willing to try using three to four drops of 100% peppermint essential oil (a natural stimulant) on the shower wall (staff applied) during his morning shower and again in the afternoon via a deep-breathing inhalation to increase alertness and feel less lethargic (Buckle, 2003). By Day 3, Alex also began using beanbag tapping 3 times per day during groups, followed by isometric exercises affording joint compression as another part of his sensory diet, to continue to decrease feelings of emotional numbing and to feel more alive and grounded bodily, all with good results.

Alex was introduced to and often requested to use the sensory modulation room, affording his ability to try other sensory modulation strategies in a sensory-supportive physical environment. Over time, the use of sensory modulation interventions, training in how to use them mindfully (Kabat-Zinn, 2005), and the use of self-rating scales and biofeedback methods increased his ability to recognize and track his progress. Providing a range of sensory modulation interventions for stabilization, in a safe therapeutic environment, helped establish the initial conditions for empowerment and the ability to engage in meaningful occupations. Over time, for example, Alex was able to increase social participation in a range of activities with staff and peers.

Within his first few days at the program, Alex had collaboratively created and begun to implement his sensory diet, and before his release he developed a modified version as part of his discharge plan. With the skilled use of a sensory diet, in addition to other supports (attending AA, seeing a cognitive–behavioral therapist regularly, medication follow through, and the decision to try neurofeedback), Alex was able to increase participation in meaningful life roles and activities with increased hopefulness and without feelings of suicidality or alcohol abuse (Gillman, Gable-Rodriguez, Sutherland, & Whitacre, 1996).

Intervention Precautions: Child and Adult Considerations

It is important to identify sensory processing, trauma-related, and SIB factors that may adversely influence development, functional performance, therapeutic exchanges, and the ability to meet targeted goals. For example, touch that is not self-initiated is often problematic for people with trauma histories; however, teaching safe and healthy forms of touch is essential, particularly among children, who need healthy forms of touch for development (Champagne & Caldwell, 2007b; Schore, 1994). For instance, when working with children, the individualized and skilled use of therapy balls, weighted ball massages, hand hugs, and play activities affording safe forms of touch (e.g., wheelbarrow races) may help to create a bridge and a tolerance for the use of touch in ways that may feel less intimidating. Attention must be paid, however, to the frequency, intensity, and duration of the activities provided because clients with trauma histories can easily become overwhelmed or triggered if the type or intensity of stimulation is perceived as too much, if the pace is too fast, or if the stimulation is similar to the trauma experience. Moreover, sensory modulation interventions can be used to help children and parents engage in ways that feel safe by learning comfortable ways to use touch, as well as stimulation strategically offered to other sensory systems, to enhance self-regulation, bonding, formation of healthy attachments, and affective attunement (Hughes, 2004, 2006, 2007; Kinniburgh, Blaustein, Spinazzola, & van der Kolk, 2005).

Whenever possible, particularly with older adolescents and adults, it is important to teach strategies that clients can do for themselves in addition to identifying strategies that may be performed with others. In this way, helpful interventions may be used whether a caregiver or therapist is present or not. Additionally, although traditional relaxation, guided imagery, mindfulness, and breathing techniques are helpful in some cases, caution must be used with people with trauma histories because of the potential to activate the stress response (Levine, 1997). Additionally, having the client keep his or her eyes open during therapeutic interventions often lessens the possibility of becoming triggered or overwhelmed. Luxenburg et al. (2001) also promoted the idea that once the client is feeling more stabilized, approaches should not be used solely for distraction or avoidance of distressful sensations or emotions, especially when the person is feeling stable enough to begin working on distress tolerance and other therapeutic goals.

Conclusion

The role of the occupational therapist in mental health practice includes working with high-risk populations; therefore, occupational therapists must be skilled in risk assessment, prevention, and crisis deescalation interventions. Occupational therapists use evidence-based practices when working with high-risk populations, and the integration of innovative, sensory processing–related assessments and interventions has significant and wide-ranging applications. Given the current political support and growing body of evidence, advanced occupational therapists practicing in the area of mental health must take a leadership role in promoting the national culture shift toward more nurturing and healing interventions and environments of care, in keeping with the *Centennial Vision* (Moyers, 2007). Sensory modulation interventions, in additional to the broad range of traditional occupational therapy approaches used with populations at high risk, provide innovative tools to support the achievement of this goal.

References

Alcoholics Anonymous. (2001). *Alcoholics Anonymous: The story of how many thousands of men and women have recovered from alcoholism* (4th ed.). New York: Alcoholics Anonymous World Services.

American Occupational Therapy Association. (2008). Occupational therapy practice framework: Domain and process (2nd ed.). *American Journal of Occupational Therapy, 62,* 625–683.

Atchinson, B. (2007). Sensory modulation disorders among children with a history of trauma: A frame of reference for speech–language pathologists. *Language, Speech, and Hearing Services in Schools, 38,* 109–116.

Ayres, A. J. (1979). *Sensory integration and the child.* Los Angeles: Western Psychological Services.

Barry, K. (1999). *Brief interventions and brief therapies for substance abuse* (DHHS Pub. No. SMA–99–3353). Rockville, MD: Substance Abuse and Mental Health Services Administration.

Beck, A., Wright, F., Newman, L., & Liese, B. (1993). *Cognitive therapy of substance abuse.* New York: Guilford.

Boriskin, J. (2004). *PTSD and addiction: A practical guide for clinicians and counselors.* Center City, MN: Hazelden.

Brockelman, P. T. (2002). Habits and personal growth: The art of the possible. *Occupational Therapy Journal of Research, 22*(Suppl.), 18S–30S.

Brodsky, B., Cloitre, M., & Dulit, R. (1995). Relationship of dissociation to self-mutilators and childhood abuse in borderline personality disorders. *American Journal of Psychiatry, 152,* 1788–1792.

Brown, C., Cromwell, R., Filion, D., Dunn, W., & Tollefson, N. (2002). Sensory processing in schizophrenia: Missing and avoiding information. *Schizophrenia Research, 55*(1–2), 187–195.

Brown, C., & Dunn, W. (2002). *The Adolescent/Adult Sensory Profile manual.* San Antonio, TX: Psychological Corporation.

Brown, C., Tollefson, N., Dunn, W., Cromwell, R., & Filion, D. (2001). The Adult Sensory Profile: Measuring patterns of sensory processing. *American Journal of Occupational Therapy, 55,* 75–82.

Brown, G. K., Ten Have, T., Henriques, G. R., Xie, S. X., Hollander, J. E., & Beck, A. T. (2005). Cognitive therapy for the prevention of suicide attempts: A randomized controlled trial. *JAMA, 294,* 563–570.

Buckle, J. (2003). *Clinical aromatherapy: Essential oils in practice*. New York: Churchill Livingstone.

Capra, F. (1996). *The web of life*. New York: Anchor Books.

Center for Substance Abuse Treatment. (2006a). *Addiction counseling competencies: The knowledge, skills, and attitudes for professional practice* (Technical Assistance Pub. Series 21). Rockville, MD: Substance Abuse and Mental Health Services Administration.

Center for Substance Abuse Treatment. (2006b). Identifying and helping patients with co-occurring substance use and mental disorders: A guide for primary care providers. *Substance Abuse in Brief Fact Sheet, 4*(2).

Champagne, T. (2003a). Creating nurturing environments and a culture of care. *ADVANCE for Occupational Therapy, 19,* 50.

Champagne, T. (2003b). *Sensory modulation and environment: Essential elements of occupation*. Southampton, MA: Champagne Conferences & Consultation.

Champagne, T. (2006a). Creating sensory rooms: Environmental enhancements for acute inpatient mental health settings. *Mental Health Special Interest Section Quarterly, 29*(4), 1–4.

Champagne, T. (2006b). *Sensory modulation and environment: Essential elements of occupation* (2nd ed.). Southampton, MA: Champagne Conferences & Consultation.

Champagne, T. (2007). Physical environment. In J. LeBel & N. Stromberg (Eds.), *Developing positive cultures of care: Resource guide* (pp. 273–289). Boston: Massachusetts Department of Mental Health.

Champagne, T. (2008a). *Activities for dynamic living: Companion workbook for the Sensory Modulation Program*. Southampton, MA: Champagne Conferences & Consultation.

Champagne, T. (2008b). *Sensory modulation and environment: Essential elements of occupation* (3rd ed.). Southampton, MA: Champagne Conferences & Consultation.

Champagne, T., & Caldwell, B. (2007a). Nurturing interventions. In J. LeBel & N. Stromberg (Eds.), *Developing positive cultures of care: Resource guide* (pp. 155–164). Boston: Massachusetts Department of Mental Health.

Champagne, T., & Caldwell, B. (2007b). Touch. In J. LeBel & N. Stromberg (Eds.), *Developing positive cultures of care: Resource guide* (pp. 248–272). Boston: Massachusetts Department of Mental Health.

Champagne, T., Ryan, J., Saccomando, H., & Lazzarini, I. (2007). A nonlinear dynamics approach to exploring the spiritual dimensions of occupation. *Emergence: Complexity and Organization, 9,* 29–43.

Champagne, T., & Stromberg, N. (2004). Sensory approaches in inpatient psychiatric settings: Innovative alternatives to seclusion and restraint. *Journal of Psychosocial Nursing, 42,* 35–44.

Chiel, H. J., & Beer, R. D. (1997). The brain has a body: Adaptive behavior emerges from interactions of nervous system, body and environment. *Trends in Neuroscience, 20,* 553–557.

Chopra, D. (2004). *The book of secrets: Unlocking the hidden dimensions of your life*. New York: Harmony Books.

Drake, R., Mueser, K., Brunette, M., & McHugo, G. (2004). A review of treatments for people with severe mental illness and co-occurring substance abuse disorders. *Psychiatric Rehabilitation Journal, 27,* 360–374.

Duberstein, P. R., Conwell, Y., Seidlitz, L., Denning, D. G., Cox, C., & Caine, E. D. (2000). Personality traits and suicidal behavior and ideation in depressed inpatients 50 years of age and older. *Journals of Gerontology, Series B: Psychological Sciences, 55B,* 18–26.

Dunn, W. (1997a). Implementing neuroscience principles to support habilitation and recovery. In C. Christiansen & C. Baum (Eds.), *Occupational therapy: Enabling function and well-being* (pp. 183–232). Thorofare, NJ: Slack.

Dunn, W. (1997b). Neuroscience constructs that support the routines of daily life. In C. Royeen (Ed.), *Neuroscience and occupation: Links to practice* (pp. 1–15). Bethesda, MD: American Occupational Therapy Association.

Dunn, W. (1999). *Sensory Profile: User's manual*. San Antonio, TX: Psychological Corporation.

Dunn, W. (2001). The sensations of everyday life: Theoretical, conceptual, and pragmatic considerations. *American Journal of Occupational Therapy, 55,* 608–620.

Felitti, V. J., Anda, R. F., Nordenberg, D., Williamson, D. F., Spitz, A. M., Edwards, V., et al. (1998). Relationship of childhood abuse and household dysfunction to many of the leading causes of death in adults: The Adverse Childhood Experiences (ACE) Study. *American Journal of Preventative Medicine, 14,* 245–258.

Francis, S. (1998). Chaos, complexity, and psychophysiology. In L. L. Chamberlain & M. R. Bütz (Eds.), *Clinical chaos: A therapist's guide to nonlinear dynamics and therapeutic change* (pp. 147–158). Philadelphia: Taylor & Francis.

Gillman, J., Gable-Rodriguez, J., Sutherland, S. M., & Whitacre, R. J. (1996). Pastoral care in a critical care setting. *Critical Care Nursing Quarterly, 19,* 10–20.

Gleick, J. (1987). *Chaos: Making a new science.* New York: Penguin.

Gould, M. S., Greenberg, T., Velting, D. M., & Shaffer, D. (2003). Youth suicide risk and preventive interventions: A review of the past 10 years. *Journal of the American Academy of Child and Adolescent Psychiatry, 42*(4), 386–405.

Hodgson, S., Lloyd, C., & Schmid, T. (2001). The leisure participation of clients with a dual diagnosis. *British Journal of Occupational Therapy, 64,* 487–492.

Hubble, M., Duncan, B., & Miller, S. (1999). *The heart and soul of change: What really works in therapy.* Washington, DC: American Psychological Association.

Huckshorn, K. A. (2004). Reducing seclusion and restraint use in mental health settings. *Journal of Psychosocial Nursing, 42,* 22–33.

Hughes, D. (2004). An attachment-based treatment of maltreated children and young people. *Attachment and Human Development, 6,* 263–278.

Hughes, D. (2006). *Building the bonds of attachment* (2nd ed.). Northvale, NJ: Jason Aronson.

Hughes, D. (2007). *Attachment-focused family therapy.* New York: W. W. Norton.

Inaba, D., & Cohen, W. (2007). *Uppers, downers, all arounders: Physical and mental effects of psychoactive drugs* (6th ed.). Medford, OR: CNS.

Jennings, S. (2004). *The damaging consequences of violence and trauma: Facts, discussion points, and recommendations for the behavioral health system.* Alexandria, VA: National Association of State Mental Health Program Directors.

Kabat-Zinn, J. (2005). *Coming to our senses: Healing ourselves and the world through mindfulness.* New York: Hyperion.

Kessler, R. C., Borges, G., & Walters, E. E. (1999). Prevalence of and risk factors for lifetime suicide attempts in the National Comorbidity Survey. *Archives of General Psychiatry, 56,* 617–626.

Khantzian, E. (2008). Addiction: Why are some of us are more vulnerable than others? *Counselor, 5*(9), 10–16.

Kinnealey, M., & Fuiek, M. (1999). The relationship between sensory defensiveness, anxiety, depression, and perception of pain in adults. *Occupational Therapy International, 6*(3), 195–206.

Kinnealey, M., Oliver, B., & Wilbarger, P. (1995). A phenomenological study of sensory defensiveness in adults. *American Journal of Occupational Therapy, 49,* 444–451.

Kinniburgh, K., Blaustein, M., Spinazzola, J., & van der Kolk, B. A. (2005). Attachment, self-regulation, and competency: A comprehensive intervention framework for children with complex trauma. *Psychiatric Annals, 35,* 424–430.

Lane, S. (2002). Sensory modulation. In A. Bundy, S. Lane, & E. Murray (Eds.), *Sensory integration: Theory and practice* (pp. 101–137). Philadelphia: F. A. Davis.

Lane, S. J., Miller, L. J., & Hanft, B. E. (2000). Toward a consensus in terminology in sensory integration theory and practice: Part 2: Sensory integration patterns of function and dysfunction. *Sensory Integration Special Interest Section Quarterly, 23*(2), 1–3.

Levine, P. (1997). *Waking the tiger: Healing trauma.* Berkeley, CA: North Atlantic Books.

Linehan, M. (1986). Suicidal people: One population or two? *Annals of the New York Academy of Sciences, USA, 487,* 16–33.

Linehan, M. (1993). *Skills training manual for treating borderline personality disorder.* New York: Guilford.

Linehan, M. (1999). Standard protocol for assessing and treating suicidal behaviors for patients in treatment. In D. G. Jacobs (Ed.), *The Harvard Medical School guide to suicidal assessment and interventions* (pp. 146–187). San Francisco: Jossey-Bass.

Luxenberg, T., Spinazzola, J., Hidalgo, J., Hunt, C., & van der Kolk, B. (2001). Complex trauma and disorders of extreme stress (DESNOS) diagnosis, part two: Treatment. *Directions in Psychiatry, 21,* 373–392.

MacLachlan, J., & Stromberg, N. (2007). Safety tools. In Massachusetts Department of Mental Health (Ed.), *Developing positive cultures of care: Resource guide* (pp. 1–21). Boston: Editor.

Meyers, R., Miller, R., Hill, D., & Tonigan, J. (1999). Community reinforcement and family training (CRAFT): Engaging unmotivated drug users in treatment. *Journal of Substance Abuse, 10,* 1–18.

Miller, L., Cermak, S., Lane, S., Anzalone, M., & Koomar, J. (2004, Summer). Developing a new taxonomy: Differentiating the disorders and interventions from the theory of sensory integration. *S.I. Focus,* pp. 6–8

Miller, L., Reisman, J., McIntosh, D., & Simon, J. (2001). An ecological model of sensory modulation. In S. Smith Roley, E. Blanche, & R. Schaaf (Eds.), *Understanding the nature of sensory integration with diverse populations* (pp. 57–82). San Antonio, TX: Therapy Skill Builders.

Miller, M., Azrael, D., Hepburn, L., Hemenway, D., & Lippmann, S. J. (2006). The association between changes in household firearm ownership and rates of suicide in the United States, 1981–2002. *Injury Prevention, 12,* 178–182.

Miller, W. R., & Rollnick, S. R. (1991). *Motivational interviewing: Preparing people to change addictive behavior.* New York: Guilford.

Moore, K., & Henry, A. (2002). Treatment of adult psychiatric patients using the Wilbarger protocol. *Occupational Therapy in Mental Health, 18,* 43–63.

Moscicki, E. K. (1997). Identification of suicide risk factors using epidemiologic studies. *Psychiatric Clinics of North America, 20,* 499–517.

Moscicki, E. K. (2001). Epidemiology of completed and attempted suicide: Toward a framework for prevention. *Clinical Neuroscience Research, 1,* 310–323.

Moyers, P. (1997). Occupational meanings and spirituality: The quest for sobriety. *American Journal of Occupational Therapy, 51,* 207–214.

Moyers, P. (2007). A legacy of leadership: Achieving our *Centennial Vision. American Journal of Occupational Therapy, 61,* 622–628.

Mullen, B., Champagne, T., Krishnamurty, S., Dickson, D., & Gao, R. (2008). Exploring the safety and therapeutic effects of deep pressure stimulation using a weighted blanket. *Occupational Therapy in Mental Health, 24,* 65–89.

Najavits, L. (2002). *Seeking safety: A treatment manual for PTSD and substance abuse.* New York: Guilford.

National Executive Training Institute. (2003). *Creating violence free and coercion free mental health treatment environments for the reduction of seclusion and restraint.* Alexandria, VA: National Technical Assistance Center for State Mental Health Planning.

National Institute of Mental Health. (2008a). *Issues to consider in intervention research with persons at high risk of suicidality.* Retrieved January 28, 2009, from www.nimh.nih.gov/health/topics/suicide-prevention/issues-to-consider-in-intervention-research-with-persons-at-high-risk-for-suicidality.shtml#9

National Institute of Mental Health. (2008b). *Suicide in the U.S.: Statistics and prevention* (NIH Pub. No. 06-4594). Retrieved July 5, 2008, from www.nimh.nih.gov/health/publications/suicide-in-the-us-statistics-and-prevention.shtml

O'Carroll, P. W., Berman, A. L., Maris, R. W., Moscicki, E. K., Tanney, B. L., & Silverman, M. M. (1996). Beyond the tower of Babel: A nomenclature for suicidology. *Suicide and Life-Threatening Behavior, 26,* 237–252.

Ogden, P., Minton, K., & Pain, C. (2006). *Trauma and the body: A sensorimotor approach to psychotherapy.* New York: W. W. Norton.

Owens, D., Harrocks, J., & House, A. (2002). Fatal and non-fatal repetition of self-harm: Systematic review. *British Journal of Psychiatry, 181,* 193–199.

Petronis, K. R., Samuels, J. F., Moscicki, E. K., & Anthony, J. C. (1990). An epidemiologic investigation of potential risk factors for suicide attempts. *Social Psychiatry and Psychiatric Epidemiology, 25*(4), 193–199.

Pfeiffer, B., & Kinnealey, M. (2003). Treatment of sensory defensiveness in adults. *Occupational Therapy International, 10,* 175–184.

President's New Freedom Commission on Mental Health. (2003). *Achieving the promise: Transforming mental health care in America* (Final Report, DHHS Pub. No. SMA–03–3832). Rockville, MD: Author.

Prochaska, J., & DiClemente, C. (1982). Transtheoretical therapy: Toward a more integrative model of change. *Psychotherapy: Theory, Research, and Practice, 19,* 276–288.

Prochaska, J., Norcross, J., & DiClemente, C. (1994). *Changing for good: A revolutionary six-stage program for overcoming bad habits and moving your life positively forward.* New York: Avon Books.

Ralph, R. (2000). *Review of recovery literature: A synthesis of a sample of recovery literature 2000.* Alexandria, VA: National Association of State Mental Health Program Directors.

Roush, S. (2008). Occupational therapy and co-occurring disorders of mental illness and substance abuse. *Mental Health Special Interest Section Quarterly, 31(4),* 1–4.

Sansone, R., Wiederman, M., & Sansone, L. (1998). The Self-Harm Inventory (SHI): Development of a scale for identifying self-destructive behaviors and borderline personality disorder. *Journal of Clinical Psychology, 54,* 973–983.

Saxe, G., Chawla, N., & van der Kolk, B. (2002). Self-destructive behavior in patients with dissociative disorders. *Suicide and Life-Threatening Behavior, 32,* 313–320.

Schore, A. (1994). *Affect regulation and the origin of the self: The neurobiology of emotional development.* Hillsdale, NJ: Erlbaum.

Schroeder, S., Rojahn, J., & Reese, R. (1997). Brief report: Reliability and validity of instruments for assessing psychotropic medication effects on self-injurious behavior in mental retardation. *Journal of Autism and Developmental Disorders, 27,* 89–102.

Siegel, D. (1999). *The developing mind: How relationships and the brain interact to shape who we are.* New York: Guilford.

Stoffel, V., & Moyers, P. (2005). Occupational therapy and substance abuse disorders. In E. Cara & A. MacRae (Eds.), *Psychosocial occupational therapy: A clinical practice* (2nd ed., pp. 446–469). Clifton Park, NY: Thomson Delmar Learning.

Suchman, A. (2006). A new theoretical foundation for relationship-centered care: Complex responsive process of relationship. *Journal of General Internal Medicine, 21*(Suppl. 1), S40–S44.

Suicide Prevention Action Network. (2001). *Suicide prevention: Prevention effectiveness and evaluation.* Washington, DC: Author.

Suicide Prevention Resource Center. (2001). *Risk and protective factors for suicide.* Newton, MA: Education Development Center, Suicide Prevention Resource Center, Substance Abuse and Mental Health Services Administration. Retrieved January 25, 2009, from www.sprc.org/suicide_prev_basics/index.asp

U.S. Public Health Service. (2001). *National strategy for suicide prevention: Goals and objectives for action.* Rockville, MD: Author.

Substance Abuse and Mental Health Services Administration. (2005). *National consensus statement on mental health recovery.* Rockville, MD: National Mental Health Information Center. Retrieved January 27, 2009, from http://mentalhealth.samhsa.gov/publications/allpubs/sma05-4129/

van der Kolk, B. (2002). The psychobiology and psychopharmacology of PTSD. *Human Psychopharmacology, 16*(S1), S49–S64.

van der Kolk, B. (2005). Developmental trauma disorder: Toward a rational diagnosis for children with complex trauma histories. *Psychiatric Annals, 35*(3), 401–408.

van der Kolk, B. (2006). Clinical implications of neuroscience research and PTSD. *Annals of the New York Academy of Sciences, 1071,* 277–293.

Wilbarger, J., & Wilbarger, P. (2002). The Wilbarger approach to treating sensory defensiveness. In A. Bundy, S. Lane, & E. Murray (Eds.), *Sensory integration: Theory and practice* (pp. 339-341). Philadelphia: F. A. Davis.

Wilbarger, P. (1984). Planning an adequate sensory diet—application of sensory processing theory during the first years of life. *Zero to Three, 5,* 7–12.

Wilbarger, P. (1995). The sensory diet: Activity programs based upon sensory processing theory. *Sensory Integration Special Interest Section Quarterly, 18*(2), 1–4.

Wilbarger, P., & Wilbarger, J. (1991). *Sensory defensiveness in children: 2–12: An intervention guide for parents and other caretakers.* Santa Barbara, CA: Avanti Education Programs.

Wilbarger, P., & Wilbarger, J. (1997). *Sensory defensiveness: A comprehensive treatment approach.* Workshop presented in New York.

Wilcock, A. (1998). *An occupational therapy perspective of health.* Thorofare, NJ: Slack.

Williams, M., & Shellenberger, S. (1996). *"How does your engine run?": A leader's guide to the alert program for self-regulation.* Albuquerque, NM: Therapy Works.

Zuckerman, M. (1994). *Behavioral expression and biosocial basis of sensation seeking.* Cambridge, England: Cambridge University.

CHAPTER 13

Therapeutic Relationships in Difficult Contexts: Involuntary Commitment, Forensic Settings, and Violence

Roxanne Castaneda, MS, OTR/L

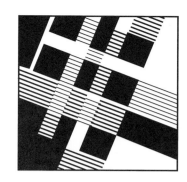

Learning Objectives

After reading this material and completing the examination, readers will be able to

- Identify how therapeutic relationships are established and maintained in ordinary or traditional circumstances,

- Identify factors in extraordinary circumstances that impede the development and maintenance of therapeutic relationships, and

- Identify techniques and best practices to overcome the difficulties that permit a comprehensive look at a client's clinical needs.

Our goal as occupational therapists is to work toward client choice, empowerment, and recovery. An effective therapeutic relationship is essential in achieving this goal. However, therapists often meet clients with severe and challenging reputations, such as residents of forensic mental health maximum security or state behavioral health hospitals or facilities. Such clients have mental illness and have been criminally charged or may be awaiting evaluation and adjudication for an alleged offense through their state's insanity plea. They may be violent or sociopathic.

In such situations, occupational therapists are faced with multifaceted, complex mental health issues that challenge the conventional health care delivery system. These challenging clients can create interpersonal difficulties that make it hard for occupational therapists to enter into a therapeutic relationship.

This chapter examines the circumstances that impede the development of such relationships and suggests ways to possibly resolve the difficulty and facilitate effective practice. It is important to begin by reviewing the following question: How are therapeutic relationships established and maintained in typical or traditional practice settings?

Therapeutic Use of Self and Clinical Reasoning

Occupational therapists working in mental health place importance on introspection and insight into interactions with clients, consumers, patients, and staff. In his Eleanor Clark Slagle Lecture, Christiansen (1999) said, "Personal identity can be defined as the person we think we are. It is the self we know. . . . [It] is not the same as self-concept nor is it the same as self-esteem, although these important concepts are related to identity" (p. 548). He further said that "identity is the pathway by which people, through daily occupations and relationships with others, are able to derive meaning from their lives" (p. 556).

Early training requires occupational therapists to reflect on their personal identity, life journey, and professional experiences that may influence their helping style. How therapists think about what they do is crucial to clinical decision making and is an inevitable part of what shapes therapeutic relationships. In a discussion on the interactive reasoning process, Schwartzberg (2002, as cited in Ward, 2003) described the way of thinking used to understand clients in the therapeutic situation as including "(1) active listening, (2) being genuine and empathetic, (3) building an alliance, (4) observing cues and clarifying meaning, (5) giving and receiving information, and (6) reality testing" (p. 626). Further discussion (Nodding, 1984, as cited in Ward, 2003) indicated that "[c]aring involves stepping out of one's own personal frame of reference into the others. . . . A fundamental existential of the life world is relationships, human connection. People with serious mental illness have trouble connecting with other people in a gratifying way" (p. 631). Piaget (1988, as cited in Ward, 2003) further described that "[c]linical intention aims at the care of others. It is purposeful and grounded activity of sentient and aware beings. The intention to care for others is manifested as attention: perceiving, apprehending and analyzing phenomena" (p. 631). To foster a therapeutic relationship that matches people's needs, therapists must pay close attention to an array of communication styles and their components (e.g., conflict resolution, listening skills), symptoms (e.g., hearing voices), cultural differences (e.g., fasting during Ramadan), and environmental issues (e.g., maximum security) with both clients and staff.

The importance of knowing oneself in relation to another person and the environment or systems in which both exist is important. This trilevel approach is essential to evaluating and interpreting the information needed in formulating the therapeutic interaction.

Taylor (2008) studied the intentional use of self in therapists working in a variety of practice areas all over the world. Although all participants had different personalities and abilities, each was nominated by his or her peers as having excellent interpersonal therapeutic ability. These therapists brought different innate abilities, strengths, and weaknesses to the therapy process. Taylor (2008) found that "each of the therapists understood what was needed and had the self awareness and self control to enact it" (p. 38).

Typical or Traditional Settings and Practice in Different Contexts

Typical or traditional mental health practice settings can be characterized by the presence of clients, consumers, or patients (B. Wise, personal communication, March 17, 2008) who are voluntary and somewhat active participants in treatment.

This is evidenced by medication compliance; regular attendance at inpatient or outpatient programs for mental health or substance abuse issues or both; relatively stable psychiatric symptoms; and the ability to demonstrate some insight into their illness. They typically have minimal to no legal issues (i.e., parking tickets, misdemeanors), exhibit no violent behavior, and are responsive to redirection.

Many clinical internship sites in occupational therapy are located at these types of facilities. On occasion, some academic institutions are able to partner with maximum security forensic mental health hospitals, prisons, jails, and homeless shelters where their students engage in fieldwork. Such placements, however, remain the minority and are considered nontraditional. Hence, many occupational therapists' early exposure to people with mental health issues is in traditional settings, usually without issues of significant noncompliance, violence, sociopathy, or court involvement. Occupational therapy employment in such nontraditional facilities is equally as limited.

This situation has recently changed, however. People in psychiatric care clinical settings are increasingly court involved, are acutely aggressive, or have a history of violence and sociopathy. They may be discharged or released back into the community—that is, the criminal justice system—or admitted to a state psychiatric hospital. First contact usually occurs in an emergency room or on admission to a short-term psychiatric service (B. Wise, personal communication, April 2007). Many state behavioral health hospitals accustomed to treating people who are under civil commitments have admitted more and more patients with current, alleged criminal charges. Depending on state law, these patient–defendants may be court ordered for evaluation of competency to stand trial and both competency and criminal responsibility. They may subsequently require some form of court-ordered discharge into the community. Some of the same facilities also serve as "step-down" transitional treatment areas for prison mental health units or hospitals.

Supporting Therapeutic Relationships

Therapeutic relationships in both traditional and nontraditional contexts are usually maintained by using a multilevel approach to understanding the use of self, interactive clinical reasoning, and supervision. Cara and MacRae (1998) summarized the nature of these relationships as

> defined in terms of: the therapist and the conscious use of self as a tool, the collaborative, interactive process and the therapist's communication skills, challenges brought up by the attitudes and personality qualities in the client, and understanding of the client's world and the meanings clients convey to us. (p. 10)

Clinical supervision addresses all of these components. Supervision is essential in the process of obtaining feedback and learning. It begins during an occupational therapy student's clinical fieldwork and continues throughout practice. In some cases, it can be the cornerstone of advanced practice in different or difficult practice areas. Costa (2007) described the

> skills of clinical supervisors [as] communication . . . feedback, listening skills, developing and maintaining relationships, openness to learning, ethical

conduct, multicultural competence, legal issues, confidentiality, and flexibility. . . . Communication and feedback are critical components of any supervisory relationship. (p. 6)

Entry-level occupational therapy training provides the basic tools to work effectively with mental health clientele in traditional settings. In those settings, therapists are likely able to make social connections with most of their clients. Interactions are eased when there is compliance, active participation, and motivation to heal and engage in familiar occupations. Extraordinary circumstances and issues, however, may impede the development and maintenance of therapeutic relationships. How do occupational therapists begin to understand the complexities affecting people who are not in treatment by choice? How do those issues affect one's capacity to establish a therapeutic relationship? How does a practitioner "treat" in environments that may not support his or her safety and security needs or those of the client?

One must begin with an understanding of the client and his or her environment and point of entry into the mental health system. This understanding could include the criminal justice system (i.e., jails, prisons, mental health courts) and mental health maximum security forensic hospitals. Forensic clients could include defendants (before trial or on evaluation), inmates (after conviction, jail, prison), or "insanity acquittees" (those acquitted on the basis of an insanity defense). They typically have mental illness and often also have an additional diagnosis such as mental retardation or substance abuse.

Legal concepts and statutes pertaining to insanity acquittees, sex offender registries, parole and probation, conditional release, victim notification, and county and state judicial operation are important to the life circumstances, treatment, and outcomes of people with mental illness and forensic involvement. The law can determine their level of freedom, choice, and community involvement (i.e., where one can live and with or near whom, mandatory compliance with medication).

Public Safety Issues That Affect the Therapeutic Relationship

The issue of public safety generally involves protection of people and property from physical or psychological harm from a variety of dangers. Potential dangers might include felony crimes (e.g., arson, assault with a deadly weapon, kidnapping, murder), sex offenses (e.g., pedophilia, rape), intentional transmission of infectious diseases, and acts of terrorism (Castaneda, 2002).

Enforcement of public safety usually involves

- Laws (e.g., restraining orders, parole and probation, drinking and driving),
- Rules (e.g., curfew, public conduct), and
- Regulations (e.g., housing authority requires zero tolerance for substance abuse).

The outcome of enforcement could result in deterrence through incapacitation and incarceration of the offender. Typically, people who come to psychiatric care settings from the criminal justice system or who are in forensic mental health facilities have presented a danger to public safety. They usually meet admission criteria set forth by the state legislature and criteria for civil and criminal commitment mandated by the public mental health system (i.e., mental health civil commitment laws).

The dilemma for the clinician lies in developing an intervention plan and approach that balances client–defendant choice and public safety. This dilemma is made more difficult by individual behavior that indicates a lack of interest in the promotion of recovery, release, or discharge. In a discussion on occupational therapy in the criminal justice system, Snively and Dressler (1998, as cited in Cara & MacRae, 1998) listed challenges for people working in this area: "developing and maintaining relationships with patients who are impaired in their ability to trust and cooperate with others, find it difficult to express their thoughts and feelings, and are unable to interact in a socially acceptable manner" (p. 544). Antisocial personality and other personality disorders are commonly encountered in the criminal justice system. In the United Kingdom (Sainsbury Centre for Mental Health, 2009), it is estimated that

> 60–80% of male prisoners and 50% of female prisoners have a personality disorder diagnosis compared with 6–15% of the general population. Of those identified, antisocial personality disorder represents by far the highest prevalence of any category, with 63% of male remand prisoners, 49% female sentenced and 31% female prisoners. (p. 3)

Occupational therapy treatment at its best focuses on client inclusion, personal choice, and empowerment. Smith-Gabai (2007) identified the therapist's role in assisting clients to develop problem-solving skills and to increase their awareness of their own strengths and barriers to occupational performance. Therapists help clients generate strategies and solutions that will foster their empowerment and assist them in achieving their stated goals. However, in the case of the clients described here, the opportunity for true choice is limited by the parameters dictated by the judiciary, the client's concomitant sociopathy, and the rules and regulations of forensic and other mental health facilities (i.e., integrated civil and forensic hospitals).

In a recent survey (Taylor, Lee, Kielhofner, & Ketkar, 2007, as cited in Taylor, 2008), a high percentage of occupational therapists (82%–90%) reported that their clients' difficult interpersonal behavior had a negative impact on therapy outcomes. Difficult behaviors included manipulative behavior, resistance, emotional disengagement and denial, difficulty with rapport and trust, and hostility (Taylor, 2008). Therapists who work in environments in which such behavior occurs daily are faced with the greater challenge of developing a positive therapy outcome.

Moral and Ethical Dilemmas

Treating such clients raises moral and ethical dilemmas. Are the concepts of choice, recovery, and public safety mutually incompatible in those cases? What is the therapist's goal in engaging the client in a therapeutic relationship? How does a therapist move a client with complex issues from refusal to negotiation to acceptance of treatment suggestions?

Violence is perhaps one of the most difficult behaviors or symptoms to work with. The MacArthur Violence Risk Assessment Study (MacArthur Research Network on Mental Health and the Law, 2001; Steadman et al., 1998) indicated that mental illness in and of itself does not lead to violence. However, a subsection of people, by virtue of substance abuse, environment (i.e., prison), or antisocial personality disorder, may continue to engage in violent, aggressive behavior toward people or property. The research, which focused on people with mental illness who had been hospitalized and were discharged to their community, found that this group is not "a homogeneous group in relation to violence in the community. The prevalence of community violence by people discharged from acute psychiatric facilities varies considerably according to diagnosis and, particularly, co-occurring substance abuse diagnosis or symptoms" (Steadman et al., 1998). Steadman et al. observed that "substance abuse symptoms significantly raised the rate of violence in both the patient and the comparison groups" and that "violence in both patient and comparison groups was most frequently targeted at family members and friends, and most often took place at home."

In a comment on media reaction to violence and people with mental illness, Pies (2008) wrote,

> Recent events have shown us that anyone may become the victim of a violent person with severe mental illness. And yet, we must put the violence–mental illness link into perspective. The patient who assaulted me more than 25 years ago was 1 in 1,000. Nearly all those I have treated since have been nonviolent. Most have coped heroically with unspeakable sorrow and pain. In truth, I would trust many of them with my life. (p. 2)

Elbogen, Van Doren, Swanson, Swartz, and Monahan (2006) reported that as self-reported adherence to outpatient psychiatric treatment increases, which typically includes a combination of case management, pharmacotherapy, and psychotherapy or group therapy, violence decreases.

Occupational therapists who choose to work in environments that have a higher probability of engaging people with a violent history or active violent symptoms must develop an understanding of possible etiology, learn how to manage aggressive behavior, and become a part of the multiple-treatment approach mentioned earlier. Each facility, agency, maximum security hospital, jail, or prison has its own department-sanctioned (e.g., Department of Mental Health, Department of Corrections) programs or protocols to manage aggressive behavior toward peers and staff. Most programs working with people with mental health issues focus on defensive moves with an emphasis on deescalating the aggression and keeping both parties safe. Training is usually available and in some cases mandatory for all staff who have direct patient contact. In some facilities, formal programs assist staff after assault, including completing documentation (i.e., variances, first report of injury), a drive to the medical clinic, debriefing, and support for as long as the employee is in need.

Working with the consumers described in this chapter can challenge one's level of professionalism and adherence to the profession's code of ethics. Demonstrating a concern for recipients' safety and well-being (beneficence) and the ability to maintain therapeutic relationships free of exploitation (nonmaleficence) may be affected by threats of physical and psychological violence. Negative feelings (fear, anger, disgust, resentment) regarding patients may develop because of the nature of the crimes with which they are charged (e.g., child molestation). Patient abandonment, "blacklisting" (i.e., off-the-record lists of difficult clients not to be admitted for treatment), refusal to treat, termination without alternatives, and filing charges against a patient after an assault (physical or verbal, as long as the recipient feels his or her safety has been threatened) are some of the dilemmas a therapist may face. Although it is considered an individual, personal right to seek the assistance of the judicial system (i.e., filing charges against a client), the question of possibly perpetrating the cycle of incarceration and hospitalization has been raised as a concern for people who work in this area of practice.

Patient abandonment is another moral and ethical issue for therapists. Terminating treatment or the therapeutic relationship without options should be avoided at all costs (D. Cash, personal communication, August 2008). If a therapist and client cannot agree on a treatment plan, termination of the therapeutic relationship must be recommended with alternatives. A list of other clinics, therapists, or day programs would be important. In an inpatient setting, a client or therapist may request to work with a different treatment team. Some facilities have internal mediation services and patients' rights advisors that both client and staff can access to help resolve breaches in therapeutic process.

Case Example

Mr. D. G., age 35, was readmitted to a 350-bed state psychiatric facility. He was arrested for alleged assault and battery and possession of drug paraphernalia. The judge ordered an inpatient pretrial evaluation for competency to stand trial. Mr. D. G. has a history of bipolar disorder, polysubstance abuse, verbal and physical threats and aggression, and antisocial personality disorder. He spends most of his time body building and exercising and appears physically menacing (e.g., he often wears tank tops showing his muscular build). Other times, he dresses impeccably and is often mistaken for a hospital staff member. He takes every opportunity to socialize with staff and more vulnerable (i.e., unassertive, passive) patients. Subsequently, some staff are seduced by his charm and allow him special favors (e.g., extra time in the fitness center when he is scheduled for group therapy).

The occupational therapist sets a limit when Mr. D. G. attempts to go to the gym rather than his scheduled occupational therapy group. Mr. D. G. threatens physical harm if the occupational therapist makes another comment. The occupational therapist continues to set the limit verbally. Mr. D. G. lunges at her, screaming that he is going to beat her up. Other staff in the area assist in physically restraining Mr. D. G. while the occupational therapist is ushered out of the room. For the next 6 months, Mr. D. G. becomes verbally and physically aggressive toward the occupational therapist whenever he sees her. He also makes frequent efforts to contact her immediate supervisor, ordering her to fire the occupational therapist. The therapist has 20 years of experience but is beginning to feel self-doubt and fear. She and Mr. D. G. had previously worked together, but the incident was the first time she had set limits on his behavior.

Did the occupational therapist make the right clinical decision to set limits? What circumstances should be present before challenging a difficult client? What should the therapist do at this point? Can a therapeutic relationship be built? The following sections describe possible interventions to ameliorate this situation.

Clinical Supervision

In a case such as this one, the therapist should consider seeking immediate supervision with his or her superior. It is difficult or close to impossible to work with someone you fear. Threats of physical and psychological harm should not be tolerated in any setting. Patients like Mr. D. G. intentionally test the boundaries of the therapeutic relationship to control and intimidate the therapist (Taylor, 2008). In this case, the therapist sought immediate supervision with her superior. The initial suggestion was to minimize contact with the patient and avoid solitary contact. The therapist's schedule was adjusted to allow for this, and all coworkers and nursing staff were made aware of the issue. In supervision, it was agreed that the therapist exercised appropriate clinical judgment when questioning the client's attempt to attend programming other than that prescribed. The therapist and her supervisor scheduled weekly meetings to monitor progress. The patient worked with his treatment team on anger management and his difficulty with perceived authority figures (i.e., staff) questioning his actions. The patient continued to have difficulty with other staff he perceived as "telling him what to do" for the remainder of his hospitalization.

Change in Clinical Duties

Opportunities for advice, planning, and collaboration are important during "empathic breaks" (Taylor, 2008, p. 123), which occur when the therapist or client fails to understand the intended communication and is perceived by the latter as hurtful or insensitive. For example, Mr. D. G. perceived the therapist's question as more than just a question. He felt disrespected by a young woman who in his mind had no right to question his whereabouts or set limits on his actions. This disrespect angered him and prompted a verbal and physical threat. The therapist in turn was unable to redirect her interactions to facilitate a therapeutic outcome, resulting in a serious empathic break. In this case, it was necessary to request temporary or permanent reassignment. Remember that termination of occupational therapy treatment should not occur without viable alternatives that meet the patient's needs.

In this case example, all agreed that no therapeutic relationship was possible. The therapist was afraid for her personal safety secondary to continuous verbal and physical threats. The patient continued treatment with his designated hospital team and as mentioned earlier continued to have difficulty with other staff over similar issues.

Clinical Judgment and Knowledge of the Law

Several additional issues should be considered in overcoming difficulties and treating clients who are adjudicated or in forensic settings. Those issues include knowledge of the law, which must be used when making clinical decisions.

Clinical judgment is essential in making daily practice decisions. It requires the ability to integrate supervisory suggestions, knowledge of applicable law, and awareness of environmental conditions and conflicts and the underlying pathology a patient may be experiencing. As mentioned earlier, each state and jurisdiction within it is subject to laws that dictate and instruct activity and sanctions for people who violate the law. Most states have statutes that include disposition for people who are found not criminally responsible or not competent to stand trial because of mental illness, mental retardation, or both. It is important for the occupational therapist working with clients affected by those laws to understand the laws and their possible implications for treatment and program planning, which may include restrictions on mobility (inside or outside of the hospital, supervised home or work); limited access to treatment modalities that involve contraband (e.g., sharps of all kind); and written court permission for community trips and off-grounds employment. Information on state and federal criminal and mental health laws is usually available through the Internet (e.g., Westlaw) or the legal or forensic office working with the hospital or agency.

Another issue to consider in treating difficult clients is the ability to have critical self-awareness and interpersonal self-discipline. Taylor (2008) described two key principles fundamental to effective, intentional use of self. She stressed that ongoing critical self-awareness is important and includes one's verbal and nonverbal communication (tone, content, word choice, stance, and gestures) and what is withheld or not communicated (e.g., cancellation of a patient's day pass). In the case of Mr. D. G., the therapist was faced with feelings of self-doubt and fear despite her many years of professional experience. Daily verbal and physical threats can cause a feeling of hypervigilance that may extend to therapeutic approaches with other clients. This insecurity may lead to decreased effectiveness and may affect the therapist's ability to provide a safe treatment environment for him- or herself, clients, and cotherapists. Interpersonal self-discipline (Taylor, 2008) allows a therapist "to develop stable predictable relationships with clients...it involves knowing the types of clients and situations that are most likely to test your interpersonal resolve and emotional perspective" (p. 58). Taylor (2008) further cautioned that therapists need to avoid viewing the relationship with "interpersonally difficult clients as a source of self esteem or a barometer by which to measure their own interpersonal competence" (p. 59). Perhaps a more disciplined response to those feelings would be to recognize the interpersonal dynamic, take responsibility for aspects of the relationship that may have been perceived by the patient as provocation, depersonalize the emotions, seek out clinical supervision or peer support, and develop a more disciplined response to the therapeutic relationship.

When treating difficult clients, it is important to know the history or possible cause of the patient's behaviors. A comprehensive intake history (B. Wise, personal communication, March 2008) is important. This information often gives the clinician necessary insight into the course of difficulty or encounters with the law, types and responses to various treatment, and relationships with various people and systems. Therapists are often plagued with time constraints resulting from numerous work demands (e.g., large caseloads; multiple, consecutive treatment groups; evening, weekend, and holiday treatment), which sometimes makes it difficult to spend adequate time with charts reviewing past history or interviewing important sources (caregivers, parole officers, friends, and family) for collateral information. Samenow (2004) suggested that it is important to focus on "errors in thinking" (pp. 16–17), meaning thought patterns developed and intensified since childhood that contribute to a radically different worldview from that of people who are basically responsible. He further stated that because behavior is a product of thinking, a fundamental change in lifelong thinking patterns must occur.

Returning to the case of Mr. D. G., what are his "errors in thinking" and what might be the therapist's possible stance or response? Mr. D. G. demonstrates a lack of the concept of injury to others. He does not stop to think about how his actions harm others. He is unable to put himself in another's place and shows no empathy unless he is trying to con someone. The therapist's suggested stance or response is to "point out how he is injuring others, asking him how he would like to be treated in this way, and give him examples of how you put him in place of others" (Samenow, 2004, pp. 16–17).

Confidentiality is an important issue to examine when treating adjudicated clients or clients in forensic settings. In addition to the requirements of the Health Insurance Portability and Accountability Act (see U.S. Department of Health and Human Services, n.d.), occupational therapists must remember to divulge only the minimum amount of information necessary to accomplish the task (to people authorized to have the information) and to always have permission to do so from the client–defendant in writing (D. Cash, personal communication, August 2008). Constant collaboration, reevaluation, permission to disclose information, and immediate documentation of conversations and interactions with clients around those issues is imperative.

For example, in assisting a client in obtaining a library card at the community public library, the therapist was called on by the client to answer questions. The client introduced the therapist as "her staff." The librarian proceeded to ask the therapist for a current address and telephone number. The therapist gave the hospital as the address and the unit nursing station's phone number. A breach of confidentiality had occurred. The therapist could have stopped the interaction, asked the client to step out of line to a quiet spot, discussed what information was about to be disclosed, and asked the client for permission to do so on her behalf. Or the therapist and client could have had this conversation before leaving the hospital, and a record of permission to disclose sensitive information could have been documented.

In most criminal commitments, information about the "instant offense" (original reason for arrest) and its particulars is public record. Such is the case with most sex offender registries. However, psychiatric hospitalization and treatment received is not public information. Therapists should take care to remember that it is considered sensitive and should be treated as such.

Therapeutic Jurisprudence

Therapeutic jurisprudence is the "study of the law as a therapeutic agent" (Wexler, 1999, p. 1). It has also been described as using the judicial process to help the client progress therapeutically (D. Cash, personal communication, August 2008). Examples may include explaining the attorney's role or encouraging the client to contact an attorney if needed. Depending on the work setting, occupational therapists may be directly or indirectly involved with assisting clients in negotiating the justice system. The occupational therapist should seek administrative permission or clearance before becoming involved. In most cases, the hospital, agency system and its staff and, in rare cases, private practitioners are considered only as interested parties and not as a part of the criminal or civil case brought against the client. In other words, unless court ordered, therapists are under no legal obligation to provide assistance to the clients.

In most situations, the legal case is between the state or federal courts and the occupational therapist's client, so any therapeutic involvement or assistance rendered must not interfere with this relationship. One example could be a person civilly involuntarily committed to an inpatient hospital. This person has been in treatment with the occupational therapist in an independent living skills group. Budgeting, money management, bill payment, cooking, and grocery shopping are some of the areas covered. While in the hospital, the client is served papers for failure to pay rent and is in danger of losing his apartment. His public defender is seeking information and a possible witness to testify in court as to his ability to manage money and pay rent. He requests access to the client's records, including the occupational therapist's progress notes, and has asked whether the therapist could accompany them to court in case he needs testimony. The occupational therapist may be required to appear in court as a treating clinician or advocate or in some cases in response to or to avoid a subpoena (a written legal order summoning a witness).

Victim Notification

Some states may have victim notification and victim's rights advocates. The occupational therapist should know whether a client–defendant with whom he or she is working is under this restriction. If a victim or alleged victim has requested through the court to be notified every time the client–defendant leaves the hospital grounds, the therapist must factor in that requirement before any off-grounds activity or community trip. Failure to do so could cause further restrictions or possible legal action against the client–defendant, hospital, or agency. Again, the therapist's clinical judgment must include all pertinent somatic, psychiatric, and legal information that may have an impact on a client's treatment, interpersonal contact, and movement within a treatment facility or in community life.

Risk Assessment, Risk Management

Risk assessment has been increasingly important in light of the frequency and type of difficult behavior, forensic issues, and possible violence one might encounter in various mental health settings. Creek (2002, p. 507), referring to Rowgowski (2002), provided the following strategies:

- Be aware of situations and factors that could be confrontational.
- Use disturbance alarms, walkie-talkies, personal alarm devices.
- Be careful in one-to-one situations, especially when in the community with no staff support.
- Be aware of where you are in a room (e.g., where the exits are).
- Be aware of the depth at which the conversation is pitched. It may be less appropriate to converse at a deep level when alone in the community, when strong emotions may be aroused in the patient and boundaries provided by the unit are not present.
- Use a calm tone of voice and body language (e.g., minimal arm, head, and body movements). Eye contact should be steady but not overly intense.
- Evaluate individual situations; sometimes it may be better to keep some distance between yourself and a patient. At other times it is helpful to get closer and perhaps make appropriate physical contact.
- Be aware of how much attention is being given to individual group members. Do not include too many patients in a group.

- If coleaders are unavailable, consider downsizing the group and include clients who are more familiar to the therapist.
- As a last resort, you may have to cancel the group and do a one-to-one session instead.
- Keep a balance between having patients the therapists know well and introducing new patients to the session.
- Be aware of conflict; negative transference from a specific patient to a specific staff member or between two patients may occur.
- Decisions have to be made regarding whether patients should attend different groups or both are present with extra staff, being aware of where the patients will sit.

- Have a minimum amount of potentially dangerous equipment or tools during therapeutic sessions.
- All sharps should be under careful inventory and kept under lock and key.
- Sign-out systems should be in place for use of tools and sharps at all times.
- Management of incidents will involve other members of the multidisciplinary team. It may include time-out or control-and-restraint procedures approved by the respective facility.

It is important to be up to date on the patient's forensic status, privilege level, and clinical picture. The therapist must be ready to reevaluate patient participation in hospital treatment and community activities for every treatment event. This approach can create environments in which the client–defendant is less likely to reoffend, additional assistance could be mobilized, and increased symptoms can be managed.

Duty to Protect–Warn

Although the duty to protect–warn is not often used, it is important that clinicians be aware of the tenets of state law in their area of practice. For example, in the state of Maryland, this duty applies to any clinician (e.g., occupational therapist, psychologist, psychiatrist, nurse; "Maryland Reporting Obligations," 2006). This state has enacted laws that require clinicians to report a client–defendant who presents a clear danger or harm to another person. Disclosure of harmful intent usually occurs during treatment. Notification of the police and intended victim and measures to admit the person to the hospital must occur immediately (C. D. Barton, personal communication, September 2008). In some states, such as Illinois, the mental health code provides liability exemption for practitioners who have made a "good-faith effort" to fulfill the duty to warn (Whitted, Cleary, & Takiff, 2009).

Summary

Are the concepts of choice, recovery, and public safety for client–defendants mutually incompatible? What becomes the goal of the occupational therapist in engaging the client–defendant in a therapeutic relationship? How does the therapist move a client with complex issues from refusal to negotiation to acceptance of treatment suggestions?

It is difficult to answer any of these questions with complete certainty. However, it is possible to incorporate ethics, clinical judgment, and knowledge of the law and risk management to assist clients in different contexts to accept treatment.

In most cases, an inherent conflict will remain between self-determination and outside control and compliance required by the law. It is important to remember one of the profession's basic tenets: "We are viewing the client, not as an object or thing to be manipulated, controlled, or made to conform but as a unique individual whose very humanness entitles him to choices in determining his own destiny" (Yerxa, 1967, pp. 6–7).

Clinical decisions involving the clients–defendants discussed in this chapter highlight the struggle between maintaining choice and public safety (Castaneda, 2002). Choice is characterized by the freedom to do what you want, with whom you want, where you want, when you want. Happiness and self-determination are usually associated with this process. Public safety involves the consideration of

- History of violent crime or behavior;
- History of or current involvement in the criminal justice system;
- Mental illness or substance abuse, mental retardation, head injury, and so forth;
- Chronic institutionalization;
- Fear of liability;
- Fear of injury to staff and others;
- Fear of implications to community agencies; and
- Fear of adverse reputation in the community.

Clinicians practicing in this area make decisions that may affect public safety by virtue of participation in community reintegration trips or events and discharge planning. The continued challenge for occupational therapists working in different contexts is to integrate knowledge and experience of

- The tenets of therapeutic relationships;
- Clinical decision making;
- Laws and regulations (civil and criminal);
- Risk management;
- Client-centered practice;
- Choice and public safety; and
- Recovery.

Regardless of clients–defendants' forensic background, history of violence, aggression, or sociopathy, as occupational therapists we must abide by our code of ethics and obligation to provide treatment to those in need of our services. The ability to provide effective therapeutic relationships in difficult contexts will continue to be required in this growing practice area.

Acknowledgments

Special thanks to the following people for their interviews and mentorship, which contributed greatly to this chapter: Beverly F. Wise, LCSW–C, administrative director, Medical Services Division, Circuit Court for Baltimore City, and adjunct faculty, Department of Psychiatry and Nursing, University of Maryland at Baltimore; Charles D. Barton, MD, MBA, assistant professor and clinical director, Department of Psychiatry and Behavioral Sciences, Johns Hopkins Hospital, and former chief executive officer, Clifton T. Perkins Hospital, a maximum security facility located in Jessup, Maryland; and Charles David Cash, JD, LLM, senior risk management attorney and former public defender, based at a state behavioral health hospital, Ellicott City, Maryland. I also thank my lifelong mentors Leah and Alfred Shulman, who taught me that when in doubt, always be human.

References

Article—Health—General. (n.d.). Retrieved March 30, 2008, from http://mlis.state.md.us/asp/web_statutes.asp?ghg&10-701

Cara, E., & MacRae, A. (1998). *Psychosocial occupational therapy: A clinical practice.* Albany, NY: Delmar.

Castaneda, R. (2002, April). *Choice and public safety: A rehabilitation professional's role in seeking to resolve the apparent conflict.* Paper presented at the World Federation of Occupational Therapists Conference, Stockholm, Sweden.

Christiansen, C. H. (1999). Defining lives: Occupation as identity: An essay on competence, coherence, and the creation of meaning (Eleanor Clarke Slagle Lecture). *American Journal of Occupational Therapy, 53*(6), 547–558.

Costa, D. M. (2007, September 10). Fieldwork Issues—A fieldwork training course for entry-level students. *OT Practice, 12*(16), 23, 26. Retrieved September 20, 2008, from www.aota.org/nonmembers/area7/links/link01.asp

Creek, J. (2002). *Occupational therapy and mental health.* London: Harcourt.

Elbogen, E., Van Doren, R., Swanson, J., Swartz, M., & Monahan, J. (2006). Treatment engagement and violence risk in mental disorders. *British Journal of Psychiatry, 189,* 354–360.

Health Insurance Portability and Accountability Act of 1996, Pub. L. 104–191.

MacArthur Research Network on Mental Health and the Law. (2001). *MacArthur Violence Risk Assessment Study.* Retrieved September 11, 2008, from www.macarthur.virginia.edu/risk.html

Maryland reporting obligations that may apply to investigators or other members of the research team. (2006, May). Retrieved September 24, 2008, from http://irb.jhmi.edu/Guidelines/reportingobligations.html

Pies, R. (2008, February 25). Mentally ill unfairly portrayed as violent. *The Boston Globe.* Retrieved September 21, 2008, from www.boston.com/news/health/articles/2008/02/25/mentally_ill_unfairly_portrayed_as_violent/

Samenow, S. E. (2004). Treating the resistant/antisocial client. *Paradigm, 9*(4), 16–17.

Sainsbury Centre for Mental Health. (2009). *Personality disorder: A briefing for people working in the criminal justice system.* London: Author. Retrieved April 4, 2009, from www.scmh.org.uk/publications/personality_disorder_briefing.aspx?ID=591

Smith-Gabai, H. (2007). Perspectives: Client empowerment. *OT Practice, 12*(13), 23–25.

Steadman, H., Mulvey, E., Monahan, J., Robbins, P., Appelbaum, P., Grisso, T., et al. (1998). Violence by people discharged from acute psychiatric inpatient facilities and by others in the same neighborhoods. *Archives of General Psychiatry, 55,* 393–401. Retrieved February 22, 2010, from http://archpsyc.ama-assn.org/cgi/content/full/55/5/393?ijkey=788e445ca41f502a62e3413990b1154549fe8fb8

Taylor, R. R. (2008). *The intentional relationship: Occupational therapy and use of self.* Philadelphia: F. A. Davis.

U.S. Department of Health and Human Services. (n.d.). *Health information privacy.* Retrieved March 22, 2008, from www.hhs.gov/ocr/hipaa

Ward, J. D. (2003). The nature of clinical reasoning with groups: A phenomenological study of an occupational therapist in community mental health. *American Journal of Occupational Therapy, 57*(6), 625–634.

Whitted, B., Cleary, L., & Takiff, N. (2009). *Breaking confidentiality: Duty to warn.* Retrieved October 6, 2009, from www.wct-law.com/CM/Publications/publications13.asp

Wexler, D. B. (1999, October 29). *Therapeutic jurisprudence: An overview.* Retrieved October 22, 2008, from www.law.arizona.edu/depts/upr-intj/

Yerxa, E. (1967). Authentic occupational therapy. *American Journal of Occupational Therapy, 21*(1), 1–9.

Resources

Castaneda, R. (1999). Creating community capacity for persons with dual diagnosis and forensic issues. *Mental Health Special Interest Section Quarterly, 22*(3), 1–3.

Davis, J. C. (2004). *Ethical reflection for OT Week.* Retrieved March 27, 2008, from www.leedsmet.ac.uk/health/osot/features/ethicalreflection1.htm

Doyle, M., & Dolan, M. (2006). Predicting community violence from patients discharged from mental health services. *British Journal of Psychiatry, 189,* 520–526.

Eklund, M. (2007). Perceived control: How is it related to daily occupation in patients with mental illness living in the community. *American Journal of Occupational Therapy, 61,* 535–542.

Ewing, C. P. (2005, July/August). Judicial notebook: *Tarasoff* reconsidered. *Monitor on Psychology, 36*(7), 112. Retrieved September 21, 2007, from www.apa.org/monitor/julaug05/jn.html

Flannery, R., Fisher, W., Walker, A., Littlewood, K., & Spillane, M. (2001). Nonviolent psychiatric inpatients and subsequent assaults on community patients and staff. *Psychiatric Quarterly, 72,* 19–27.

Forchuk, C., Reynolds, W., Sharkey, S., Martin, M. L., & Jensen, E. (2007, April). Transitional discharge based on therapeutic relationships: State of the art. *Archives of Psychiatric Nursing, 21*(2), 80–86. doi: 10.1016/j.apnu.2006.11.002

Gilliland, J. C. (2005, April 19). *Patient abandonment.* Retrieved March 15, 2008, from http://gillilandmarkette.com/docs/PatientAbandonmentwlogo.pdf

Gutheil, T. G. (1999). A confusion of tongues: Competence, insanity, psychiatry, and the law. *Psychiatric Services, 50,* 767–773.

Harris, G. H. (1984). The criminal personality: A dialogue with Stanton Samenow PhD. *Journal of Counseling and Development, 63,* 227–229.

Hodgins, S., Cree, A., Alderton, J., & Mak, T. (2007). From conduct disorder to severe mental illness: Associations with aggressive behavior, crime and victimization. *Psychological Medicine, 38,* 975–987. doi: 10.1017/S0033291707002164

Junginger, J., Claypoole, K., Laygo, R., & Crisanti, A. (2006). Effects of serious mental illness and substance abuse on criminal offenses. *Psychiatric Services, 57,* 879–882.

Lohman, H. (2003).Critical analysis of a public policy: An occupational therapist's experience with the patient bill of rights. *American Journal of Occupational Therapy, 57*(4), 468–472.

Martin, J. P. (1998, February 27). The insanity defense: A closer look. *The Washington Post.* Retrieved March 22, 2007, from www.washingtonpost.com/wp-srv/local/longterm/aron/qa227.htm

Massachusetts Victim Bill of Rights. (n.d.) Retrieved March 20, 2009, from www.mass.gov/mova/page89.html

Mulvey, E. P., & Fardella, J. (2000). Are the mentally ill really violent? *Psychology Today.* Retrieved March 20, 2008, from www.psychologytoday.com/articles/200011/are-the-mentally-ill-really-violent

Neeleman, J., & Watts, V. (1996). Preventing the admission of difficult psychiatric patients: A questionnaire survey. *Journal of the Royal Society of Medicine, 89,* 141–151.

Owen, C., Tarantello, C., Jones, M., & Tennant, C. (1998). Violence and aggression in psychiatric units. *Psychiatric Services, 49,* 1452–1457.

Peloquin, S. M. (2006). Occupations: Strands of coherence in life. *American Journal of Occupational Therapy, 60*(2), 236–239.

Sparr, L. F., Rogers, J. L., Beahrs, J. O., & Mazur, D. J. (1992). Disruptive medical patients. Forensically informed decision making. *Western Journal of Medicine,156*(5), 501–506. Retrieved September 21, 2007, from www.pubmedcentral.nih.gov/picrender.fcgi?artid=1003312&blobtype=pdf

Stewart, P., & Craik, C. (2007). Occupation, mental illness and medium security: Exploring time-use in forensic regional secure units. *British Journal of Occupational Therapy, 70*(10), 416–425.

Substance Abuse and Mental Health Services Administration. (2005). *National consensus statement on mental health recovery.* Rockville, MD: National Mental Health Information Center. Retrieved March 20, 2008, from http://mentalhealth.samhsa.gov/publications/allpubs/sma05-4129/

Vatne, S., & Hoem, E. (2008). Acknowledging communication: A milieu-therapeutic approach in mental health care. *Journal of Advanced Nursing, 61*(6), 690–698. doi: 10.1111.j.1365-2648.2007.04565.x

West, J. (2008). *A brief look into the history and current trends in mental health court.* Tucson: University of Arizona Roger's College of Law, Therapeutic Jurisprudence.

Wood, W. (2004). The heart, mind, and soul of professionalism in occupational therapy. *American Journal of Occupational Therapy, 58*(3), 249–256.

Wood, W. (2005). A Firm Persuasion in Our Work—Associate editor's note—Celebrating the bridge makers. *American Journal of Occupational Therapy, 59,* 475.

CHAPTER 14

Trauma, Mental Health Care, and Occupational Therapy Practice

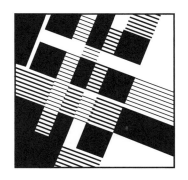

Tina Champagne, MEd, OTR/L, CCAP, and
Diane B. Tewfik, MA, OTR/L

Learning Objectives

After reading this material and completing the examination, readers will be able to

- Identify the pervasive impact of trauma on occupational performance,

- Recognize the necessity of trauma-informed and recovery-focused care,

- Recognize how the therapeutic alliance and collaborative practice facilitate autonomy and choice,

- Identify the clinical reasoning used to provide different sensory supportive interventions among varied populations with trauma histories,

- Differentiate the occupational therapist's leadership role in trauma-informed care initiatives across client types (person, organization, population), and

- Recognize the centrality of cultural context and its impact on occupational performance.

Consumers of mental health services are known to have a high incidence of trauma experiences (National Executive Training Institute [NETI], 2003, 2006). The National Association of State Mental Health Program Directors (NASMHPD) and the Substance Abuse and Mental Health Services Administration (SAMHSA) "have longstanding commitments to the study of trauma, violence, trauma-informed care and to establishing best practices to address its consequences" (Jennings, 2004, p. v). Nationally, it has been determined that a trauma-informed transformation in mental health care must be addressed at the public policy, educational, and practice levels to effectively promote recovery among people with trauma histories (Jennings, 2004). Trauma-informed care includes evidence-based and promising best practices that directly address trauma and its sequelae to facilitate recovery and to decrease and prevent future public health problems (NASMHPD, 2000; National Center for Trauma-Informed Care, 2008). Consequently, national initiatives in mental health include those focused on ensuring that mental health care organizations provide services that do not further traumatize people with mental illness (e.g., seclusion and restraint reduction). This chapter reviews trauma, trauma-informed care initiatives, and occupational therapy's leadership role in this time of transformation and culture change.

Impact of Trauma and Disorders of Extreme Stress

Trauma: An Experiential Process

Trauma is not an event; it is an experiential process, and what may be perceived as traumatic to one person may or may not seem traumatic to another (NETI, 2003, 2006). Perception is influenced by a host of variables (e.g., age, personality, life experience, ethnicity), and a person's perceived degree of control during the traumatic event has a significant impact on the ability to cope (Levine, 2005; van der Kolk, 2006). If people believe that they can do something during a traumatic event, even if their degree of control is relatively low, the trauma experience's severity is often lessened (Levine, 2005; van der Kolk, McFarlane, & Weisaeth, 1996). People can become traumatized, therefore, by any event that is perceived to be life threatening or out of their control (consciously or unconsciously; Levine, 2005).

Traumatic Events

Trauma may occur as a single event or continue over time. Traumatic events include

- Emotional, sexual, or physical abuse;
- Violent assault, automobile accidents, and physical injuries;
- Neglect, betrayal, or abandonment;
- Witnessing violence or restraint and seclusion;
- Rape;
- Invasive medical or dental procedures;
- Natural disasters; and
- Death or illness of a family member or close friend and loss of related caregiving responsibilities.

According to the *Diagnostic and Statistical Manual of Mental Disorders* (*DSM–IV*; American Psychiatric Association [APA], 2000), traumatic events can be reexperienced in, for example, recurrent and intrusive thoughts of the event, recurrent and distressing dreams, flashbacks, and dissociation.

Research has revealed that people with trauma histories are vulnerable to being triggered by sensory stimulation, actions, and thoughts related to the traumatic event (van der Kolk, 2006). Evidence has shown that people often find it difficult to modulate sensations and organize behavior when they feel overwhelmed by emotions (Damasio, 1999; Damasio, Grabowski, & Bechara, 2000), which sets into motion hormonal secretions and subcortical (intentional and emotional) and cortical (conceptual) responses from which the following may emerge:

- Heightened arousal and physiological reactivity, such as the fight-or-flight response
- Psychological distress

- Persistent anxiety
- Hypervigilance
- Difficulty communicating
- Integration and coordination of sensory–motor systems
- Modulation of arousal
- Difficulty identifying and modulating emotions
- Difficulty concentrating or paying attention
- Difficulty being present and reality oriented
- Hypersensitivities
- Avoidant behavior
- Numbing
- Self-injurious behaviors
- Paranoia
- Risk-taking and sensory-seeking behaviors.

Hence, it is not surprising that children and adults with trauma histories become disregulated and have difficulty participating in meaningful life roles and activities. This knowledge has important implications for occupational therapy interventions.

Chronic Stress and Trauma Responses

The stress response is characterized by an increase in autonomic arousal, a feeling of alarm, orienting to the concern, and a defensive fight-or-flight response—or freezing, if neither fight nor flight is effective (Levine, 1997, 2005). The person typically discharges energy, marked by trembling and temperature change, and then rests because of exhaustion related to the intensity of the stressor (Levine, 2005). Chronic stress can lead to stress-related disorders and, when overwhelming, can become traumatic.

Posttraumatic Stress Disorder

Posttraumatic stress disorder (PTSD) stems from isolated, discrete traumatic events in which the "person experienced, witnessed, or was confronted with an event or events that involved actual or threatened death or serious injury, or a threat to the physical integrity of self or others" (APA, 2000, p. 467). Symptoms of PTSD can be acute (less than 3 months in duration), chronic (3 months or more in duration), or delayed in onset (6 months or later; APA, 2000). Symptoms may include reexperiencing the trauma through intrusive memories or nightmares; avoiding thoughts, conversations, activities, people, or places associated with the trauma; or feeling detached or unable to have intimate relations. Other symptoms include a heightened arousal of the nervous system, often leading to insomnia, irritability, exaggerated startle responses, and hypersensitivities (APA, 2000).

PTSD can lead to serious emotional pain and impairment in functioning and warrants careful diagnosis and individualized intervention. Chronic traumatization often has a significant and pervasive influence on the developmental process and may affect occupation across the lifespan. The term *complex trauma* has been adopted and widely promoted by the traumatic stress field to represent "the experience of multiple, chronic and prolonged, developmentally adverse traumatic events, most often of an interpersonal nature (e.g., sexual or physical abuse, war, domestic and community violence) and early-life onset" (van der Kolk, 2005, p. 402).

Childhood Trauma

Trauma experiences that occur during childhood influence the development of the brain, one's sense of self, emotion regulation, and the ability to develop healthy attachments (Schore, 1994, 2003a, 2003b). More recently, van der Kolk (2005) has advocated for the addition of developmental trauma disorder to more specifically identify and target interventions specific to people whose trauma occurs in childhood. Children who feel safe and secure learn how to flexibly trust, which shapes their perceptions, intuitions, and capacity to form healthy relationships over time. The ability to identify and modulate thoughts, emotions, and arousal is a learned skill, and the ability to cope with daily stressors and traumatic events is mitigated by a personal sense of security, self-esteem, identity, and self-control. Cole and Putnam (1992) emphasized that a person's core perception of self is largely defined by the ability to self-regulate and function when experiencing distress.

One of the primary issues in trauma is how it affects the ability to process and come to terms with the trauma experience. If the trauma experience becomes overwhelming or persistent, systemwide changes occur. In those cases, anxiety, feelings of fragmentation (dissociative tendencies), somatic symptoms, retraumatization, and the tendency to minimize or catastrophize feelings, thoughts, and emotions often emerge and can become persistent patterns (Luxenberg, Spinazzola, Hidalgo, Hunt, & van der Kolk, 2001; van der Kolk, 2006).

Childhood trauma often leads to pervasive mental health issues, physical manifestations, and difficulty establishing competence in social relationships, in part because of profound difficulty with intimacy and emotion regulation, which is often linked to chronic anxiety and depression, engagement in self-injurious behaviors (e.g., eating disorders, substance abuse, self-mutilation), and suicidal ideation (Felitti et al., 1998; Saxe, Chawla, & van der Kolk, 2002; Schore, 2003a, 2003b; van der Kolk, 2006). Thus, childhood trauma often has a negative impact on occupational performance skills and patterns.

Case Example: Svetlana

Svetlana is a 12-year-old child from Moldova, a former republic of the Soviet Union and one of the poorest nations in Europe, with severe shortages of mental health services (Tewfik, Divale, & Moldovan, 2007). Svetlana was adopted by an American couple and brought to the United States after her mother died and her father was unable to care for her alone. In Moldova, she had been hospitalized 3 times for issues related to aggression and mild retardation. She was also described as being "nervous, with eye problems and headaches" and demonstrated symptoms of mild tactile defensiveness. At school in the United States, Svetlana would rarely speak and was described as being intrusive and oppositional. When asked in Russian what she most liked to do, however, she often replied "play" and would reply only to very few questions.

An individualized education plan (IEP) was created with Svetlana, her adoptive parents, and the members of the IEP team. Coming from extreme poverty, neglect, and negative environmental influences (lead poisoning and sensory deprivation), Svetlana responded well to an occupational therapy intervention plan of activities that she found positive, comfortably stimulating, and fun. The occupational therapist recommended that the primary therapeutic attitude with Svetlana emulate the PACE Model (*p*layfulness, *a*cceptance, *c*uriosity, and *e*mpathy), promoted for working with children with complex trauma (Hughes, 2004, 2006, 2007).

Svetlana began to thrive and speak more spontaneously shortly after occupational therapy services were introduced. The occupational therapist provided evidence-based, culturally competent, meaningful, and purposeful activities that were motivating to Svetlana. Demonstrating symptoms of tactile defensiveness, Svetlana avoided being touched but was observed to enjoy engaging in activities that included materials that were soft and smooth. She loved items that were brightly colored and handicrafts that did not require getting her hands "sticky." She could not get enough of making things for herself, initially choosing simple projects, completing them quickly, and then immediately gesturing to make another. She related to sunflowers and lavender because they reminded her of Moldova and her friends when they played in the fields. She was encouraged by the occupational therapist to complete projects that were graded from simple to more challenging, such as first sorting lavender blossoms and sunflower seeds and then partially hand sewing a velvet bag for the blossoms and a second bag for the seeds.

Positive, comfortable, preparatory, and purposeful sensory–motor activities provided opportunities for Svetlana to engage in play in a nonthreatening manner, which helped her to stabilize and start connecting with others. Over time, additional activities were promoted to foster praxis skills, increased tolerance for different textures, and emotion regulation and to help Svetlana become more comfortable in the presence of her peers. A change in one performance skill often influences change in others, a phenomenon that was evidenced by Svetlana's increasing ability to further engage in age-appropriate school roles (student, friend) and occupation-based interventions over time.

Svetlana's tactile defensiveness further complicated the ability to establish a strong parent–child bond. The PLACE model (*p*layfulness, *l*oving, *a*cceptance, *c*uriosity, and *e*mpathy) was recommended to foster the relationship between Svetlana and her adoptive parents (Hughes, 2007). The occupational therapist explained and modeled how to provide and engage in safe, comfortable, and fun activities to facilitate the parenting process, integrating the PLACE and sensory integration-related theory and interventions, with positive results. One example is the bedtime rituals and routine (part of a sensory diet) that were collaboratively established. The occupational therapist trained Svetlana and her parents in safely using weighted ball massage, the weighted blanket, seamless cotton clothing and bed linens, and lavender oil on a cotton ball under Svetlana's pillowcase as part of her bedtime routine to enhance bonding and sleep. Svetlana enjoyed all of these interventions. Over time, the collaborative partnership and use of evidence-based practices offered hope and cultivated the conditions for adaptation, as evidenced by improved sleep and increases in emotion regulation and parent–child bonding.

Trauma-Informed Interventions

Trauma-informed care is mental health care that is grounded in and directed by a thorough understanding of the neurological, biological, psychological, and social effects of trauma, violence, and their prevalence among people who receive mental health services (NETI, 2003, 2006). Given the prevalence of trauma in mental health consumer populations, trauma-informed care requires that therapists also be knowledgeable of trauma-informed therapeutic practices to best meet clients' specific needs and goals.

Establishing the Therapeutic Alliance

People with trauma histories, mental health symptoms, or both often perceive entering into a therapeutic relationship as threatening. Thus, staff attitudes and the therapeutic use of self are central to the person's ability to feel safe and less vulnerable (Bloom, 2002). Consequently, the principles of trauma-informed care require both a relationship-centered and a client-centered philosophy of practice. *Relationship-centered care* refers to a clinical philosophy emphasizing partnership, increased self-awareness by both consumer and therapist, and shared decision making (Suchman, 2006). *Client-centered care* focuses on the centrality of the consumer to all aspects of care delivery and the individualization of interventions to ensure utmost effectiveness (American Occupational Therapy Association [AOTA], 2008). By integrating relationship-centered care and client-centered care philosophies, clinicians are able to establish the initial conditions necessary to build trust and support empowerment through collaborative processes.

Trauma Assessment and Advance Directives

In 1996, Carmen et al. published a groundbreaking report providing a comprehensive review of consumer revictimization experiences in a variety of mental health settings. They indicated that practice improvements must include

- The use of trauma assessments at admission to identify other potential areas in need of assessment (e.g., sensory processing, dissociation),
- The collaborative development of trauma-informed intervention plans,
- The collection of data to better understand the needs of people with trauma histories (e.g., trauma-related symptoms, Adolescent/Adult Sensory Profile [Brown & Dunn, 2002]), and
- The development and use of deescalation plans (also known as *safety tools* or *personal deescalation plans*) that are updated over time.

The safety tool was specifically developed to serve as a consumer advance directive and proactive deescalation plan to help decrease the need for the use of seclusion and restraint and increase the ability to provide trauma-informed care (NETI, 2003). The safety tool is used to collect some of the following information on admission or initial intake: trauma history, warning signs, triggers, helpful strategies, specific preferences in the event of increasing anxiety or crisis, and preferences if restraint is necessary (e.g., preferred medications; MacLachlan & Stromberg, 2007; NETI, 2003). The information obtained must be used in the intervention planning process for prevention and when the person is experiencing increased symptoms of distress or crisis. Safety tools are now used internationally across a wide range of mental health care settings, and their completion is typically part of the initial evaluation process in inpatient settings (Champagne & Stromberg, 2004). Safety tools provide valuable information to the occupational therapy chart review and evaluation process. Psychiatric advance directives have become increasingly more popular as a means for consumers to have greater involvement in their own care. They are written or verbal instructions for health care, should the consumer be incapable of making or unable to make decisions regarding his or her own mental or physical health care treatment (Bazelon Center for Mental Health Law, 2008; Swartz, 2008).

Linking Assessment to Intervention Planning and Implementation

Therapists must review information from trauma assessment and advance directive documents, participate in the trauma assessment process, and include relevant information in the occupational therapy profile and intervention plan. An analysis of occupational performance includes the implementation of assessment tools used to "observe, measure, and inquire about factors that support or hinder occupational performance" (AOTA, 2008, p. 669). Thus, it is within the scope of occupational therapy practice to administer formal and informal assessments focusing more specifically on trauma history, risk assessment, related symptoms, and the impact on occupational skills and patterns. Cognitive and sensory processing issues may preexist, coexist, or become further affected by trauma and other medical or mental health symptoms. Occupational performance issues may unfold in myriad ways over time and must be explored during the development of the occupational therapy profile and through the use of other applicable assessments of occupational performance. Cognitive, sensory, mood, self-injurious behavior, and dissociation screening tools are examples of additional assessments that may assist in collaboratively determining the most effective intervention plan with people with trauma histories. Additionally, readiness for change (Prochaska, Norcross, & DiClemente, 1994), the Disorders of Extreme Stress Not Otherwise Specified (DESNOS) three-phase model (Luxenberg et al., 2001), and sensory supportive interventions (Champagne 2005, 2008) help ensure that intervention planning is trauma informed. (For more information on the DESNOS model and sensory supportive interventions, refer to Chapter 12.)

Case Example: Tony

Tony is a 33-year-old Marine veteran of two tours in Iraq. Wounded when a land mine exploded, he sustained shrapnel wounds to his legs, arms, and chest and lost 85% of the vision in his left eye. When referred to occupational therapy services, he was experiencing symptoms of depression and PTSD and engaging in alcohol and drug abuse.

When he was injured, Tony was forced to take a medical leave and felt lost and rejected. He began drinking excessive amounts of alcohol and described symptoms of depersonalization: "I don't feel like I am ever really present in my body." He became extremely aggressive and was getting into fights with his family and friends. One night his family called the police, and he was taken to the acute inpatient unit, where he presented with anxiety, depression, depersonalization, and poor sleep because of frightening nightmares and recurring thoughts of being in combat. He admitted to taking large doses of painkillers for pain related to his injuries and as sleep aids.

The collaborative creation of the occupational profile (AOTA, 2008) included a comprehensive examination of Tony's occupational history and experiences. He completed a safety tool on admission, which shed light on his occupational performance facilitators and barriers. Given Tony's initial values, goals, and needs and in accordance with the DESNOS model's stabilization phase, preparatory interventions were first warranted.

After developing a therapeutic alliance through the initial interview, Tony was assessed using the Allen Cognitive Level (ACL; Allen, Earhart, & Blue, 1992) screening, on which he scored 5.2, suggesting mild cognitive impairment. Weekly assistance to help monitor home safety, participation in instrumental activities of daily living, and follow-through with recommended medical and therapeutic services are among the recommendations at this cognitive level, and those recommendations were taken into account during intervention planning and implementation (Allen, Earhart, & Blue, 1992). From initial observations, Tony was able to perform all activities of daily living independently. He mentioned, however, that he startled easily from noises, was highly sensitive to smells, and ate only bland and uninteresting foods. Tony also demonstrated sensitivity to touch. All of these symptoms affected his ability to feel safe and comfortable in the therapeutic milieu and intimate relationships. The Adolescent/Adult Sensory Profile (Brown & Dunn, 2002) was administered to explore global sensory modulation patterns. Results revealed high scores in sensory sensitivity and sensory avoiding. The therapist explained how the information obtained from the assessments could help Tony make informed choices and described the benefits of creating and using a sensory diet to support Tony's ability to feel safe and engage in meaningful activities in the therapeutic milieu. Tony commented on how the strategies gave him a sense of control over his feelings and how knowing that he could actively do to something to understand, overcome, and better cope with his symptoms increased his hope.

Collaboratively, Tony and the therapist identified initial sensory modulation-related activities and modalities that afforded distracting, grounding, and relaxing influences for prevention and crisis-deescalation purposes. Developing an initial sensory diet included a routine of sit-ups and push-ups 30 minutes before meals in the general milieu (grounding–preparatory), the use of a weighted vest during group sessions on difficult topics (grounding–preparatory), and doodling and the use of certain music selections as positive forms of distraction when feeling triggered (purposeful activities). To help prepare for sleep, Tony decided to try a hot shower 60 minutes before bedtime, reading, and the use of the weighted blanket to help him fall asleep and potentially stay asleep.

With the continued help of the occupational therapist and increased self-awareness, Tony expressed a desire to identify educational and vocational options that would provide the needed structure and socialization that he enjoyed in the Marine Corps. The Social Profile (Donohue, 2007) was used in group sessions, verifying that once Tony felt more stabilized, his role was always as the leader or facilitator in groups. Tony quickly came to realize that an important part of his recovery was the structure and activities afforded by the unit and attendance and participation in self-help groups on addiction and self-reflection. Tony chose to also participate in the unit's tai chi classes. Additionally, a revised sensory diet for use on discharge was co-created during the final days of his admission.

Through engagement in addiction-related counseling, support groups, and sensory modulation interventions (Champagne, 2008; Precin, 1999), Tony realized that he had been self-medicating with substances. Through sharing experiences in groups, he developed more self-awareness of his triggers, warning signs, and helpful strategies. He learned that his PTSD symptoms were a typical response to traumatic events and learned alternative ways to cope and change over time. His cognition improved over the course of the admission, and he became motivated to go back to school. He met new friends who were motivated to stay clean and sober, and he continued to shape his sensory diet over the course of the admission to include purposeful and occupation-based activities, including both prevention and crisis-intervention strategies. Tony formulated a discharge plan that included a structured sensory diet, including a daily exercise plan; a sobriety kit with items to use to distract and ground him; a relaxing bedtime routine; and the use of a heavy quilt. He created a list of where he would go and whom he would call if he felt the urge to use drugs or alcohol. He also was able to identify environmental triggers to avoid, such as crowded areas and bars and restaurants where he could readily find drinking buddies. He also created a list of warning signs, triggers, and alternative environments and activities to help decrease the risk of relapse.

According to Tony, and validated by his ACL screening score of 5.6 before discharge, he demonstrated the cognitive ability to follow through with discharge recommendations and referrals, with the supports collaboratively identified and established before discharge (e.g., support groups and sober friends, sensory diet and structured routine, therapist, psychiatrist).

Seclusion and Restraint Reduction

In 1998, the *Hartford Courant* reported a series of articles on deaths resulting from seclusion and restraint, citing annual estimates of 50 to 150 deaths nationwide (Weiss, Altimari, Blint, & Megan, 1998; NMHA, 2006). This series led to further research and mounting legislative concerns, including a call by the U.S. Congress to focus on making the decreased use of seclusion and restraint a national public health priority (Huckshorn, 2004; NETI, 2003, 2006). Occupational therapists must be aware of national initiatives and the impact of their role when working with consumers with mental illness and mental health systems of care. Accordingly, occupational therapists must actively participate in developing trauma-informed and recovery-focused tools and systems of care that specifically address the need to decrease the use of intrusive and violent interventions such as seclusion and restraint (NASMHPD, 1999, 2000; NETI, 2003, 2006).

> The use of violent or coercive interventions, such as seclusion and restraint, with people with trauma histories leads to the high probability of retraumatization for clients and staff, compounding the problems that led the client to get help in the first place. It is evident that additional interventions that are humane, trauma informed, and recovery focused are necessary. Occupational therapists must recognize and partake in leadership roles to help promote the work of mental health stakeholders in this and other national mental health initiatives to effect wide-scale culture change at national, state, and local levels. Great care must be taken to protect the dignity and psychological well-being of mental health consumers and to provide safe, nurturing, and recovery-focused interventions for people with mental illness and trauma histories (NMHA, 2006).

Public Health Prevention Model

The public health prevention model (PHPM) serves as a guideline for the provision of services that help to decrease the need for the use of seclusion and restraint. The PHPM promotes the use of the public health constructs of primary, secondary, and tertiary prevention interventions (LeBel et al., 2004; NASMHPD, 1999), as outlined in Table 14.1. One example of how occupational therapists can contribute to the promotion of the PHPM is by taking a leadership role in helping organizations shape the provision of trauma-informed approaches across the categories outlined in Table 14.2 (Champagne, 2003; Champagne & Caldwell, 2007). Trauma-informed care is necessary not only across mental health care settings but also in rehabilitation and skilled nursing practice settings, as evidenced by the case of Mr. Evans.

Case Example: Mr. Evans

Mr. Evans is 84 years old and was admitted to an acute care inpatient medical unit after falling and hitting his head, resulting in severe bruising, concussion, generalized weakness, and muscle deterioration. Mr. Evans is a veteran and had a history of chronic obstructive pulmonary disease and diabetes and ongoing problems with balance. Frustrated and fearful about being in the hospital again, Mr. Evans was becoming increasingly depressed, angry, and belligerent, especially when needle

Table 14.1. Public Health Prevention Model and Seclusion and Restraint Reduction

Public Health Construct	Applications to Seclusion and Restraint Reduction	Intervention Examples
Primary	Development of an administrative and clinical treatment environment that • Creates systems that support decreased occurrences of conflict; • Performs analysis of and ongoing revisions to related policies and procedures; and • Ensures use of risk assessments and early intervention.	• Create a clear leadership plan. • Establish and communicate the vision and mission, and outline roles and responsibilities of staff. • Create systems supporting the use of prevention and deescalation strategies. • Implement workforce development. • Enhance the physical environment. • Integrate consumer roles. • Use systems evaluation and inform staff of progress.
Secondary	Effective use of early interventions to mitigate conflict or aggression that • Foster staff attitudes, activities, and physical environments that decrease the potential for conflict and • Inclusion the integration and use of prevention and deescalation interventions.	• Implement staff training related to trauma-informed care, risk assessment, and sensory modulation–related assessment tools and interventions. • Create competencies and monitor and ensure the skilled and responsible use of sensory modulation interventions. • Review and enhance the programmatic structure and activities provided. • Create and use sensory rooms and other sensory supportive, environmental enhancements.
Tertiary	Use of the most effective ways to mitigate the damage done to staff, consumers, and others who witness seclusion and restraint events: • Debriefing activities • Analysis of factors related to incidences of seclusion and restraint • Inclusion of consumer roles.	• Reestablish the therapeutic alliance. • Encourage the use of helpful strategies. • Assist staff with coping with vicarious traumatization. • Debrief consumers and staff. • Use data to inform practice.

Sources. LeBel et al. (2004); National Association of State Mental Health Program Directors (1999).

sticks were required for the blood draws necessary for his care. Staff were considering the use of restraints because he would become extremely agitated and repeatedly attempted to hit the technician during blood draws.

Seen at the bedside by the occupational therapist, Mr. Evans quickly responded to the therapist's acknowledgment of his fears and anxiety. The therapist proposed some simple strategies, such as breathing techniques and positioning in bed, that would provide him with more comfort and feelings of security. The therapist placed pillows under his knees and feet, providing him with a supportive environment so that he could relax and focus on an efficient breathing pattern (Sabel & Gallagher, 2007). Additionally, the occupational therapist explained that lavender essential oil is often used to decrease the pain involved in needle sticks and for its calming influence (Buckle, 2003). With an empathetic approach, the use of clinical aromatherapy, and simple breathing and positioning techniques, Mr. Evans felt more secure and in control of his environment, became calm, and allowed the technician to draw his blood, demonstrating the integration of secondary public health prevention interventions. In addition to traditional rehabilitation interventions, occupational therapy sessions included a continuation of breathing techniques for relaxation and simple positioning principles of restorative yoga (Sabel & Gallagher, 2007).

Discharge planning included helping Mr. Evans understand how formulating a psychiatric advance directive would ensure that his wishes for care would be understood should he become incapable of making decisions for himself. Over time, he became much more receptive to care delivery and ultimately to being transferred to a skilled nursing facility for further rehabilitation.

This case illustrates the importance of ensuring the client's centrality and feelings of safety and instilling control in decision making related to care planning and delivery; it also illustrates how this approach helps decrease the potential for retraumatization from the use of violent or coercive interventions, such as restraints. Although important to all consumers of mental health services, fostering increased feelings of control and safety through collaboration is crucial when working with people with a history of trauma to enable engagement in occupation-based interventions.

Table 14.2. Nurturing Intervention Categories

Category	Example
Therapeutic use of self	All verbal and nonverbal interactions and interventions by staff send the message that they care and believe in resiliency and recovery.
Development of positive and supportive peer relationships	Individual, group, and community efforts to help each client respect and support peers' efforts toward recovery, healing, and learning
Program practices and interventions	Practices and interventions are modified on the basis of client factors, needs, values, and spirituality and provide a range of holistic and evidence-based activities that are part of the daily routine.
Providing a nurturing physical environment	The physical environment of care is comfortable and supportive of client's sensory needs and offers alternative spaces to meet those needs (e.g., a sensory modulation room, an indoor gym, enhancements to the general physical environments).

Source. From "Nurturing Interventions," by T. Champagne and B. Caldwell, in *Developing Positive Cultures of Care: Resource Guide,* p. 156, by J. LeBel and N. Stromberg (Eds.), 2007. Boston: Massachusetts Department of Mental Health. Adapted with permission.

Sensory Modulation and Mindfulness

As demonstrated in each of the cases in this chapter, sensory modulation is part of the human condition, and sensory modulation interventions are often used when working with people with trauma histories (Brown, 2001; Champagne, 2003, 2006, 2007, 2008; Champagne & Stromberg, 2004; Kinnealey & Fuiek, 1999; Moore, 2005; Moore & Henry, 2002; NETI, 2003, 2006). Sensory modulation approaches include the therapeutic use of self, evaluation, sensory–motor activities, modalities, environmental modifications, and sensory diet (Wilbarger, 1984, 1995). They may be used as preparatory interventions, purposeful activities, and occupation-based interventions and for individual, group, and systemwide applications (Champagne, 2008; Nackley, 2001). Moreover, sensory modulation interventions are promoted for use throughout the DESNOS three-phase treatment model. For more information on sensory modulation approaches, refer to Chapter 12.

Benson (1975, 2001) emphasized that the relaxation response is most readily achieved when focusing on a sensory cue in a quiet environment (e.g., use of a sensory room and a specific item to focus on). The relaxation response is promoted for decreasing stress and stress-related illness and is often appropriate for use with consumers with complex trauma histories and symptoms of mental illness. At times, however, relaxation exercises can bring about an increase in the sympathetic nervous system response when used with people with trauma histories. During times of stress, the sympathetic nervous system activates the adrenal gland to increase the secretion of additional neurotransmitters, which influence an increase in heart rate and feelings of anxiety or panic. Therefore, when using any intervention with people with trauma histories, it is important to continuously and collaboratively assess effectiveness.

Mindfulness is "the capacity for self-awareness and self-knowing" (Kabat-Zinn, 2005, p. 11), which is cultivated by being present in the moment. Mindfulness is a method that helps people to feel more centered, grounded, and relaxed. Dialectical behavior therapy is an example of an evidence-based approach created specifically for use with people with trauma histories, integrating mindfulness as a core skill to be developed (Linehan, 1993), in addition to interpersonal effectiveness, emotion regulation, and distress tolerance. Additionally, non-Western cultures have long appreciated the healing qualities of spiritual and integrative activities, such as tai chi, yoga, meditation, and qigong, for the purposes of cultivating the ability to be present and to enhance the ability to self-regulate (van der Kolk, 2006). Other examples of therapies used with people with trauma histories that have focused on the spirit–mind–body–world interconnection include clinical aromatherapy (Buckle, 2003), eye movement desensitization and reprocessing (Shapiro, 2001), neurofeedback (Fisher, 2007), somatic experiencing (Levine, 1997, 2005), sensory–motor psychotherapy (Ogden, Minton & Pain, 2007), the Sensory Modulation Program (Champagne, 2003, 2006, 2008), and a wide range of expressive and integrative therapies.

In each case study presented in this chapter, the occupational therapist was comfortable with the terminology of the *Occupational Therapy Practice Framework* (AOTA, 2008), understood the goals of national mental health initiatives, and integrated evidence-based and emergent best practices. The therapist recommended trauma-informed, recovery-focused, and culturally competent interventions to help engage each client in activities that brought meaning back into his and her life and instilled hope, self-regulation, and responsibility for engagement in interventions as part of the personal recovery process. For example, Svetlana became a more functional, active, and precocious 12-year-old girl through the consistent use of the PACE, PLACE, and sensory supportive approaches (including a sensory diet), which included meaningful occupation-based, purposeful, and preparatory activities over time. She and her adoptive parents were able to significantly enhance their relationship through interventions discovered in occupational therapy sessions. Tony's recovery began with developing an alliance with the occupational therapist, creating and implementing a meaningful sensory diet, acquiring information about PTSD and addictions, and drawing support from others. Over time, he was able to put his experiences into perspective with the help of the occupational therapist and other people who had similar experiences. He continued to engage in activities that supported his recovery process and helped maintain hope for his future. Mr. Evans recovered and eventually returned home and to his local American Legion group, where he enjoyed spending much of his time with friends and engaged in community support activities.

Conclusion

In this "time of rapid and unpredictable change . . . in an era of hyperchange" (Hinojosa, 2007, p. 629), occupational therapists must continue to help people advocate for themselves and navigate an often unfriendly and complicated era of managed care (Baum, 2007; Hinojosa, 2007; Moyers, 2007; Scott, 1998). Recovery from mental illness typically requires learning new strategies to cope with symptoms, stress, illness, interpersonal conflicts, disaster, and war. Along with poverty and the stigma of mental illness and its causes, many people in recovery work daily to organize their lives and find meaning and hope through occupation (Christiansen, Baum, & Haugen, 2004; Kielhofner, 2002).

Occupational therapists need to understand and enhance practice patterns related to the national initiatives of trauma-informed care, seclusion and restraint reduction, the recovery movement, and related interventions that enable occupation. Only by using a client-centered, relationship-centered, holistic, and sensory-supportive practice that includes cultural competence (Wells & Black, 2000), spiritual occupation (Champagne, 2008; Rosenfeld, 2000), and competencies in evidence-based practice can the profession ultimately fulfill its new vision for the future (AOTA, 2007). By partnering with experts in the fields of trauma, restraint/seclusion reduction, wellness, and recovery, occupational therapy can play a multidimensional and vital role in collaborating with people with mental illness, mental health organizations, and governmental bodies dedicated to changing the culture of care across mental health service delivery.

References

Allen, C. K., Earhart, C. A., & Blue, T. (1992). *Occupational therapy treatment goals for the physically and cognitively disabled.* Rockville, MD: American Occupational Therapy Association.

American Occupational Therapy Association. (2007). AOTA's *Centennial Vision* and executive summary. *American Journal of Occupational Therapy, 61*(6), 613–614.

American Occupational Therapy Association. (2008). Occupational therapy practice framework: Domain and process (2nd ed.). *American Journal of Occupational Therapy, 62,* 625–683.

American Psychiatric Association. (2000). *Diagnostic and statistical manual of mental disorders* (4th ed., text rev.). Washington, DC: Author.

Baum, C. M. (2007). Achieving our potential (Farewell Presidential Address). *American Journal of Occupational Therapy, 61,* 615–621.

Bazelon Center for Mental Health Law. (2008). *Issue: Advance directives.* Retrieved May 15, 2008, from www.bazelon.org/issues/advancedirectives/advdir1.htm

Benson, H. (1975). *The relaxation response* (Rev. ed.). New York: Morrow.

Benson, H. (2001, May/June). The science of meditation. *Psychology Today,* pp. 56–60.

Bloom, S. (2002). Creating sanctuary. In National Technical Assistance Center for State Mental Health Planning (Ed.), *Networks* (p. 1). Alexandria, VA: National Association of State Mental Health Program Directors.

Brown, C. (2001). What is the best environment for me? A sensory processing perspective. *Occupational Therapy in Mental Health, 17,* 115–125.

Brown, C., & Dunn, W. (2002). *The Adolescent/Adult Sensory Profile manual.* San Antonio, TX: Psychological Corporation.

Buckle, J. (2003). *Clinical aromatherapy: Essential oils in practice.* New York: Churchill Livingstone.

Carmen, E., Crane, W., Dunncliff, M., Holochuck, S., Prescott, L., Reiker, P., et al. (1996). *Task force on the restraint and seclusion of persons who have been physically or sexually abused: Report and recommendations.* Boston: Massachusetts Department of Mental Health.

Champagne, T. (2003). Creating nurturing environments and a culture of care. *Advance for Occupational Therapy, 19,* 50.

Champagne, T. (2005, March). Expanding the role of sensory approaches for acute inpatient psychiatry. *Mental Health Special Interest Section Quarterly, 1,* 1–4.

Champagne, T. (2006). *Sensory modulation and environment: Essential elements of occupation* (2nd ed.). Southampton, MA: Champagne Conferences & Consultation.

Champagne, T. (2007). Sensory approaches. In J. LeBel & N. Stromberg (Eds.), *Developing positive cultures of care: Resource guide* (pp. 206–247). Boston: Massachusetts Department of Mental Health.

Champagne, T. (2008). *Sensory modulation and environment: Essential elements of occupation* (3rd ed.). Southampton, MA: Champagne Conferences & Consultation.

Champagne, T., & Caldwell, B. (2007). Nurturing interventions. In J. LeBel & N. Stromberg (Eds.), *Developing positive cultures of care: Resource guide* (pp. 155–164). Boston: Massachusetts Department of Mental Health.

Champagne, T., & Stromberg, N. (2004). Sensory approaches in inpatient psychiatric settings: Innovative alternatives to seclusion and restraint. *Journal of Psychosocial Nursing, 42,* 35–44.

Christiansen, C. H., Baum, C. M., & Haugen, J. B. (2004). *Occupational therapy: Performance, participation, and well-being* (3rd ed.). Thorofare, NJ: Slack.

Cole, P., & Putnam, F. (1992). Effect of incest on self and social functioning: A developmental psychopathology perspective. *Journal of Consulting and Clinical Psychology, 60,* 174–184.

Damasio, A. R. (1999). *The feeling of what happens: Body and emotion in the making of consciousness.* New York: Harcourt.

Damasio, A. R., Grabowski, T. J., & Bechara, A. (2000). Cortical and subcortical brain activity during the feeling of self-generated emotions. *Nature Neuroscience, 3,* 1049–1056.

Donohue, M. V. (2007). Interrater reliability of the Social Profile: Assessment of community and psychiatric group participation. *Australian Occupational Therapy Journal, 54,* 49–58.

Felitti, V. J., Anda, R. F., Nordenberg, D., Williamson, D. F., Spitz, A. M., Edwards, V., et al. (1998). Relationship of childhood abuse and household dysfunction to many of the leading causes of death in adults: The Adverse Childhood Experiences (ACE) study. *American Journal of Preventative Medicine, 14*(4), 245–258.

Fisher, S. (2007). Neurofeedback, affect regulation, and attachment: A case study and analysis of anti-social personality. *International Journal of Behavioral Consultation and Therapy, 3,* 109–117.

Hinojosa, J. (2007). Becoming innovators in an era of hyperchange. *American Journal of Occupational Therapy, 61,* 629–637.

Huckshorn, K. A. (2004). Reducing seclusion and restraint use in mental health settings. *Journal of Psychosocial Nursing, 42,* 22–33.

Hughes, D. (2004). An attachment-based treatment of maltreated children and young people. *Attachment and Human Development, 6,* 263–278.

Hughes, D. (2006). *Building the bonds of attachment* (2nd ed.). Northvale, NJ: Jason Aronson.

Hughes, D. (2007). *Attachment-focused family therapy.* New York: W. W. Norton.

Jennings, S. (2004). *The damaging consequences of violence and trauma: Facts, discussion points, and recommendations for the behavioral health system.* Alexandria, VA: National Association of State Mental Health Program Directors.

Kabat-Zinn, J. (2005). *Coming to our senses: Healing ourselves and the world through mindfulness.* New York: Hyperion.

Kielhofner, G. (2002). *A Model of Human Occupation: Theory and application.* Baltimore: Williams & Wilkins.

Kinnealey, M., & Fuiek, M. (1999). The relationship between sensory defensiveness, anxiety, depression, and perception of pain in adults. *Occupational Therapy International, 3,* 195–206.

LeBel, J., Stromberg, N., Duckworth, K., Kerzner, J., Goldstein, R., Weeks, M., et al. (2004). Child and adolescent inpatient restraint reduction: A state initiative to promote strength-based care. *Journal of the American Academy of Child and Adolescent Psychiatry, 43,* 37–45.

Levine, P. (1997). *Waking the tiger: Healing trauma.* Berkeley, CA: North Atlantic.

Levine, P. (2005). *Healing trauma: A pioneering program for restoring the wisdom of your body.* Boulder, CO: Sounds True.

Linehan, M. (1993). *Skills training manual for treating borderline personality disorder.* New York: Guilford Press.

Luxenberg, T., Spinazzola, J., Hidalgo, J., Hunt, C., & van der Kolk, B. (2001). Complex trauma and disorders of extreme stress (DESNOS) diagnosis, part two: Treatment. *Directions in Psychiatry, 21,* 373–392.

MacLachlan, J., & Stromberg, N. (2007). Safety tools. In Massachusetts Department of Mental Health (Ed.), *Developing positive cultures of care: Resource guide* (pp. 165–205). Boston: Editor.

Moore, K. (2005). *The sensory connection program: Activities for mental health treatment: Manual and handbook.* Framingham, MA: Therapro.

Moore, K., & Henry, A. (2002). Treatment of adult psychiatric patients using the Wilbarger protocol. *Occupational Therapy in Mental Health, 18,* 43–63.

Moyers, P. A. (2007). A legacy of leadership: Achieving our *Centennial Vision. American Journal of Occupational Therapy, 61,* 622–628.

Nackley, V. (2001). Sensory diet applications and environmental modifications: A winning combination. *Sensory Integration Special Interest Section Quarterly, 24*(1), 1–4.

National Association of State Mental Health Program Directors. (2000). Reducing the use of seclusion and restraint: Findings, strategies, and recommendations. *Emergency Psychiatry, 6,* 7–13.

National Association of State Mental Health Program Directors, Medical Directors Council. (1999). *Reducing the use of seclusion and restraint.* Alexandria, VA: National Association of State Mental Health Program Directors.

National Center for Trauma-Informed Care. (2008). *Healing from trauma.* Retrieved September 6, 2008, from http://mentalhealth.samhsa.gov/nctic/healing.asp#trem

National Executive Training Institute. (2003). *Creating violence free and coercion free mental health treatment environments for the reduction of seclusion and restraint* (Workshop Presentation, Las Vegas, NV). Alexandria, VA: National Technical Assistance Center for State Mental Health Planning.

National Executive Training Institute. (2006). *Creating violence free and coercion free mental health treatment environments for the reduction of seclusion and restraint* (Workshop Presentation, Boston). Alexandria, VA: National Executive Institute for State Mental Health Planning.

National Mental Health Association. (2006). *Position Statement 24: The use of restraining techniques and seclusion.* Retrieved March 23, 2008, from www.mentalhealthamerica.net/go/position-statements/24

Ogden, P., Minton, K., & Pain, C. (2007). *Trauma and the body: A sensorimotor approach to psychotherapy.* New York: Norton.

Precin, P. (1999). *Living skills recovery workbook.* Boston: Butterworth-Heinemann.

Prochaska, J., Norcross, J., & DiClemente, C. (1994). *Changing for good: A revolutionary six-stage program for overcoming bad habits and moving your life positively forward.* New York: Avon Books.

Rosenfeld, M. (2000, January 17). Spiritual agent modalities for occupational therapy practice. *OT Practice, 5,* 17–21.

Sabel, R., & Gallagher, B. (2007). Restorative yoga: An integrative approach to promote occupational performance. *OT Practice, 12*(19), 16–21.

Saxe, G., Chawla, N., & van der Kolk, B. (2002). Self-destructive behavior in patients with dissociative disorders. *Suicide and Life-Threatening Behavior, 32*(3), 313–320.

Schore, A. (1994). *Affect regulation and the origin of the self: The neurobiology of emotional development.* Hillsdale, NJ: Erlbaum.

Schore, A. (2003a). *Affect disregulation and the disorders of the self.* New York: W. W. Norton.

Schore, A. (2003b). *Affect regulation and the repair of the self.* New York: W. W. Norton.

Scott, A. H. (1998). *New frontiers in psychosocial occupational therapy.* New York: Haworth Press.

Shapiro, F. (2001). *Eye movement desensitization and reprocessing (EMDR): Basic protocols, principles, and procedures* (2nd ed.). New York: Guilford Press.

Suchman, A. (2006). A new theoretical foundation for relationship-centered care: Complex responsive process of relationship. *Journal of General Internal Medicine, 21*(Suppl. 1), S40–S44.

Swartz, M. (2008). *Psychiatric advance directives: A tool for patients and clinicians.* Retrieved May 19, 2008, from www.miwatch.org/2008/04/psychiatric_advance_directives.html

Tewfik, D., Divale, W., & Moldovan, V. (2007). Promoting partnerships in Moldova. In *New York State annual conference presentation.* New York: United Nations.

van der Kolk, B. (2005). Developmental trauma disorder: Toward a rational diagnosis for children with complex trauma histories. *Psychiatric Annals, 35*(3), 401–408.

van der Kolk, B. (2006). Clinical implications of neuroscience research and PTSD. *Annals of the New York Academy of Sciences, 1071*(1), 1–17.

van der Kolk, B., MacFarlane, A., & Weisaeth, L. (1996). *Traumatic stress: The effects of overwhelming experience on mind, body, and society.* New York: Guilford.

Weiss, E. M., Altimari, D., Blint, D., & Megan, K. (1998, October 11–15). Deadly restraints: A nationwide pattern of death. *The Hartford Courant.*

Wells, S. A., & Black, R. M. (2000). *Cultural competency for health professionals.* Bethesda, MD: American Occupational Therapy Association.

Wilbarger, P. (1984, September). Planning an adequate sensory diet—Application of sensory processing theory during the first years of life. *Zero to Three,* pp. 7–12.

Wilbarger, P. (1995, June). The sensory diet: Activity programs based upon sensory processing theory. *Sensory Integration Special Interest Section Quarterly, 18*(2), 1–4.

Consumer-Centered Practice

CHAPTER 15

Lived Experience: Recovery and Wellness Concepts for Systems Transformation

Margaret Swarbrick, PhD, OTR, CPRP

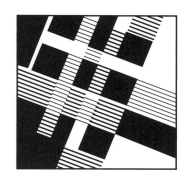

Learning Objectives

After reading this material and completing the examination, readers will be able to

- Recognize social and political factors influencing mental health system reform and the shift toward a recovery vision,
- Delineate 10 components of recovery,
- Identify types of peer-delivered service models,
- Identify benefits of peer-operated services and self-help groups, and
- Recognize roles and opportunities for occupational therapy practice.

Occupational therapy practice is client centered in its roots; however, the profession is challenged to reexamine how it can more effectively engage people in recovery and, when appropriate, their families and relevant others as full collaborators and partners in the design, delivery, and evaluation process. This chapter illustrates how people in recovery have made strides toward shifting the mental health service delivery system toward a recovery and wellness orientation. It defines the recovery and wellness framework, provides an overview of the peer-delivered service model, and suggests implications for occupational therapy practice.

System Reform and Transformation

Early System Reformers

A growing cohort of people with mental illness have become influential leaders in efforts to reform and transform the mental health service delivery system. They have designed self-help groups and peer-operated services as a complementary and alternative service model and have been leaders in efforts to transform the delivery system from a traditional model of care to a recovery and wellness model.

Historically, a person with a mental illness was relegated to an institutional environment and had limited expectations for returning to the community (Goffman, 1961). Social reformers, researchers, and sociologists revealed the detrimental effects of those environments (Goffman, 1961; Grob, 1983). An early reformer was Elizabeth Packard, who wrote pamphlets about the treatment her husband forced her to undergo. In the 1860s, she founded the Anti-Insane Asylum Society to rally public opinion as a means of stopping unjust incarceration of the "insane" (Grob, 1983). Clifford Beers was another early reformer who encountered firsthand the need for progressive change when he experienced episodes of confused thinking, agitation, and depression that caused him to be placed in a mental hospital (Beers, 1953; Dain, 1989). After his recovery in 1909, Beers wrote an autobiographical account of his experiences in the mental hospital titled *A Mind That Found Itself* (Beers, 1953). Through Beers, the mental health reform movement built momentum, and he organized the National Committee on Mental Hygiene, which later became the National Mental Health Association,[1] an organization focused on advocacy, promotion of mental health, and prevention of mental illness (Dain, 1989; Grob, 1983).

During the late 1960s through the early 1980s, people who had experienced the inadequacies of traditional mental health care settings and the indignities those settings engendered organized to form a mental health consumer–survivor movement. This movement has continued to affect the transformation efforts of federal and state mental health systems.

In 1977, the National Institute of Mental Health, under the U.S. Department of Health and Human Services, launched the Community Support Program. The Community Support Program was an initiative focused on assisting and empowering people with long-term mental illness to meet their needs and develop their personal potential without being unnecessarily isolated or excluded from their communities. The Community Support Program strengthened the active involvement of key stakeholders, including people in recovery and family members. These stakeholders became influential in the development of a peer-operated service model starting in the 1980s, systems transformation efforts toward recovery in the late 1990s, and wellness in the new millennium. Although divergent in their origins and motives, all have assumed a role in the efforts to transform the mental health service delivery system.

Family members of people with mental illness formed the National Alliance on Mental Illness (NAMI). They became influential stakeholders as they advocated for the needs of family members and aimed to reform the system by creating more and better services for their family members. NAMI's mission promotes research, public education, advocacy for better mental health services, and a national health plan that it believes should provide mental health insurance coverage on par with coverage for somatic illnesses (mental health parity). NAMI continues to make significant impact on federal and state policy development. In 2008, NAMI was part of a broad coalition of mental health advocates, including the American Occupational

---

[1]The National Mental Health Association is now called Mental Health America.

Therapy Association, that successfully lobbied for passage of federal mental health parity legislation.

People in recovery as stakeholders have been influential in terms of advocacy, services innovation, and systems transformation. Psychiatric survivors, who also refer to themselves as *ex-patients* and *ex-inmates,* tend to focus on advocacy. Many survivors view the mental health care system as dehumanizing and unresponsive to individual needs, and some insist on complete liberation from psychiatry because they reject the medical model of mental illness, professional control, and forced treatment. Psychiatric survivors initially organized in the 1970s on the East and West Coasts: the Insane Liberation Front in Portland, Oregon; the Mental Patients Liberation Project in New York, Boston, and San Francisco; and the Madness News Network and the Network Against Psychiatric Assault, both in San Francisco (Chamberlin, 1978, 1984). These groups oppose involuntary commitment and interventions such as electroconvulsive therapy and antipsychotic medications and have limited involvement with the traditional mental health system, which they view as coercive (Everett, 1994).

People in recovery have become leaders in terms of service innovation and systems transformation efforts. They have influenced the development of the consumer- or peer-operated service model and spearheaded efforts to move the system toward a recovery and wellness orientation.

Service Innovation: Self-Help

Peer-run self-help groups are another example of a consumer-operated service model in which people in recovery have assumed leadership roles that have affected systems transformation. The term *self-help group* has also been used to distinguish member-run support groups from professionally run support groups. Self-help groups are a valuable source of ongoing support, education, and connection to a community for people in recovery. Self-help groups have become a major legitimate and important means of providing a cost-effective adjunct to the traditional mental health service system. They can be more appropriately described as *mutual-help support groups* because peers helping one another is the primary dynamic.

Self-help groups are widely available for many different kinds of difficult life experiences including most illnesses, addictions, disabilities, bereavement situations, abuse experiences, parenting problems, and other stressful life problems. Self-help is based on the idea that people facing the same problem learn from and support one another when they share their experiences and strengths with an understanding and accepting community of peers. A tremendous number and variety of member-run self-help groups have evolved since the formation of Alcoholics Anonymous (AA) in 1935. The first national self-help group for mental health consumers was Recovery Inc., started in 1937 by psychiatrist Abraham A. Low. Self-help groups for peers in recovery include Schizophrenics Anonymous, the Depression and Bipolar Support Alliance, GROW, Double Trouble in Recovery, and many local grassroots groups that have been independently initiated by people in recovery. Peers supporting peers provides an informal structure that can enhance social support and social networks.

Groups are typically held outside the conventional mental health system in informal local community settings. In addition to often being geographically accessible, groups are more financially accessible because they charge no fees and may have only minimal dues, if any. Groups can serve as bridges to professional treatment through provision of referral information from peers.

Over the past decade, people have been participating in online self-help groups, many of which were developed independently over the years by people in recovery. Most of the national self-help groups now have their own online message boards, e-mail discussion groups, or scheduled real-time chat meetings. Online self-help networks eliminate many barriers that previously kept people from participating in a community group, including the lack of any local support group or the lack of transportation.

Self-help groups offer an excellent resource for people in recovery who are seeking ongoing support and education. Occupational therapists should be aware of available local and national self-help groups. Occupational therapists can advocate for or initiate self-help groups in hospital settings, where they most likely are not happening, and promote such groups to people being discharged from these settings.

Innovation: Peer-Operated Services

A significant contribution of people in recovery has been service innovation, in particular the design and delivery of the peer-operated service model. The Substance Abuse and Mental Health Service Administration's (SAMHSA's) Center for Mental Health Services (CMHS) funded demonstration projects in the 1980s to examine the feasibility of peer-operated services, and a variety of services has evolved over the years, including peer-run housing programs, consumer businesses, self-help groups, peer support programs, case management, and drop-in centers (Salzer, 2001; Van Tosh & del Vecchio, 2000). Roles for occupational therapists in these programs have been proposed (Swarbrick & Duffy, 2000; Swarbrick & Pratt, 2006).

Clay (2005) organized peer-operated services into three clusters: (1) drop-in centers, which provide varied services such as meals and housing assistance for members, as well as a place to meet friends and relax; (2) peer-support programs, consisting of self-help groups and peer-support systems in which people in recovery provide services to one another; and (3) education programs, which include training programs during which consumers learn recovery or advocacy skills (Clay, 2005). Eight successful programs from the CMHS demonstration project have been described in depth (Clay, 2005).

Peer-operated services are based on the notion that past and present recipients of mental health services can provide a unique perspective on and expertise to design and implement services to improve peers' quality of life. Core principles are as follows: (1) People in recovery develop, control, and provide the services; (2) participation is completely voluntary; (3) the emphasis is on strengths and competencies; and (4) the goal is mutuality among members. People in recovery assume a lead role in the development and provision of services. Members participate of their own volition rather than being required or coerced to attend. Many of these principles are congruent with the components of the National Consensus Statement on Mental Health Recovery (peer support, strength based, holistic, self-direction, and empowerment; SAMHSA, 2005).

Peer-operated services offer a setting that fosters empowerment by creating opportunities for all members to participate in an inclusive, democratic process of shared decision making (Swarbrick, 2005). The consumer operators control whether nonpeers or professionals are included (Solomon & Draine, 2001 Some services are entirely peer managed; others incorporate nonpeer professionals in certain areas of planning, implementation, and evaluation (Solomon, 2004). Such services are referred to as a *consumer–professional partnership*. The Vet-to-Vet program is an example of a consumer–professional partnership model in which consumer services are embedded in a mental health system (Resnick, Armstrong, Sperrazza, Harkness, & Rosenheck, 2004). Vet-to-Vet is an open meeting facilitated by peers during times of the day when there are no competing staff-led activities.

Research on peer-operated services has mainly offered descriptive reports that illustrate participant and program characteristics, service usage, and program outcomes (Chamberlin, Rogers, & Ellison, 1996; Davidson et al., 1999; Salzer, 2001; Solomon, 2004; Swarbrick, 2007a, 2007b), but more recently fidelity measures[2] have been developed (Clay, 2005; Holter, Mowbray, Bellamy, MacFarlane, & Dukarski, 2004). Peer-operated services seem to offer a tolerant, flexible, and supportive environment. They provide a network of natural supporters, and many people have reported that they provide family-like supports and environments (Swarbrick, 2005).

In 1998, CMHS funded a multisite research study designed to examine the extent to which peer-operated services, when used as an adjunct to traditional mental health services, effectively improve outcomes of adults with serious and persistent mental illness (SAMHSA, 1998). The Consumer Operated Service Programs Initiative was a 4-year project using a multisite, random-assignment experimental design aimed at generating empirical data to provide a more in-depth understanding of peer-operated programs and services. This study is the largest such to date, with more than 1,800 consumer participants. The Consumer Operated Service Programs Initiative investigated the extent to which peer-operated services are effective in improving self-empowerment, employment, housing, social inclusion, and satisfaction with services (Clay, 2005). The peer services involved in this study are described in *On Our Own, Together: Peer Programs for People With Mental Illness* (Clay, 2005). The findings of the Consumer Operated Service Programs Initiative are also being developed by SAMHSA into an evidence-based practice tool kit to be published in the future.

Formal individual assessment of participants attending peer-operated services is challenging. Participation is voluntary, and no formal assessments are used to include or exclude members. Efforts are being made to assess specific peer-operated service programs using standardized fidelity measures. Fidelity measures rate programs against an agreed-on list of components within a program model. The Consumer Operated Service Programs Initiative led to the development of the Fidelity Assessment Common Ingredients Tool (FACIT; Campbell & Adkins, 2007). Another instrument, the Fidelity Rating Instrument (FRI), was developed in Michigan by Holter et al. (2004) on the basis of a review of literature and expert feedback. Both the FRI and the FACIT include structural and process components and capture the following values and beliefs: consumerism, control and choice, opportunities for decision making, voluntary participation (absence of coercion), and respect for members. These instruments provide descriptions of the common program

---

[2]*Fidelity measures* examine the extent to which a program's implementation is true to the program model.

ingredients of a consumer service model, and both are at initial phases in terms of evaluating and establishing their psychometric properties. Fidelity instruments can be used for program development or program improvement and research.

Occupational therapists can help mobilize grassroots consumer or family groups to start and form a peer-operated service. It is important for therapists to refer people served to peer-operated services for socialization, support, education, and other needs those services fulfill. Occupational therapists have roles in leadership development and training of peer-operated service leaders, and occupational therapy researchers should consider partnering with consumer groups to conduct needed evaluation of this service model (Swarbrick & Pratt, 2006).

Recovery and Wellness Framework

Recovery Vision

People in recovery have assumed leadership roles in the attempt to transform the medical model of care's traditional orientation into a wellness and recovery orientation. As a result of their efforts—and those of prominent practitioners in the field of psychiatric rehabilitation—recovery and wellness are now considered organizing principles for the mental health services delivery system. The vision of recovery was influenced strongly by Anthony (1991, 1993) and Deegan (1988) and by those involved in the President's New Freedom Commission on Mental Health (2003) final report. A significant, ground-breaking study by Harding, Brooks, Ashikaga, Strauss, and Breier (1987a, 1987b) demonstrated that even people with severe mental disorders can live full and productive lives in the community. Harding and colleagues followed people 30 years after they left an institutional setting and found that a high percentage of them were living successfully in the community with little or no access to formal mental health services. No matter how long a person has experienced symptoms of mental illness or how severe the symptoms appear to be, people can and often do recover.

People with mental illness want the same things that many people in society desire: a sense of belonging, an adequate income, and a decent place to live. They aspire to fulfill various life roles and contribute to their community at large. Recovery is a personal, unique process of (re)gaining physical, spiritual, mental, and emotional balance after one encounters illness, crisis, or trauma. For some people, recovery is the ability to work, to live in housing of their own choice, to have friends and intimate relationships, and to become contributing members of their community. Recovery, therefore, is a process of healing and restoring health and wellness during episodes of illness and life stress. Some debate has occurred regarding a clear definition of *recovery,* although Davidson, O'Connell, Tondora, Lawless, and Evans (2005) provided a summary of common elements of recovery, including renewing hope, overcoming stigma, assuming control, managing symptoms, becoming empowered, and exercising citizenship.

Research, personal experience, and strong advocacy by the consumer movement promoted the notion of recovery, now endorsed and on the national agenda. The President's New Freedom Commission on Mental Health (2003) defined *recovery* as a process in which people are able to live, work, learn, and participate fully in their communities. For some people, recovery is the ability to live a fulfilling and productive life despite a disability. For others, recovery implies the reduction or complete remission of symptoms. A group of stakeholders, including people in recovery, wrote a National Consensus Statement on Mental Health Recovery, which is endorsed by SAMHSA (2005). The 10 components of the National Consensus Statement on Mental Health Recovery and their implications for occupational therapists can be summarized as follows:

1. *Hope:* Hope is the catalyst of the recovery process; without it, situations involving psychological distress can deteriorate rapidly. Therapists must be hopeful that people living with mental illness, regardless of its severity, can realize personal goals and dreams and must convey that to the people they serve. Therapists can help people develop the skills they need to live, work, learn, and contribute to their communities of choice. When one is in the midst of emotional distress, it can be difficult to hold onto the hope that things can change. Occupational therapists can play an important role in fostering hope in terms of interpersonal interaction, programs, services, and environments.

2. *Nonlinear:* Recovery is a nonlinear process; as such, it is based on continual growth, occasional setbacks, and learning from experience. Occupational therapists should offer interventions that enhance coping and relapse prevention skills and not allow relapse or setbacks to interfere with the belief in the recovery process.

3. *Strengths based:* Focusing on strengths rather than deficits is an integral part of the recovery process. It is important to view people as the individuals they are, complete with their own unique strengths and challenges. People living with mental illness sometimes feel denigrated by those who are attempting to help because they infantilize them, disregard their strengths, and concentrate solely on attempting to ameliorate weaknesses or challenges. Rather than viewing the person as broken and in need of fixing, the recovery paradigm focuses on valuing and building on that person's strengths, capacities, resiliencies, talents, coping abilities, and inherent worth. Occupational therapists should use a strengths-based perspective to cultivate coping skills and enhance self-esteem.

4. *Peer support:* Peer and mutual support, including the sharing of experiential knowledge and skills, is an important aspect of recovery. Self-help groups and friendships are extremely valuable, and steering a person in distress toward sources of peer support can enhance the therapeutic process. Support groups can be an important adjunct or alternative to formal mental health treatment. People can establish social networks that may prevent isolation, promote health, and possibly reduce the incidence, or severity, of illness. Support can reduce the stigma associated with mental illness and foster early detection of other related health issues. Occupational therapists can assume an important role by linking people to self-help groups and peer-operated services.

5. *Self-direction.* Recovery is a process that must be directed by the person, who defines his or her own life goals and designs a unique path toward

those goals. Recovery is possible when people assume personal responsibility for their own self-care, learning coping strategies and seeking support. The person living with the illness or emotional challenge knows himself or herself best and ultimately makes the decisions about what to do. The psychiatric advance directive is an effective tool to ensure that one's wishes for care are carried out in the event that one is unable to make those decisions in a time of crisis. Occupational therapists can facilitate the development of the advance directive as part of the plan for enhancing self-care skills.

6. *Responsibility:* People must all assume personal responsibility for their own self-care and journeys of recovery. Taking steps toward goals may require great courage. *Recovery* includes understanding and giving meaning to one's experiences and identifying coping strategies and healing processes that can enhance personal wellness. Occupational therapists should effectively partner with people in recovery to help them develop the motivation, knowledge, and skills to assume personal responsibility for wellness.

7. *Holistic.* Recovery encompasses a person's whole life—mind, body, spirit, and community. Recovery embraces all aspects of life, including housing, employment, education, mental and physical health care treatment and services, complementary and naturalistic services, addictions treatment, spirituality, creativity, family supports, social networks, and community participation as determined by the person. Occupational therapists must examine how these factors influence healing and health when planning assessments and interventions. Occupational therapists' focus on the mind–body connection and their knowledge of physical health issues make them particularly effective in enhancing this aspect of recovery.

8. *Individualized and person centered.* Each person's vision of recovery, and therefore journey of recovery, is unique and based on his or her personal needs, preferences, experiences—including past trauma—and cultural background. What it means to be "mentally healthy" is subject to many different interpretations that are rooted in value judgments that may vary across cultures. Reactions to distress and seeking help also have significant cultural implications. When engaging someone in treatment, occupational therapists must see the situation from the person's viewpoint and help to define recovery goals.

9. *Empowerment:* Consumers have the authority to choose from a variety of options and to participate in all decisions, including the allocation of resources that will affect their lives, and are to be educated and supported in doing so. This participation includes the assumption of legal power and authority to control resources. An aspect of empowerment is the willingness and ability to join with other peers to collectively and effectively speak for themselves about their needs, wants, desires, and aspirations. Through empowerment, a person gains control of his or her own destiny and influences the organizational and societal structures affecting his or her life. Occupational therapists should offer people in recovery a range of options and the opportunity to participate in all decisions that affect their recovery and wellness. Occupational therapy training should include a

focus on the shared decision-making model in mental health practice (del Vecchio, 2008).

10. *Respect:* Crucial to recovery is societal acceptance and appreciation of people, including protecting their rights and eliminating discrimination and stigma. Self-acceptance and regaining belief in one's self are particularly vital. Respect ensures the inclusion and full participation of consumers in all aspects of their lives.

The recovery vision cannot happen without changing the way in which the mental health service delivery system is designed, delivered, and funded. It continues to need an overhaul in terms of creating a culture that is based on self-determination, empowerment of relationships, and opportunities for people in recovery to fully participate in all facets of community living. The National Consensus Statement on Mental Health Recovery (SAMHSA, 2005) needs to be operationalized to fully transform the mental health service delivery system. Occupational therapists are challenged to examine how its 10 components can be operationalized in terms of interpersonal interactions (therapeutic use of self), services, and program environment.

Wellness Model

The transformation of the mental health system also includes a focus on wellness. The notion of wellness was initially introduced within public health in the late 1990s and has been proposed as an important component of mental health practice (Copeland, 1997, 2001; Copeland & Mead, 2004; Hutchinson, 2000; Hutchinson et al., 2006; Swarbrick, 1997, 2006). *Wellness is* a conscious, deliberate process that requires a person to become aware of and make choices for a more satisfying lifestyle (Swarbrick, 1997, 2006). A *wellness lifestyle* includes a balance of health habits, including adequate sleep, rest, and good nutrition; productivity and exercise; participation in meaningful activity; and connections with supportive relationships (Swarbrick, 1997, 2006).

Wellness views a person holistically (more than just mental and emotional well-being) and includes physical, intellectual, social, environmental, and spiritual dimensions. In terms of mental health recovery, a person can regain mental and emotional balance by concentrating on the various wellness dimensions (e.g., social support; spiritual connections; taking care of one's physical health through rest, sleep, and adequate nutrition). Research has revealed the health benefits of physical exercise on mental and emotional well-being (Hutchinson, Skrinar, & Cross, 1999) as well as the value of social support and social determinants of health.

Wellness is the process of creating and adapting patterns of behavior that lead to improved health in the various dimensions including physical, spiritual, social, environmental, intellectual, occupational, and financial (Figure 15.1). People's strengths are a focal point rather than solely an emotional imbalance. For many, spirituality can inspire hope when they experience distress or despair, and self-defined spiritual practices can help them manage or prevent a personal crisis. The Wellness Model focuses on good health and personal control as motivators.

Peer support resources are an excellent means of promoting the notion of wellness. Examples include a peer-delivered wellness curriculum delivered at state

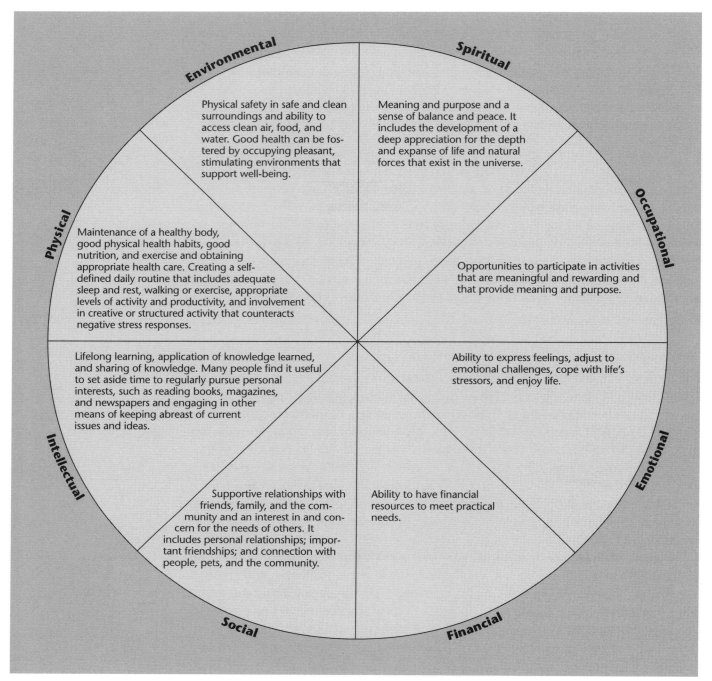

Figure 15.1. Wellness dimensions.

psychiatric hospitals (Swarbrick & Brice, 2006) and the Wellness Recovery Action Plan (WRAP; Copeland, 1997, 2001). WRAP is a structured self-monitoring system for managing uncomfortable and distressing symptoms and enhancing personal wellness (Copeland, 2001), and many of its core principles and components are aligned with the components of the National Consensus Statement on Mental Health Recovery (SAMHSA, 2005): person centered, self-directed, peer support, and strengths based. The "wellness toolbox" in particular helps a person identify the things he or she does to stay well. WRAP helps a person establish and maintain balanced routines and habits that are, ideally, within the realm of occupational therapy practice. Occupational therapists can support people in recovery either individually or in groups to create and update a personal WRAP.

The physical dimension of wellness has become more prominent because recent data have indicated that on average, people with serious mental illness die 25 years earlier than the general population (Parks, Svendsen, Singer, Foti, & Mauer, 2006). Unfortunately, many people living with serious mental illness (even under the care of the mental health system) are dying much sooner than the general population or are living with chronic health conditions that negatively affect their quality of life. Although suicide is a factor, premature mortality is primarily the result of conditions such as diabetes, infectious and pulmonary diseases, and cardiovascular disease. Cardiac events alone account for more deaths than suicide. The mental health system routinely screens for suicide risk and develops suicide response plans but does relatively little to screen for or respond to other diseases that affect a person's life expectancy.

The mental health system clearly does not adequately address physical health, and the primary health care system often does not treat people in recovery who seek medical care equitably. It is noteworthy that a core physical health concern that affects people in recovery are the medications prescribed for their psychiatric conditions. Compelling data have revealed how medications prescribed to ameliorate the symptoms of mental illness can produce many serious health issues, including the metabolic syndrome, diabetes, dyslipidemia, obesity, osteoporosis, periodontal disease, and sexual dysfunction (Joukamaa et al., 2006; Meltzer, 2005). The Clinical Anti-Psychotic Trials of Intervention Effectiveness (CATIE) study found that people who take olanzapine are at higher risk for abnormal glucose and lipid metabolism than those taking conventional antipsychotics (Lieberman et al., 2005). The CATIE findings also indicated that most people who develop these complications are not treated for them or are treated for them inadequately (Nasrallah et al., 2006). The National Association of State Mental Health Program Directors has published a resource paper that describes medical conditions people encounter that shorten their lifespan (Parks et al., 2006).

A clear need exists to help people in recovery make more informed choices and for professionals to monitor and treat cardiovascular risk factors in people prescribed psychotropic medication. Routine screening for metabolic syndrome must be a standard practice whenever someone is prescribed an atypical antipsychotic. Additionally, occupational therapists need to advocate for shared decision making as a standard mental health practice. Shared decision making is an interactive collaborative process between a practitioner and client (Deegan, 2006, 2007; Schauer, Everett, & del Vecchio, 2007) and involves decision aids that bridge scientific evidence, personal values, and quality-of-life considerations (Deegan, 2006).

In September 2007, CMHS sponsored a National Wellness Summit for People With Mental Illness (Manderscheid & del Vecchio, 2008). The summit gathered together a broad range of stakeholders to develop plans to deal with the considerably shortened life expectancy and reduced quality of life associated with living with a serious mental illness. Many of the papers presented there are available on a single repository Web site (www.bu.edu/cpr/resources/wellness-summit/index.html).

Items discussed at the summit were health risk factors and barriers; key principles and elements of and barriers to wellness; promoting wellness on an individual level; the health promotion efforts of the National Council for Community Behavioral Healthcare; promoting wellness at academic and research settings; integrating physical and mental health care; and federal initiatives on improving health. An exciting outcome of the summit was the development of "The Pledge for Wellness":

> *We envision* a future in which people with mental illnesses pursue optimal health, happiness, recovery, and a full and satisfying life in the community via access to a range of effective services, supports, and resources.

> *We pledge* to promote wellness for people with mental illnesses by taking action to prevent and reduce early mortality by 10 years over the next 10-year time period. (Manderscheid & Delvecchio, 2008, p. 7)

It seems apparent that "taking the pledge" is the first step in a long journey. Occupational therapists will need to grapple with difficult issues, such as

- What do we and the people we serve need to know to make this pledge a reality, and how do we get and disseminate that knowledge?
- How do we help everyone involved to implement a wellness focus on an individual level and at the same time support organizational efforts and initiatives?
- How do we deal with conflicts that may arise between an existing medically oriented service approach and one focused on wellness?
- How do we help people who are pursuing mental health recovery overcome years of poor health habits that have resulted in debility and health risk factors?
- How do we help every member of our community overcome a history of being encouraged to place more importance on symptom management than on wellness?

Health Promotion Models

Federal mandates are pressuring the mental health system to transform its approach to mental health care to ensure that services support the full recovery of mental health consumers and include an emphasis on health promotion and improved access to and interface with physical and mental health (CMHS, 2005; Koyanagi, 2004; Mental Health America, 2007; U.S. Department of Health and Human Services, 2005). The need to develop and research integrated health models is increasingly being recognized (Begley et al., 2008). Many different models exist, including colocating primary care and mental health services, collaborative care, referral to specialty providers, and the Primary Care Behavioral Health Model (Hogg Foundation for Mental Health, n.d.).

The lifestyle habits such as overeating and poor nutritional choices, physical inactivity, tobacco use, and substance abuse that contribute to the nation's poor health (U.S. Department of Health and Human Services, 2000) equally affect people living with serious mental illness. The staggering lack of a wellness lifestyle has been a powerful contributor to the disability experience and the recovery efforts of people who live with mental illness (Hutchinson et al., 2006). Significant numbers of people living with mental illness are unemployed and live in poverty, experience homelessness, or both, which also contribute to poor physical health.

The good news is that all of these factors are controllable through lifestyle. Educating and empowering people in recovery to develop healthy routines and habits is an important focus for occupational therapy practice. Helping people to seek gainful employment and pursue a career can go a long way in helping them create good health habits and transcend the negative effects of poverty.

Occupational therapy practice focusing on wellness should embrace health promotion principles. Hutchinson et al. (2006) offered several health promotion principles that are relevant to occupational therapy practice: (1) Health promotion recognizes the potential for health and wellness for mental health consumers; (2) active participation of mental health consumers in health promotion activities is ideal; (3) health education is the cornerstone of health promotion for mental health consumers; and (4) health promotion for consumers addresses the characteristics of the environments in which people live, learn, and work (Hutchinson et al., 2006). Occupational therapists can play an important role in empowering people in recovery by designing and delivering services on the basis of these health promotion principles (Hutchinson et al., 2006) and the wellness approaches presented in this chapter (Copeland, 1997, 2001; Swarbrick, 1997, 2006).

Conclusion

Wellness and recovery are possible, and people who experience mental health problems and disorders can and do live full lives, often with limited or even no professional intervention. People may experience a diagnosable condition resulting from myriad reactions to life's stressors. However, people are resilient and capable of leading productive lives. This chapter has described the tremendous impact that people in recovery have had and continue to have in the needed transformation of the mental health service delivery system. People with lived experience have played a role in advocacy and service innovation and helping to move the service delivery system toward a recovery and wellness framework. This chapter also illustrates how occupational therapists can partner collaboratively with people in recovery and other health care professionals, which is vital to shifting to a recovery and wellness orientation. Occupational therapists can play a pivotal role in the design of innovative approaches, based on recovery components, to empower people in recovery to achieve goals and dreams and to maintain a personally defined level of wellness.

References

Anthony, W. (1991). Recovery from mental illness: The new vision of service researchers. *Innovation and Research, 1,* 13–14.

Anthony, W. (1993). Recovery from mental illness: The guiding vision of the mental health service system in the 1990's. *Psychosocial Rehabilitation Journal, 16,* 11–23.

Beers, C. W. (1953). *A mind that found itself.* New York: Doubleday.

Begley, C. E., Hickey, J. S., Ostermeyer, B., Teske, L. A., Vu, T., Wolf, J., et al. (2008). Integrating behavioral health and primary care: The Harris County community behavioral health program. *Psychiatric Services, 59*(4), 356–358.

Campbell, J., & Adkins, R. E. (2007). *Fidelity assessment common ingredients tool e-FACIT workbook users' guide.* St. Louis: Missouri Institute of Mental Health, Behavioral Health Division, Program in Consumer Studies and Training.

Center for Mental Health Services. (2005). *Building bridges: Mental health consumers and primary care representatives in dialogue*. Rockville, MD: Center for Mental Health Services, Substance Abuse and Mental Health Services Administration.

Chamberlin, J. (1978). *On our own: Patient-controlled alternatives to the mental health system*. New York: McGraw-Hill.

Chamberlin, J. (1984). Speaking for ourselves: An overview of the ex-psychiatric inmates' movement. *Psychiatric Rehabilitation Journal, 2,* 56–63.

Chamberlin, J., Rogers, S. E., & Ellison, M. L. (1996). Self-help programs: A description of their characteristics and their members. *Psychiatric Rehabilitation Journal, 19,* 33–42.

Clay, S. (Ed.). (2005). *On our own, together: Peer programs for people with mental illness*. Nashville, TN: Vanderbilt University Press.

Copeland, M. E. (1997). *Wellness recovery action plan*. Brattleboro, VT: Peach Press.

Copeland, M. (2001). Wellness recovery action plan: A system for monitoring, reducing, and eliminating uncomfortable or dangerous physical symptoms or emotional feelings. *Occupational Therapy in Mental Health, 17*(3/4), 127–150.

Copeland, M. E., & Mead, S. (2004). *Wellness recovery action plan and peer support: Personal, group, and program development*. West Dummerston, VT: Peach Press.

Dain, N. (1989). Critics and dissenters: Reflections on "anti-psychiatry" in the United States. *Journal of the History of Behavioral Sciences, 25,* 3–25.

Davidson, L., Chinman, M., Kloos, B., Weingarten, R., Stayner, D., & Tebes, J. (1999). Peer support among individuals with severe mental illness: A review of evidence. *Clinical Psychology: Science and Practice, 6,* 165–187.

Davidson, L., O'Connell, M., Tondora, J., Lawless, M., & Evans, A. (2005). Recovery in serious mental illness: A new wine or just a new bottle. *Professional Psychology: Research and Practice, 36*(5), 480–487.

Deegan, P. (1988). Recovering: The lived experience of rehabilitation. *Psychosocial Nursing and Mental Health Services, 31*(4), 7–11.

Deegan, P. (2006). Shared decision making and medication management in the recovery process. *Psychiatric Services, 57*(11), 1636–1639.

Deegan, P. (2007). The lived experience of using psychiatric medication in the recovery process, and a program to support it. *Psychiatric Rehabilitation Journal, 31*(1), 62–69.

del Vecchio, P. (2008). *SAMHSA's shared decision-making (SDM): Making recovery real in mental health care project*. Retrieved from http://download.ncadi.samhsa.gov/ken/msword/SDM_fact_sheet_7-23-2008.doc

Everett, B. (1994). Something is happening: The contemporary consumer and psychiatric survivor movement in historical context. *Journal of Mind and Behavior, 15*(1/2), 55–70.

Goffman, E. (1961). *Asylums: Essays on the social situation of mental patients and other inmates*. New York: Anchor Books.

Grob, G. (1983). *Mental illness and American society, 1875–1940*. Princeton, NJ: Princeton University Press.

Harding, C. M., Brooks, G. W., Ashikaga, T., Strauss, J. S., & Breier, A. (1987a). The Vermont longitudinal study of persons with severe mental illness, I: Methodology, study sample, and overall status 32 years later. *American Journal of Psychiatry, 144*(6), 718–726.

Harding, C. M., Brooks, G. W., Ashikaga, T., Strauss, J. S., & Breier, A. (1987b). The Vermont Longitudinal Study of Persons With Severe Mental Illness, II: Long-term outcome of subjects who retrospectively met *DSM–III* criteria for schizophrenia. *American Journal of Psychiatry, 144*(6), 727–735.

Hogg Foundation for Mental Health. (n.d). *Connecting mind and body: A resource guide to integrated healthcare in Texas and the United States*. Austin, TX: Author.

Holter, M., Mowbray, C., Bellamy, C., MacFarlane, P., & Dukarski, J. (2004). Critical ingredients of consumer run services: Results of a national survey. *Community Mental Health Journal, 40,* 47–63.

Hutchinson, D. S. (2000). The journey towards wellness. *Journal of NAMI California, 11*(4), 7.

Hutchinson, D. S., Gagne, C., Bowers, A., Russinova, Z., Skrinar, G. S., & Anthony, W. A. (2006). Framework for health promotion services and for people with psychiatric disabilities. *Psychiatric Rehabilitation Journal, 29,* 241–250.

Hutchinson, D., Skrinar, G., & Cross, C. (1999). The role of improved physical fitness in rehabilitation and recovery. *Psychiatric Rehabilitation Journal, 22*(4), 355–359.

Joukamaa, M., Heliövaara, M., Knekt, P., Aromaa, A., Raitasalo, R., & Lehtinen, V. (2006). Schizophrenia, neuroleptic medication, and mortality. *British Journal of Psychiatry, 188,* 122–127

Koyanagi, C. (2004). *Get it together: How to integrate physical and mental health care or people with serious mental disorders.* Washington, DC: Bazelon Center for Mental Health Law.

Lieberman, J. A., Stroup, T. S., McEvoy, J. P., Swartz, M. S., Rosenheck, R. A., Perkins, D. O., et al. (2005). Effectiveness of antipsychotic drugs in patients with chronic schizophrenia. *New England Journal of Medicine, 353*(12), 1209–1223.

Manderscheid, R., & del Vecchio, P. (2008). Moving toward solutions: Responses to the crisis of premature death. *International Journal of Mental Health, 37*(2), 3–7.

Meltzer, H. Y. (2005). Focus on metabolic consequences of long-term treatment with olanzapine, quetiapine, and risperidone: Are there differences? *International Journal of Neuropsychopharmacology, 8*(2), 153–156.

Mental Health America. (2007). *Position Statement 16: Health and wellness for people with serious mental illnesses.* Retrieved July 11, 2008, from www.mentalhealthamerica.net/go/postion-statements/16

Nasrallah, H. A., Meyer, J. M., Goff, D. C., McEvoy, J. P., Davis, S. M., Stroup, T., et al. (2006). Low rates of treatment for hypertension, dyslipidemia, and diabetes in schizophrenia: Data from the CATIE schizophrenia trial sample at baseline. *Schizophrenia Research, 6*(1–3), 15–22.

Parks, J., Svendsen, D., Singer, P., Foti, M. E., & Mauer, B. (2006, October). *Morbidity and mortality in people with serious mental illness* (Tech. Rep. 13). Alexandria, VA: National Association of State Mental Health Program Directors, Medical Directors Council. Retrieved August 12, 2008, from www.nasmhpd.org/general_files/publications/med_directors_pubs/Technical%20Report%20on%20Morbidity%20and%20Mortaility%20-%20Final%2011-06.pdf

President's New Freedom Commission on Mental Health. (2003). *Achieving the promise: Transforming mental health care in America* (Final Report, DHHS Pub. No. SMA 03–3832). Rockville, MD: Author.

Resnick, S., Armstrong, M., Sperrazza, M., Harkness, L., & Rosenheck, R. (2004). A model of consumer-provider partnership: Vet-to-vet. *Psychiatric Rehabilitation Journal, 28*(2), 185–187.

Salzer, M. (2001). *Best practice guidelines for consumer-delivered services.* Unpublished manuscript, Behavioral Health Recovery Management Project.

Schauer, C., Everett, A., & del Vecchio, P. (2007). Promoting the value and practice of shared decision making in mental health care. *Psychiatric Rehabilitation Journal, 31*(1), 54–61.

Solomon, P. (2004). Peer support/peer-provided services: Underlying processes, benefits, and critical ingredients. *Psychiatric Rehabilitation Journal, 27*, 392–402.

Solomon, P., & Draine, J. (2001). The state of knowledge of the effectiveness of consumer provided services. *Psychiatric Rehabilitation Journal, 25*, 20–27.

Substance Abuse and Mental Health Services Administration. (1998). *Cooperative agreements to evaluate peer-operated human service programs for persons with serious mental illness* (GFA No. SM 98-004). Rockville, MD: Author.

Substance Abuse and Mental Health Services Administration. (2005). *National consensus statement on mental health recovery.* Rockville, MD: National Mental Health Information Center. Retrieved January 4, 2009, from http://mentalhealth.samhsa.gov/publications/allpubs/SMA05-4129/

Swarbrick, M. (1997, March). A wellness model for clients. *Mental Health Special Interest Section Quarterly, 20*(1), 1–4.

Swarbrick, M. (2005). *Consumer-operated self-help centers: The relationship between the social environment and its association with empowerment and satisfaction.* Unpublished manuscript, New York University.

Swarbrick, M. (2006). A wellness approach. *Psychiatric Rehabilitation Journal, 29*(4), 311–314.

Swarbrick, M. (2007a). Consumer-operated self-help centers. *Psychiatric Rehabilitation Journal, 31*, 76–79.

Swarbrick, M. (2007b). Consumer-operated self-help services. *Journal of Psychosocial Nursing, 44*(12), 26–35.

Swarbrick, M., & Brice, G. (2006). Sharing the message of hope, wellness, and recovery with consumers and staff at psychiatric hospitals. *American Journal of Psychiatric Rehabilitation, 9*, 101–109.

Swarbrick, M., & Duffy, M. (2000, March). Consumer-operated organizations and programs: A role for occupational therapists. *Mental Health Special Interest Quarterly, 23*(1), 1–4.

Swarbrick, P., & Pratt, C. (2006, March 20). Consumer-operated self-help services: Roles and opportunities for occupational therapy practitioners. *OT Practice, 11*, CE-1–CE-8.

U.S. Department of Health and Human Services. (2000). *Healthy People 2010: Understanding and improving health* (2nd ed.). Washington, DC: U.S. Government Printing Office.

U.S. Department of Health and Human Services. (2005). *The Surgeon General's call to action to improve the health and wellness of persons with disabilities.* Rockville, MD: Author.

Van Tosh, L., & del Vecchio, P. (2000). *Consumer/survivor-operated self-help programs: A technical report.* Rockville, MD: U.S. Department of Health and Human Services, Substance Abuse and Mental Health Services Administration, Center for Mental Health Services.

CHAPTER 16

Client-Centered Principles and Systems

Katherine A. Burson, MS, OTR/L, CPRP, and Tina Champagne, MEd, OTR/L, CCAP

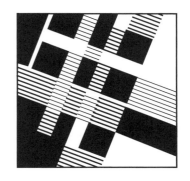

*E*mpowerment is not a program. It is a core condition for quality. You can't give, bestow, grant, authorize, delegate, or impose empowerment. You create the conditions to develop it.

—Covey (2007, p. 49)

Learning Objectives

After reading this material and completing the examination, readers will be able to

- Identify the similarities and differences between client-centered care (CCC) and relationship-centered care (RCC),

- Identify how to apply CCC and RCC principles to the treatment planning and delivery processes,

- Identify client-centered strategies that can be applied to program development and organizational change, and

- Recognize arenas where client-centered principles can be applied to organizational development.

This chapter reviews ways in which advanced occupational therapists apply client-centered and relationship-centered principles when working with systems. To facilitate this exploration, the chapter provides a brief summary of terms. According to the second edition of the *Occupational Therapy Practice Framework: Domain and Process* (American Occupational Therapy Association [AOTA], 2008), a *client* is a person, organization, or population. The Substance Abuse and Mental Health Services Administration (SAMHSA) uses the term *consumer* to refer to a client who is a person with a mental illness. The plural, *consumers*, refers to organizations or populations that use mental health services. Family members may also be considered clients or consumers. For the purposes of this discussion, the terms *consumer* and *client* may be used interchangeably. Although advanced occupational therapists often work with mental health provider organizations as clients, the client-centered and relationship-centered principles discussed in this chapter are used in reference to people with mental illness and their family members or caregivers and illustrate how occupational therapists apply these principles when working with people, programs, and organizations in delivering care; managing personnel; and developing and shaping programs, policies, and procedures.

Client-Centered and Relationship-Centered Care

Client-Centered Care

Concern for human rights and consumer empowerment in the provision of mental health care services has prompted efforts to promote client-centered models of care as an alternative to provider-centered approaches. *Client-centered care* (CCC) refers to an orientation that honors the priorities and wishes of the care recipient (AOTA, 2008). CCC was developed from the realization of the need to understand and include the client's perceptions as part of the care delivery process (Gage, 1993).

Occupational therapists use the *Framework* to organize their clinical reasoning and care delivery. A client-centered approach is viewed as pivotal to the occupational therapy process and is clearly advocated for in the *Framework* (AOTA, 2008). *Client-centered principles* are a set of values and practices that embrace the person with mental illness as central to the decision-making process in mental health care. Incorporating a client-centered approach throughout the occupational therapy process focuses all interventions on the client's priorities. Occupational engagement is by its nature intrinsically motivated and individually defined, requiring the client's active participation (AOTA, 2008); therefore, the client must be an active participant throughout the entire process. The Canadian Model of Occupational Performance is one example of an occupational therapy–based frame of reference emphasizing the necessity of the client's being an active, key participant throughout the entire occupational therapy process (Fearing, Law, & Clark, 1997; Law et al., 2005).

CCC embodies the values of occupational justice by enabling people to be active agents and participants in their care (AOTA, 2008). CCC also encompasses the need to individualize interventions on the basis of the client's goals and needs. It is worth noting, however, that the embodiment of CCC may be challenging to, or perceived as threatening by, occupational therapists who prefer rigid adherence to protocol-based approaches or the medical model approach, in which a practitioner-centered model is often viewed as most effective (Gage, 1993; National Executive Training Institute [NETI], 2003).

For many people, the concept of CCC may be relatively ambiguous because it has been applied and defined differently throughout the literature, yet the core assumption is that the care that is provided is centered around the client's needs (Gage, 1993). Hence, CCC's charge is a more holistic and empowering system of care that is not new to occupational therapy, which has historically worked to engage people in becoming active participants in care. Although CCC clearly emphasizes the centrality of the collaborative relationship, it does not fully represent the dynamic nature of the relational process in its entirety. This recognition led to the consideration of the deep significance and impact of the relational process and relationship-centered care (RCC; Tresolini & the Pew-Fetzer Task Force, 1994).

Relationship-Centered Care

RCC is a clinical philosophy and approach emphasizing the centrality of partnership and mindfulness in all aspects of the relational processes, including collaborative decision making and the emergent process of self-awareness (Suchman, 2006). RCC is a humanistic and pragmatic effort to bring to the forefront the fundamental nature of the relational process in a health care world that places great value on reductionism (Suchman, 2006). Thus, it has been recognized that a more empathic and relational approach is vital and that the combined roles of client, practitioner, and interdisciplinary team (the parts) create a partnership (the whole) that provides a degree of knowledge that each individual alone cannot (Lawrence & Weisz, 1998). RCC calls attention to the fact that the ability to form an effective working partnership requires therapists' self-reflection and ongoing self-assessment. This RCC requirement creates an emergent group process in which a core philosophical assumption is that therapists' roles may change as relationships progress (Stacey, 2001). Moreover, RCC principles support viewing care delivery as group process, or co-occupation (AOTA, 2008), in which two or more people are involved in a meaningful activity, such as collaborative engagement in treatment planning and therapeutic interventions.

Client-Centered Care and Relationship-Centered Care: A Foundation for Empowerment

CCC and RCC are used to develop and maintain processes or systems of care that are deeply rooted in the core values of respect, empowerment, and the recognition of the resilient nature of both the client and the partnering process. Historically, occupational therapists have used both CCC and RCC principles to guide practice patterns with individuals, family, programs, organizations, and the system of care. In like manner, occupational therapists are capable of helping mental health care policymakers, health care organizations, and treatment teams more clearly define, establish, and implement the principles of CCC and RCC. In this way, a foundation for empowerment and the process of recovery is more deeply anchored and understood as central to the dynamic process of care delivery and healing.

Client-Centered Care and Relationship-Centered Care: Intervention Planning

As outlined in the preceding section, CCC and RCC principles must be actualized when working with people in mental health care services, including intervention planning. This section presents some examples of the treatment planning process and treatment plans that foster the centrality of the consumer to varying degrees.

Treatment Planning Process

Becoming a valued and respected member of the treatment team requires opening up the treatment team process in ways that mindfully include consumers and

Table 16.1. Intervention Examples: Fostering Preparation and Active Participation in Treatment Team Meetings

Intervention Example	Practical Tools
Establish rapport by actively listening to client concerns and perspectives, thereby creating a relationship in which the client feels safe and comfortable.	• Ensure adequate time for the initial interview. • Structure the interview to obtain client goals, values, beliefs, concerns, perspectives, and priorities. • Continue to build rapport in subsequent individual or group sessions.
Explain to the client that this setting values and encourages active client participation throughout the treatment planning and implementation process; specify how this is achieved.	• Include this information in the client orientation materials. • Include the review of this information in the policy and procedures for the admission and treatment team processes.
Create and provide organizational materials that help to foster the process.	Provide a workbook or journal to be used to help the client organize, track, and communicate about the process.
Assist in the identification and use of individualized sensory modulation techniques.	Use sensory modulation checklists, active or assisted relaxation techniques or tools, and self-rating or biofeedback tools; collaboratively integrate strategies into client's sensory diet.
Assist with creating a list of questions and important points the client wants to cover.	Use a workbook, journal, or checklists.
After the meeting, collaboratively process how the meeting went and the effectiveness of sensory modulation strategies used, and create a list of things the client may want to do or readdress as a direct result of treatment team participation.	Use self-rating or biofeedback tools, self-reflection journal, worksheets, and checklists.
Assist the client with following through and tracking progress with the process and task-related issues that emerge.	Introduce and instruct on the use of tools that can be used as memory aids; use self-rating tools, worksheets, and checklists.

Note. This list is not exhaustive.

interdisciplinary practitioners. Creativity is often needed to identify ways to structure the team meeting and organizational processes to enable interdisciplinary practitioners to come together and meet with each consumer regularly. One example includes creating regularly scheduled treatment team times that are part of the program schedule, where clients are aware of the plan to meet with providers and are able to prepare ahead of time. Table 16.1 outlines examples of occupational therapy interventions often used to help clients prepare for and actively participate in treatment team meetings.

Treatment Plans

Treatment plans are interdisciplinary care plans that must include the consumer in both the initial development and the ongoing reassessment and discharge processes over time. One way to make a treatment plan relationship centered and strengths based is to consider it as a working document and as a worksheet to be explored with the consumer (LeBel et al., 2004; NETI, 2003). Creative ways to ensure communication, collaborative completion, and review are often necessary, particularly in the fast-paced world of acute inpatient care. However, time must be taken to recognize and engage in relational processes that support consumer inclusion, communication, and, ultimately, empowering partnerships.

Advanced Prevention and Crisis Planning

Initiatives geared toward involving consumers in the development of documents and processes are meant to increase their involvement in the care planning and delivery processes. One example is the creation of the safety tool, a deescalation tool that also serves as an advance directive. A task force of consumers and the Massachusetts Department of Mental Health (MDMH) worked together to create the safety tool (see Chapter 12), which is now used across the country and is part of the licensing requirements set by the MDMH (Champagne & Stromberg, 2004; MDMH, 2007).

Another example of a consumer-created and -directed tool is the wellness recovery action plan (WRAP) developed by Mary Ellen Copeland (1997). WRAP was created to help people identify and use specific wellness tools to relieve problematic feelings, facilitate recovery, and maintain health and wellness (Copeland, 1997). Key elements of WRAP include a daily maintenance plan, identification of triggers and an action plan, identification of warning signs and an action plan, crisis and postcrisis planning, and a wellness toolbox (Copeland, 1997).

Occupational therapists are skilled in helping consumers and interdisciplinary teams modify tools and approaches, such as those described earlier, to ensure that communication and other cognitive processing factors are addressed to fully support and enable the collaborative process.

Case Example: Lindsay

Lindsay is a 24-year-old woman admitted to an acute inpatient unit as a result of self-injury and reports of strong suicidal ideation. She has a history of physical, sexual, and emotional abuse throughout her childhood and has been diagnosed with recurrent major depression and posttraumatic stress disorder. Additionally, she has tactile defensiveness. Before admission, she had cut her abdomen, requiring 78 staples, and consumed large amounts of alcohol after a breakup with her boyfriend of 1 year. On arrival at the unit, she refused to engage in any formal evaluation processes and attempted to pull out her staples. Using a CCC and RCC approach, the psychiatrist, nurse, and occupational therapist met with her and calmly explained a few of the helpful strategies available on the unit to assist her with safety and stabilization.

Lindsay identified clinical aromatherapy and the 20-lb. weighted blanket as sensory modulation modalities that had been helpful in the past but refused to complete most of the initial evaluation processes at that time. In recognition of the degree of distress she was in and the severity of her injury, the psychiatrist, occupational therapist, and charge nurse agreed with her request for initial interventions and discussed concerns related to use of the weighted blanket. The possibility of reinjury if Lindsey tried to independently lift the weighted blanket on and off or twist to adjust it were primary concerns. Therefore, Lindsay and the team collaboratively developed a plan in which staff would assist with lifting and adjusting the weighted blanket when Lindsey wanted to use it. With Lindsay's agreement to use the weighted blanket as negotiated, the psychiatrist ordered the use of the 20-lb. weighted blanket with the specific safety instructions. Collaboratively, it was determined that because Lindsay had a significant history of restraint use, which ended with the use of the weighted blanket over the past two admissions; close supervision and careful use would validate and respect Lindsay's knowledge and experience while helping to enhance useful coping habits. Moreover, the weighted blanket, with proper use, was viewed as having the potential to help with the wound-healing processes.

Lindsay also used lavender oil on a cotton ball under her pillowcase for calming, as she requested. The primary collaborative goals of safety and stabilization and Lindsay's self-identified key strategies were outlined in the initial care plan. Lindsay was given a copy of the plan, and CCC, RCC, and the careful use of sensory modulation modalities were found to help her to stabilize. This case illustrates how CCC and RCC were used to establish the treatment plan, demonstrating the importance of the therapist–consumer relationship and of using creativity and flexibility. On Day 2 of admission, Lindsay was able to fully participate in all aspects of the evaluation, treatment team, and intervention planning. In this way, the practitioners used unconditional positive regard and relational processes to support safety, stabilization, empowerment, dignity, and respect.

Caregiver, Family, and Consumer Partnership

Caregiver Roles

Caregivers and families exist in different constellations and perform various roles. Caregivers and families include "biological families, adoptive families, stepfamilies, extended families, foster families and/or other individuals or group of individuals who play a significant role" in the consumer's life (Caldwell, LaFlair, Freedman-Gurspan, & Welles, 2007, p. 1). According to Worthington, Hernandez, Friedman, and Uzzell (2001), some of the positive outcomes associated with programs that actively partner with families and caregivers include reductions in length of stay in treatment programs, increases in caregiver satisfaction scores, increased investment in treatment and treatment outcomes, and positive sense of parental or caregiver efficacy.

Case Example: Dan

Dan is a 33-year-old man with paranoid schizophrenia who was having difficulty adhering to his medication plan. He lived alone in an apartment in the community and had weekly contact with a community services worker, quarterly meetings with a case manager from the Department of Mental Health, and daily visits from his supportive biological family members. One of the services provided by a community-based occupational therapist to address Dan's problem with taking medication as prescribed was a cognitive screen using the Allen Cognitive Level Test (Allen, Earhart & Blue, 1992). The occupational therapist received permission from Dan to engage in a family and service provider meeting. Dan and the occupational therapist relayed that Dan scored 4.6 on the Allen Cognitive Level screening, suggesting the need for daily supervision with medication management and other instrumental activities of daily living (IADLs).

Dan and all caregivers were provided with caregiver recommendations based on Dan's cognitive ability at that time. All of the participants in the meeting, including Dan, worked to create a system to help Dan remember to consistently take his medications and attend to IADLs in a manner that included his central participation. A just-right fit between client factors and available supports enabled Dan's ability to successfully achieve his goals with a level of assistance that did not minimize his abilities and fostered empowerment and dignity. Dan used a pillbox that was organized with his caseworker weekly and routinely checked by family members during daily visits. Dan was able to adhere to his medication regime when provided with the appropriate level of assistance and caregiver involvement. Dan's family valued the occupational therapy assessments and recommendations, stating how helpful it was in advocating for Dan's needs.

Consumer Advocacy and Leadership

Client-centered principles are also enacted by involving consumers and caregivers in leadership roles to help shape and reform mental health service delivery. Formal and representative roles include advocates, peers, peer specialists, and quality improvement–assurance teams. Peer support is one of the 10 fundamental components of recovery (SAMHSA, 2005). *Peer support* refers to the mutual giving and receiving of support, founded on principles of mutual agreement, shared responsibility, and respect. *Peer specialists* is the most commonly used term for consumers providing services to other consumers across a variety of mental health settings. Training programs to certify peer specialists are being conducted in numerous states (e.g., Georgia, Hawaii) in which consumers are employed and paid for their services. Payment for services delivered by peer specialists is now a optional Medicaid-covered service, should states choose this option and incorporate it into their service taxonomy.

When considering the hiring of a peer specialist, some helpful considerations include qualifications, supervision, mentorship, salary and benefits, training, and support help to facilitate positive partnerships and smooth transitions (Solomon, Jonikas, Cook, & Kerouac, 1998). The National Association of Peer Specialists is an example of a national organization of dedicated peer specialists promoting the peer specialist role and movement throughout the United States, serving as a resource to people interested in more information and support. The growth of the peer specialist movement demonstrates the legitimacy and redefinition of consumer roles, and certification of peer specialists is a growing trend. For example, the Illinois Alcohol and Other Drug Abuse Professional Certification Association (n.d.) certifies recovery support specialists, which legitimizes their role, defines domains of expertise, promotes professionalism, and ensures competency.

The Community Support Programs branch of SAMHSA fosters self-help approaches and consumer involvement in the planning, implementation, and evaluation of mental health services (SAMHSA, 2008). In 1992, the Community Support Programs branch funded the first consumer-directed self-help technical assistance centers.

In 1998, consumer supporter technical assistance centers for family members and friends of consumers were added to the program. Jointly, these technical assistance centers are now called *consumer and consumer supporter technical assistance centers*. Information on the centers is available from SAMHSA at http://mentalhealth. samhsa.gov/csp/consumers/tacs.asp.

The Protection and Advocacy for Individuals With Mental Illness program is available in every state and serves to protect the rights of people with significant mental illness who may be at risk for abuse, neglect, or civil rights violations while receiving care or treatment in a public or private residential facility. Mediation, administrative hearings, and litigation (last resort) help to ensure protection of the rights of clients with mental illness who are eligible for protection and advocacy. Clients who are not eligible for protection and advocacy may be eligible for other services from programs within their state protection and advocacy system.

Although protection and advocacy systems are necessary and valuable, they have not historically engaged consumers in the development of their own personal self-advocacy skills. In contrast, the primary goal of consumer roles such as peer specialist is to support the empowerment of people with mental health issues and to help in the efforts to improve the systems of mental health service delivery (Bluebird, 2004). People who have the lived experience of receiving mental health services can best share that experience and serve as important role models for those with similar issues, offering inspiration and hope (Bluebird, 2004). Transforming a culture of care requires participation by all people engaged in the process, particularly consumers.

Consumers and caregivers also assume administrative and leadership roles within care delivery systems. State, federal, and private entities are hiring consumers into senior management positions to help drive systems change and ensure that consumer-voiced needs are recognized and heeded. For example, Illinois has a director of recovery support services who reports directly to the director of the division of mental health. Value Options, a private, national managed-care company that specializes in disease management for all mental health and chemical dependency diagnoses, has a similar leadership position. These influential positions are key to achieving the transformational goal identified in the final report of the President's New Freedom Commission on Mental Health (2003)—that mental health care must be family and consumer driven (pp. 27–47).

Consumers and family members must be given the authority to choose from a range of treatment options and to participate in all decisions that will affect their lives. If clients are to effectively speak about their needs, wants, and desires, they must have an influential seat at the table whenever and wherever policy and practice decisions are made. Occupational therapists must advocate for consumers and family members or caregivers to be full partners at all levels and in all vehicles used to drive organizational and systems change. Advocacy must include the levels and types of support and information needed to make informed decisions and advocate for positions, which means that meetings must be structured to accommodate a range of cognitive abilities and learning and sensory processing styles. Information presented must be culturally relevant and available in auditory, visual, and written formats at appropriate comprehension and reading levels. Occupational therapists are skilled at modifying materials and methods to fully support and enable the collaborative process.

Policy, Program Development, Evaluation, and Modification

Policies and programs guide service delivery, whether within programs, units, facilities, organizations, or larger systems of care (e.g., state and federal health, education, disability, vocational rehabilitation, and workforce investment policy; private health insurance). Clients must have the authority to participate at the center of it all.

The President's New Freedom Commission on Mental Health (2003) stated, "Consumers of mental health services must stand at the *center* of the system of care. Consumers' needs must drive the care and services that are provided" (p. 27). Recommendation 2.2 of the report stated, "Involve consumers and families fully in orienting the mental health system toward recovery" (President's New Freedom Commission on Mental Health, 2003, p. 37). Consumers and family members must be able to participate in full partnership with providers and policymakers on decisions about treatment and services, and they must be able to participate in decisions about what services will be paid for under what conditions. To do this, they must have designated places and opportunities to influence policy and practice, such as membership in groups that direct transformation of statewide mental health systems. People with lived experience of mental illness were members of the President's New Freedom Commission on Mental Health, which for its final report drew on "comments from more than 2,300 consumers" (President's New Freedom Commission on Mental Health, 2003, p. 4). Moreover, states awarded SAMHSA transformation grants (5-year, multimillion-dollar infrastructure change grants) are required to have direct representation of consumer and family needs in all planning and transformation activities ("$92.5 million," 2005).

Transformation working groups in each state plan and direct the activities of the grant and are required to have consumers and family members as part of the team. Consumers and family members are provided with initial training and ongoing mentoring to perform these important leadership roles. Continuing in this vein, health insurance providers need to involve people with mental illness and their family members in coverage discussions. Locally, people with lived experience of mental illness must have designated influential roles in making decisions about program development, access, and evaluation. Thus, ongoing opportunities for consumers and family members to learn about mental health services and service delivery issues must be made available (Illinois Mental Health Collaborative for Access and Choice, n.d.).

When embedding CCC and RCC principles into policy, program development, and evaluation, it is important to pay attention to both structures and processes. The effectiveness of structures may be significantly influenced by the degree to which all parties involved have been educated on recovery principles and have validated the lived experience of consumers and caregivers. All participants must value experience, remove professional jargon, define terms, and identify and rely on their respective strengths. People with lived experience of mental illness and those who serve them share responsibility for both problems and solutions (Illinois Department of Human Services, 2007c). Hence, education of all stakeholders can improve communication, systems processes, and ultimately the effectiveness of structures and services.

An example of structures developed to improve the process by which consumers and caregivers influence systems of care is given in Table 16.2. The table details some steps taken by a statewide advisory committee to ensure that consumers are influential in policy decisions pertaining to the implementation of evidence-based supported employment. In the example, "[Involving] consumers and families fully in orienting the mental health system toward recovery" (President's New Freedom

Table 16.2. Structures Used to Promote Client Involvement: Establishing a Program Advisory Committee for Evidence-Based Supported Employment

Structure Implemented to Improve Process	Process Outcome
Step 1: Meetings are structured to accommodate a range of cognitive abilities and sensory processing styles.	Optimizes consumers' ability to contribute their expertise
Step 2: Consumers share testimony of the role of employment in the recovery process.	Establishes consumers as experts on what has facilitated resiliency and recovery
Step 3: An advisory committee is established with 50% consumer and family membership.	Establishes consumers as experts and equal partners with non–consumer advisory committee members
Step 4: All advisory committee members attend presentations about the evidence-based practice model of supported employment and the research behind it.	Establishes common knowledge of existing research, the model, language, and terms
Step 5: The advisory committee clarifies roles, ground rules, and the procedures for making and passing motions.	Establishes shared expectations and teaches the information and skills pertinent to role of an advisory committee member
Step 6: Program status reports track organization's follow-through on advisory committee recommendations.	Establishes program leadership accountability to advisory committee
Step 7: Advisory committee reviews program outcome data.	Allows advisory committee to see the impact of changes made

Commission on Mental Health, 2003, p. 37) is broken down into steps to establish clients as experts and full participants, and those steps may be applied to any agency's or program's advisory needs. Occupational therapists' understanding of the interface between contexts, activity demands, and client factors is used to identify variables and structures (interventions) that establish a working culture in which all parties contribute optimally to establishing a recovery-oriented system of care.

Various structures can be used to increase the likelihood that mental health care is client driven (i.e., by consumers and family members or caregivers as individuals, organizations, and populations). These structures include substantial client membership on advisory boards and committees, client focus groups, and clients as evaluators. Clients can also be trainers and designers of staff development activities as paid staff. Ideally, clients will be full partners on program design teams to ensure that programs maximize accessibility, flexibility, and individualized client-driven care. A strong client voice points to areas most in need of change and provides the impetus for that change.

Clients have a key role in program evaluation and modification and can be instrumental in deciding what and how to monitor and evaluate program effectiveness. Participation in analyzing and interpreting program evaluation data, as both staff and members of advisory boards, demonstrates additional inclusion roles. Full inclusion requires participation in identifying problems, making recommendations, and crafting solutions across the levels of systems analysis. Figure 16.1 provides examples of increasing client inclusion.

Sustaining Client-Centered Principles and Practices in Organizations and Systems of Care

CCC principles and practices must be embedded in organizational structures if they are to systematically influence and shape practice. Structures are intended to assist

Application 1: Consumer staff are initiators and drivers of a supported education program to enable more consumers to graduate from the Psychiatric Rehabilitation Certificate Program (Burson, 2003). The occupational therapist and executive dean of instruction assisted in building stakeholder support and program design.

Application 2: Consumer and rehabilitation leadership collaboratively develop procedures, sample methods, and questions for consumer and family focus groups for evaluating hospital-based rehabilitation services. They collaboratively facilitate focus groups, compile and interpret findings, and develop action plans (Massachusetts Department of Mental Health [MDMH], 2007; National Executive Training Institute [NETI], 2003, 2006).

Application 3: Consumer and family focus groups for Mental Health System Restructuring Initiative shaped modifications of Medicaid services and requirements and guided priorities for system change (Illinois Department of Human Services [DHS] with Parker Dennison & Associates, 2006).

Application 4: Consumers as leaders and partners train mental health providers on recovery, consumer-driven care, peer support, and so forth (Illinois DHS, 2007a, 2007b, 2007c; MDMH, 2007; NETI, 2003, 2006).

Application 5: Consumers as leaders equip other consumers with knowledge of recovery, peer support, mental health system, and service changes and terms. For example, a recovery support development team (all members are consumers) identifies training needs of consumers and arranges for or provides statewide toll-free teletraining. In Illinois, topics have included recovery principles, wellness recovery action plan, integrated mental health and substance abuse treatment, changes in the services in the state's Medicaid rule, certification for recovery support specialists, warm lines (telephone services for noncrisis peer support), orientation to consumer and family handbook, employment services, crisis plans, permanent supportive housing, and so forth (Illinois DHS, 2005, 2008; Illinois Mental Health Collaborative for Access and Choice, n.d.; MDMH, 2007; NETI, 2003, 2006).

Application 6: Consumers are partners in training police officers on crisis response.

Application 7: Establish statewide and local supported employment advisory committees with strong consumer and family representation (see Table 16.1).

Application 8: Consumers are members of an evidence-based practice technical assistance team. Conduct fidelity reviews, make recommendations, teach, and monitor for follow-through (NETI, 2003, 2006).

Application 9: People with lived recovery experience serve as members of the rehabilitation team (Medicaid Community Mental Health Services Program, 2008; MDMH, 2007; NETI, 2003, 2006).

Application 10: Consumers participate in the selection of the skills training curriculum and the schedule and structure of rehabilitation groups (Illinois DHS, 2007c).

Application 11: Consumers participate in developing a research agenda, are members of institutional review boards, define meaningful outcomes, and assist with interpreting results (National Working Group on Evidence-Based Health Care, 2008).

Figure 16.1. Consumer inclusion application examples.

the organization in meeting identified goals. For example, mission and vision statements clarify purpose and direction; strategic plans set priorities; budgets allocate financial resources according to those priorities; and personnel policies and reporting structures organize how the work will be done. These structures intentionally move an organization in a desired direction. Not all goals are met, some plans are abandoned or replaced, markets change, and events occur that may alter the path. The process of change is nonlinear and dynamic. Still, the organization moves forward. Similarly, if consumers are to be at the center of the service delivery system, organizations must operationalize and standardize CCC and RCC practices into policies, procedures, and operations.

For example, if the goal is a client-driven treatment plan, providing an in-service can facilitate progress but is unlikely to establish sustainability. After the in-service, a small portion of staff may change their practice if the requested change is viewed as valid, relevant, and feasible. Others will believe that their treatment plans are already consumer driven because they use the same language to describe staff-driven care that is customized for an individual. Others will argue that their clients are not capable of or willing to make informed decisions about their care. If this is the only

Table 16.3. Organizational Interventions to Achieve and Sustain Consumer-Driven Treatment Planning

Structure	Intervention
Mission and vision statements	Clearly spell out commitment to recovery and consumer-driven care.
Strategic plan	Includes goal of recovery-oriented and consumer-driven care.
Budget	Supports training, form modifications, computers, and so forth.
Treatment planning policy	Make a policy requirement that treatment plans state the consumer's recovery goals in his or her own words.
Treatment plan form	Designate space to cue staff to use consumer's own words (e.g., consumer's recovery goal [in his or her own words] or consumer's desired interventions [in his or her own words]).
Documentation policy	Documentation and treatment occur concurrently. Consumers participate in determining the content of progress notes and plans for next session.
Documentation format	Forms, method, tools, and equipment allow for consumer participation.
Job descriptions	Include accountability to consumer-driven treatment plans.
Competencies	Consumers participate in selecting staff evaluation methods.
Treatment team composition	Paid peer specialists are full members of the treatment team and use their life experiences to engage others in setting recovery goals and determining what is most helpful in people's recovery paths.
Quality improvement program	Consumers participate in the selection of indicators, evaluation methods, and improvement strategies.
Consumer development activities	Consumer orientation includes empowering consumers to be active participants in shaping the care they receive. Staff of all disciplines (including peer specialists) continually encourage consumer-self advocacy. Training is provided if length of engagement with organization supports it. Wellness recovery action plan is supported. Peer specialists share recovery stories and their process of becoming agents of their own care.
Staff development activities	Training developed and conducted in full partnership with consumers. Addresses relationship between client-centered care and relationship-centered care principles, goal setting, hope, and recovery. Teaches how to tie consumer recovery goals to medical necessity and reimbursable interventions. Addresses methods of engaging consumer in ongoing evaluation and modification of the effectiveness of their treatment plan.
Orientation of new staff	Recovery vision and value of consumer-driven care and the consumer voice articulated to all agency staff, regardless of position.
Required annual training	Annual refresher training developed and conducted in full partnership with consumers.

Sources. Becker, Swanson, Bond, Carlson, et al. (2008); Becker, Swanson, Bond, and Merrens (2008); Copeland (1997); Illinois Department of Human Services (2007a, 2007b); Illinois Mental Health Collaborative for Access and Choice (2008); Massachusetts Department of Mental Health (2007); Medicaid Community Mental Health Services Program (2008); National Executive Training Institute (2003, 2006); Substance Abuse and Mental Health Services Administration (2003).

intervention, it is likely that an outsider viewing the organization a year after the in-service will note minimal change.

A more systematic approach, albeit nonlinear and dynamic, is likely to effect a greater and more lasting change. A systematic approach may begin with a single intervention directed toward the goal of a client-driven treatment plan, such as an in-service. Over time, the occupational therapist might partner with consumers, family members, and invested others to advocate for a few more system interventions. Table 16.3 identifies 13 organizational structures that can be modified to increase the quality and consistency of client-driven treatment planning. Some interventions are as simple as creating a space on a form to remind staff of the requirement. Others include consumers in decision making, such as how staff competency in a given area will be measured. Others involve peer specialists on treatment teams or as trainers. As more consumers and staff gain experience with client-driven treatment planning, new strategies to improve both process and outcome will emerge. These examples illustrate how client-centered principles effect systems change. The occupational therapist's CCC and RCC orientation; skill with activity analysis, and understanding of the interactions among contexts, activity demands, and client factors are foundational to facilitating the desired outcome of consumers and family members as full partners and agents in designing and sustaining recovery-oriented systems of care.

Occupational therapy has held the longstanding tradition of valuing CCC and RCC principles, which is evident in the *Framework,* which clearly addresses the need for the client to be central in all aspects of care provision. National initiatives to transform the culture of care in mental health, and occupational therapy's core concern with occupational justice, require that occupational therapists continue to support and help create innovative opportunities for the inclusion of consumers and family members across levels of care. Occupational therapists are skilled in the ability to help identify the just-right challenge and respect the centrality of roles and routines to facilitate change. Whether meeting the charge at the level of client services, making efforts at organizational change, or working with governmental stakeholders, occupational therapists must take an active role in bringing clients to the table as partners in the change process. Collaboration is an invaluable element in the mission and vision outlined in governmental mental health initiatives (President's New Freedom Commission on Mental Health, 2003; NETI, 2003, 2006; SAMHSA, 2005) and AOTA's (2007) *Centennial Vision* across the multiple systems of mental health care delivery. Only in this way can we hope to create and sustain a client-centered culture of care that fully values and supports empowerment and the recovery process.

References

$92.5 million awarded for mental health transformation state incentive grants, USA. (2005). *Medical News Today.* Retrieved May 1, 2008, from www.medicalnewstoday.com/articles/31366.php

Allen, C. K., Earhart, C. A., & Blue, T. (1992). *Occupational therapy treatment goals for the physically and cognitively disabled.* Rockville, MD: American Occupational Therapy Association.

American Occupational Therapy Association. (2007). AOTA's *Centennial Vision* and executive summary. *American Journal of Occupational Therapy, 61*(6), 613–614.

American Occupational Therapy Association. (2008). Occupational therapy practice framework: Domain and process (2nd ed.). *American Journal of Occupational Therapy, 62*(6), 625–683.

Becker, D. R., Swanson, S. J., Bond, G. R., Carlson, L., Flint, L., Smith, G., et al. (2008). *Supported employment fidelity scale.* Lebanon, NH: Dartmouth Psychiatric Research Center. Retrieved August 27, 2008, from http://dms.dartmouth.edu/dsec/jj/supported/se_fidelity/SEfid.pdf

Becker, D.R., Swanson, S., Bond, G. R., & Merrens, M.R. (2008). *Supported employment fidelity review manual.* Lebanon, NH: Dartmouth Psychiatric Research Center. Retrieved August 27, 2008, from http://dms.dartmouth.edu/dsec/jj/supported/se_fidelity/SEManual.pdf

Bluebird, G. (2004). Redefining consumer roles: Changing culture and practice in mental health care settings. *Journal of Psychosocial Nursing, 42,* 46–53.

Burson, K. (2003). Supported education: Consumers as partners and colleagues. *Mental Health Special Interest Section Quarterly, 26*(3), 1–4.

Caldwell, B., LaFlair, L., Freedman-Gurspan, M., & Welles, D. (2007). Valuing families. In Massachusetts Department of Mental Health (Ed.), *Developing positive cultures of care: Resource guide* (pp. 85–111). Boston: Editor.

Champagne, T., & Stromberg, N. (2004). Sensory approaches in inpatient psychiatric settings: Innovative alternatives to seclusion and restraint. *Journal of Psychosocial Nursing, 42,* 35–44.

Copeland, M. (1997). *Wellness recovery action plan.* Dummerston, VT: Peach Press.

Covey, S. (2007). Giving people a voice, choice, and role. In Massachusetts Department of Mental Health (Ed.), *Developing positive cultures of care: Resource guide* (pp. 49–84). Boston: Editor.

Fearing, V. G., Law, M., & Clark, J. (1997). An occupational performance process model: Fostering client and therapist alliances. *Canadian Journal of Occupational Therapy, 64,* 7–15.

Gage, M. (1993). Reengineering or care: Opportunity or threat for occupational therapists? *Canadian Journal of Occupational Therapy, 62,* 197–207.

Illinois Alcohol and Other Drug Abuse Professional Certification Association. (n.d.). *Certified recovery support specialist.* Retrieved May 1, 2008, from www.iaodapca.org/certifications/crss/

Illinois Department of Human Services. (2005). *Huh???? Helping you understand what you Hear!!!* Retrieved May 5, 2008, from www.dhs.state.il.us/OneNetLibrary/27897/documents/Mental%20Health/HUHPamplet.pdf

Illinois Department of Human Services. (2007a). *Operational issues for implementing community support services* (Workshop presentation). Retrieved August 26, 2008, from www.parkerdennison.com/uploads/Day2ClinicalTrainingforweb.pdf

Illinois Department of Human Services. (2007b). *Rehabilitative interventions Day 1 of 2* (Workshop presentation). Retrieved November 30, 2009, from www.illinoismentalhealthcollaborative.com/provider/forums/DMH_Clinical_Training_Fall2007_Day1.pdf

Illinois Department of Human Services. (2007c). *Rule 132: New services clinical overview* (Workshop presentation). Retrieved March 23, 2010, from www.dhs.state.il/us/OneNetLibrary/27896/documents/By_Division/MentalHealth/Rule132/Master132ClinTrainfinalized4-30-07.ppt

Illinois Department of Human Services. (2008). *Recovery support services.* Retrieved May 5, 2008, from www.dhs.state.il.us/page.aspx?item=36696

Illinois Department of Human Services with Parker Dennison & Associates. (2006). *Summary of consumer focus groups: Illinois Department of Human Services/Division of Mental Health.* Retrieved May 5, 2008 from www.dhs.state.il.us/OneNetLibrary/27897/documents/Mental%20Health/ConsumerFocusGroupReport8-24-06.pdf

Illinois Mental Health Collaborative for Access and Choice. (n.d.). *Consumer education and support statewide call-in.* Retrieved September 29, 2008, from www.illinoismentalhealthcollaborative.com/consumers/consumer_education.htm

Law, M., Baptiste, S., Carswell, A., McColl, M. A., Polatajko, H., & Pollock, N. (2005). *The Canadian Occupational Performance Measure* (4th ed.). Ottawa, Ontario, Canada: CAOT Publications.

Lawrence, C., & Weisz, G. (1998). *Greater than the parts: Holism in biomedicine 1920–50.* Oxford, England: Oxford University Press.

LeBel, J., Stromberg, N., Duckworth, K., Kerzer, J., Goldstein, R., Weeks, M., et al. (2004). Child and adolescent inpatient restraint reduction: A state initiative to promote strength-based care. *Journal of the American Academy of Child and Adolescent Psychiatry, 43,* 37–45.

Massachusetts Department of Mental Health. (2007). *Developing positive cultures of care: Resource guide.* Boston: Author.

Medicaid Community Mental Health Services Program, Ill. Admin. Code tit. 59, chap. 4, pt. 132. (2008). Retrieved May 4, 2008, from www.dhs.state.il.us/OneNetLibrary/27896/documents/By_Division/MentalHealth/Rule132/JCARadopted110807.pdf

National Executive Training Institute. (2003). *Creating violence free and coercion free mental health treatment environments for the reduction of seclusion and restraint* (Workshop Presentation, Las Vegas, NV). Alexandria, VA: National Technical Assistance Center for State Mental Health Planning.

National Working Group on Evidence-Based Health Care. (2008). *The role of the patient/consumer in establishing a dynamic research continuum: Models of patient/consumer inclusion.* Retrieved August 26, 2008, from www.evidencebasedhealthcare.org

President's New Freedom Commission on Mental Health. (2003). *Achieving the promise: Transforming mental health care in America* (Final Report, DHHS Pub. No. SMA–03–3832). Rockville, MD: Author.

Solomon, M. L., Jonikas, J. A., Cook, J. A., & Kerouac, J. (1998). *Positive partnerships: How consumers and nonconsumers can work together as service providers* (2nd ed.). Chicago: University of Illinois, National Research and Training Center on Psychiatric Disability.

Stacey, R. (2001). *Complex responsive processes in organizations.* New York: Routledge.

Substance Abuse and Mental Health Services Administration. (2003). *Using General Organizational Index for evidence-based practices.* Rockville, MD: Author. Retrieved August 28, 2008, from http://download.ncadi.samhsa.gov/ken/pdf/toolkits/employment/14.SE_GOI.pdf

Substance Abuse and Mental Health Services Administration. (2005). *National consensus statement on mental health recovery.* Rockville, MD: National Mental Health Information Center. Retrieved January 4, 2009, from http://mentalhealth.samhsa.gov/publications/allpubs/SMA05-4129/

Substance Abuse and Mental Health Services Administration. (2008). *Protection and advocacy.* Retrieved April 8, 2008, from http://mentalhealth.samhsa.gov/cmhs/P&A/

Suchman, A. (2006). A new theoretical foundation for relationship-centered care: Complex responsive process of relationship. *Journal of General Internal Medicine, 21*(Suppl. 1), S40–S44.

Tresolini, C. P., & the Pew–Fetzer Task Force. (1994). *Health professionals education and relationship-centered care.* San Francisco: Pew Health Professionals Commission.

Worthington, J. E., Hernandez, M., Friedman, B., & Uzzell, D. (2001). *Systems of care: Promising practices in children's mental health, 2001 series. Volume 2: Learning from families: Identifying services strategies for success.* Washington, DC: American Institute for Research, Center for Effective Collaboration and Practice.

Mental Health Systems and Team Participation

CHAPTER 17

Mental Health Policy and Regulation

M. Beth Merryman, PhD, OTR/L

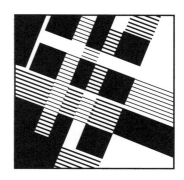

Learning Objectives

After reading this material and completing the examination, readers will be able to

- Differentiate the roles of the federal, state, and local governments relative to mental health policy-making and administration;

- Identify key stakeholders in mental health policy-making;

- Recognize current issues in mental health policy and effects on occupational therapy practice; and

- Understand funding sources for mental health.

Public policy is defined as "the basic policy or set of policies forming the foundation of public laws, especially such policy not yet formally enunciated" (*American Heritage Dictionary of the English Language,* 2000). Occupational therapists are affected in daily practice by public policies. This chapter addresses policies and regulations and mental health. It briefly discusses the roles of the federal and state governments and private insurance, including key aspects of payment systems in the public and private sectors, legislation that has an effect on mental health service delivery, and key stakeholders relative to mental health policy. It also address policy issues that affect occupational therapy practice in mental health.

Occupational therapists must be aware of how policy decisions are made at the federal, state, and local levels so that advocacy for service access can occur. Successful advocacy actions can potentially influence reimbursement, providers, and locus of treatment decisions for occupational therapy providers.

Key Stakeholders

Many stakeholders are interested in mental health policy. Occupational therapists are familiar with, at the national level, professional organizations such as the American Occupational Therapy Association and American Occupational Therapy Political Action Committee and, at the state level, licensure boards and professional organizations. In addition, occupational therapists are traditionally involved in advocating for needs of individual clients or families relative to access to services or a discharge placement, for example. Other stakeholders include people in decision-making roles, such as elected and appointed local, state, and national mental health leaders. Examples of federal mental health leadership might be key appointees to the U.S. Department of Health and Human Services (DHHS) or an elected member of Congress. Examples of state leadership include state Medicaid leaders and state mental health agency leaders. Local mental health leadership may include key people in the faith-based, school, and nonprofit human service community and advocacy group leaders. Occupational therapists need to become familiar with key contacts to effect policy change.

Historic Role of the Federal, State, and Local Governments in Mental Health Policy

Public mental health has traditionally been a state responsibility. Historically, it took the form of large state hospitals that provided only institutional care. As deinstitutionalization progressed, services moved to the community, and treatment options expanded (Frank & Glied, 2006). With the introduction of programs that support social safety nets such as Medicare, Medicaid, and Supplemental Security Income (SSI), the federal role in public mental health has increased. The federal role includes block grants to states, underwriting basic mental health research, and promoting the development of effective support strategies for community living (Smith, Kennedy, Knipper, O'Brien, & O'Keeffe, 2005). It also includes establishing a broad agenda relative to mental health policy. For example, the Surgeon General's report on mental health (DHHS, 1999) articulated the need to support the translation of research evidence into routine practice and to adopt a recovery orientation toward mental health care.

Although states must adhere to federal mandates, the design and delivery of public mental health services now has some flexibility. This flexibility results in 51 different public mental health programs as each state and the District of Columbia designs its system on the basis of both mandates and options such as eligibility, organizing structure, and services.

An ongoing complaint of the public mental health delivery system is the challenge of fragmented funding (Mechanic, 2002). Various federal, state, and local agencies are responsible for funding services across the continuum of mental health and human services. During times of economic belt tightening and, some would say, because of the social stigmatization of people using mental health and substance abuse services, funding is often reduced or attempts are made to shift costs to another part of the sector, enabled by the fragmented funding structures and lack of integrated national mental health and substance abuse policy. For example, Mechanic (2008, p. 192) described the "transinstitutionalization" of some patients discharged from state-funded hospitals to nursing homes where the federal government was responsible for at least half of the cost.

Organization, Delivery, and Payment of Mental Health Services

Medicaid

Medicaid is the single largest source of funding for the public mental health system. It is a joint federally and state-funded entitlement that is known as the "payer of last resort." Medicaid provides health and long-term care services to low-income adults and children. People must meet eligibility standards based on income and disability status to qualify for Medicaid. For example, if a person is incarcerated, he or she loses Medicaid benefits immediately. If institutionalized for more than 3 months, the person loses Medicaid eligibility. Although some categories of eligibility and services are mandatory, states are responsible for determining eligibility, establishing scope and types of services, determining payment, and administering the program. Institutional services for people younger than age 22 and older than age 65 are the only mental health benefits identified under Medicaid. Other benefits fall under general Medicaid-mandated or optional coverage categories. Physician services are mandatory, but occupational therapy, rehabilitation, clinic, and targeted case management and peer services are all optional.

According to recent survey data, 20% to 25% of nonelderly adult mental health service users received publicly funded services through Medicaid. In addition, 98% of children and adolescents receiving public mental health services obtained at least some of their care from Medicaid (Day, 2006). Thus, occupational therapists working in mental health need to be knowledgeable about Medicaid policy. For example, with the exception of early, prevention, screening, diagnostic, and treatment services for children, all other occupational therapy services provided under Medicaid are optional for inclusion into state plans. Therefore, how state mental health policy relative to Medicaid is defined is critical for occupational therapy services to be accessible to people who would benefit.

Rehabilitation Option

Outpatient mental health services offered under the Medicaid rehabilitation option are relatively flexible. Settings, providers, and services are defined broadly. For example, the locus of services can be a mental health program setting, the community, or a consumer's home. The definition of *provider* includes licensed medical and mental health providers, qualified mental health professionals, human services workers, and those providing peer services. It is noteworthy that many states do not recognize occupational therapists as qualified mental health professionals. In these states, under Medicaid occupational therapy is considered a medical profession that is typically consulted only when "medically necessary." For example, an occupational therapist would be consulted in a medical model setting for evaluation of functional decline relative to acute exacerbation of schizophrenia. Occupational therapy services are thus restricted to only assessment and consultation at the rehabilitation level of care. Skills training is considered psychiatric rehabilitation, whereas therapy is considered medical rehabilitation.

Service requirements support community integration and have as goals that rehabilitation intervention be active and based on an individualized rehabilitation plan of care in which the consumer is involved. Mental health services tend to be comprehensive and meet people's needs for non–medical model structure and supports. This distinction is an important one because rehabilitation is considered a nonmedical model of care. Because under Medicaid occupational therapy is considered a medical profession, access is severely compromised. Services under the rehabilitation option include supported employment, supportive housing, targeted case management, family education, medication management, and services for people with co-occurring disorders, such as developmental disability or substance abuse.

Clinic Option

Outpatient mental health services offered through the Medicaid clinic option tend to fall more into the medical model, as evidenced by requirements of setting, providers, and services and because a key goal is symptom stabilization. Clinic services are offered in a clinic environment by licensed medical and mental health providers, with more involvement of psychiatrists in either direct care or supervision of other licensed professionals. These services are similar to those provided to other Medicaid populations in terms of structure and type of intervention. For example, outpatient psychiatry visits are treated similarly to other medical clinic outpatient visits and held to that level of medical necessity. They are not structured specifically to meet the people's mental health needs, such as, for example, psychosocial rehabilitation. Occupational therapists would be accessed as are other medical rehabilitation professionals.

Targeted Case Management

Case management options under Medicaid include targeted case management and services case management. *Services case management* refers to the coordinating and monitoring functions that are provided when a consumer receives Medicaid-reimbursable services, such as residential or employment services. *Targeted case management* differs in that it can be restricted to a targeted group, such as people with serious and persistent mental illness or those in a specific or targeted geographic area (which does not need to be statewide in scope). It is up to the state to define the population and scope of the targeted group. Services under the targeted case management option include "planning, linking, and monitoring direct services and supports obtained from various sources" (Smith et al., 2005, p. 62). The intent of targeted case management is to assist recipients in gaining access to needed services. Services can be provided face to face, on the phone, or to link the recipient with another service. All services provided under targeted case management must directly involve the recipient. Occupational therapists may function as services case managers in employment or residential environments and may possess skills relevant to a targeted population, such as people with cognitive impairments.

Peer Services

Peer services are a component of the state rehabilitation option. State rules provide definitions of covered services and who can provide peer services. Services that states have identified for delivery by peers include social and daily living skills training, services to support housing or employment, and case management (Semansky & Koyanagi, 2001, p. 30). Medicaid and mental health policy in general are increasingly supporting consumer-directed services. Consumer-directed initiatives include those in which people with disabilities are provided an individual budget funded through Medicaid waivers to hire and manage personal assistance services. The mental health community has a growing interest in supporting self-determination through consumer-directed and peer services. Occupational therapists' embrace of client centeredness and collaboration are a good fit with this movement.

Waivers

Waivers refers to the section of the Social Security Act that is permitted to be "waived" for budget-neutral innovations of state Medicaid applications to be considered. These waivers have been in place for at least the past decade. They are designed to support innovative delivery methods to Medicaid populations and have requirements such as budget neutrality (the costs of the innovation cannot exceed usual Medicaid costs for the state) and that states cannot use waivers to expand coverage. Many waivers have been used to support state applications as they shifted to a managed care method of service delivery. In fact, managed care in state Medicaid programs has grown from 9.5% in 1991 to 59% in 2003. At this time, virtually all states have some type of Medicaid-managed care program (Monahan, Swartz, & Bonnie, 2003; Wieman & Dorwart, 1999).

Occupational therapists assist consumers in performing what they want and need to do to resume valued roles in their communities of choice. Awareness of both the waiver process and other means of serving people with disabilities in their communities is critical for occupational therapists because these services are often driven more by the client than by medical necessity. Waivers often permit broader service delivery that is more congruent with principles familiar to both occupational therapy and the recovery philosophy, such as client-directed care. Among the basic tenets of a recovery framework is that the consumer of services be integrally involved in decisions about his or her care in an informed manner that supports individual choice and preserves autonomy. Jacobson and Greenley (2001) referred to adherence to human rights, a culture of healing, and policies that support recovery as external aspects that are critical for success. These aspects are congruent with occupational therapy values and collaborative intervention approaches.

Block Grant

A block grant is a type of federal mental health and substance abuse funding, administered by the Substance Abuse and Mental Health Services Administration, that permits states to use funds within broad parameters. States decide which state agency administers the block grant program, which providers can participate, whether managed care will be used, and what type of enrollment system will be used (Mental Health America, 2007b). It is important for occupational therapists to understand the roles of key stakeholders in deciding mental health priorities and designing state delivery systems. Although the federal government establishes general guidelines and broad priorities, states have a great deal of autonomy in deciding how the system is structured and operates.

Medicare

Medicare is the primary source of reimbursement for occupational therapy services. Because Medicare is a federal program, guidelines are issued that directly affect service provisions in terms of who can provide services, what a service involves, and where it can be provided for payment to occur. Medicare is an entitlement (a type of benefit from which one cannot be excluded if one meets the criteria) that is based on age or disability status. People with mental illness who have Medicare and are younger than age 65 obtain Medicare as a result of their disability status (Social Security Disability Insurance [SSDI] benefits). Data from 1995 revealed that 37% of Medicare beneficiaries younger than age 65 qualified as a result of mental illness, mental retardation, or dementia (Foote & Hogan, 2001). Adults younger than age 65 who qualify for SSDI typically must wait 24 months after they start receiving their SSDI benefits before they are enrolled in Medicare, which is a serious challenge for people with serious mental illness because they most often do not have alternative resources for mental or physical health care.

Medicare was initially designed as a medical safety net to protect elderly people from financial ruin because of catastrophic acute illness. At the time of its design, this safety net meant inpatient acute care. Because of technological advances, people are living longer and have more chronic illnesses. In addition, costs and social influences have shifted most health care delivery to the community. Medicare policies have slowly shifted to cover nonacute care but have not kept pace with the dramatic shift from inpatient care to ambulatory care. In the area of mental health care, Medicare also continues to discriminate against people who receive outpatient mental health care versus outpatient physical care by charging mental health consumers a 50% copayment per visit and physical health consumers a 20% copayment per visit. This policy is being phased out, but it will take several years to achieve parity. Mental health care, including occupational therapy, must meet medical necessity criteria for reimbursement to occur. It is important to note that the entitlement aspect of Part A Medicare does not address outpatient care, so if a consumer does not have alternative funding, coverage has limits. Medicare is a primary reimbursement source for occupational therapy; however, this is not the case with outpatient mental health because of strict medical necessity criteria and population served.

Supplemental Security Income and Social Security Disability Income

SSI and SSDI are forms of social insurance. SSI was created in 1972. It is a federal needs-based income-support program for people with disabilities. Most states link SSI receipt to Medicaid eligibility. Some say that the creation of the SSI support program, and later amendments that enabled people with serious mental illness to more easily qualify for it, were the most instrumental policies in supporting deinstitutionalization and community integration (Sharfstein, Boronow, & Dickerson, 1999).

SSI provides cash support for people with disabilities who have little income. The income that is afforded to people who meet the criteria enables them to live in the community. A challenge continues to be the lack of affordable housing and general increased cost of living compared with the cost of living allowance that recipients receive.

SSDI differs from SSI in that it is available only to people who have paid into the Social Security system through employment. In most cases, SSDI is available to people who have worked for a certain period of time and become unable to work because of an illness or disability. People with serious mental illness may be included, although many people with debilitating, persistent forms of mental illness may not have the work history and so only can qualify for SSI. It is noteworthy that 40% of people qualifying for SSDI also qualify for SSI because they do not have enough earnings history to receive enough SSDI to equal what they would get under SSI, which is addressed by providing SSI funds to equal that amount (Whittaker, 2005).

Knowledge of SSI and SSDI is increasingly important for occupational therapists because 35% of SSI recipients are disabled by mental illness, and 27.4% of recipients of SSDI are disabled by mental illness (Frank & Glied, 2006). As indicated earlier, people who qualify for SSI also receive Medicaid, and those with disability as result of mental illness have been one of the fastest-growing groups to receive SSI (Mashow & Reno, 1996; Mechanic, 2007). Also of significance is that if people are institutionalized or incarcerated for more than 30 days, their SSI is suspended.

Children may also qualify for SSI. In 2005, 1 million children qualified, approximately two-thirds as a result of a mental disorder (Institute of Medicine, 2007). Children reaching transition age must be reevaluated to determine continued qualification for SSI.

Occupational therapists in mental health practice address daily life with consumers. Income source and poverty are often identified in the literature as structural barriers to recovery. These considerations are important in treatment.

Other Funding That Supports Community Living for People With Mental Illness

Three types of programs are part of the mental health safety net, although they were not developed with the needs of this population in mind. They include human service programs, such as vocational rehabilitation; public housing supports, such as vouchers for reimbursement for providing units for low-income people with disabilities; and criminal justice funds such as jail diversion, treatment during incarceration, and intervention to support reintegration to the community. According to the National Governors Association (2001), several DHHS optional programs address employment and community barriers for people with mental illness. Those programs include

- *Social Services Block grants* to support mental health activities for low-income people in the pursuit of self-sufficiency;
- *Personal Responsibility and Work Opportunity Reconciliation Act of 1996,* welfare reform that replaced the traditional form of welfare with the Temporary Assistance for Needy Families (TANF) block grant (and also limited TANF to 5 years); and
- *Welfare to Work Block grants,* which target especially hard-to-serve people, such as those with mental illness (Brown, 2001; see the Work and Employment Support section for more information).

Housing Support

The U.S. Department of Housing and Urban Development offers federal grants to support homeless or disabled people. States use the federal grants to offer housing or wraparound services. Housing and Urban Development programs that may support people with mental illness include

- *Section 8 Fair Housing,* which provides rental assistance in the form of vouchers to eligible low-income people to find housing in the private market;
- *Section 811 Supportive Housing for the Disabled,* which states use to build, operate, or lease housing units or support services for low-income people with disabilities; and
- *Continuum of Care (McKinney) Grants,* which provide funding for states to develop innovative systems to address homelessness and can target specific populations, such as people with mental illness (U.S. General Accounting Office [GAO], 2000b).

It is noteworthy that affordable housing is an issue in many areas across the country and is most pressing for people on a fixed income, such as those with serious mental illness receiving SSI or SSDI. Occupational therapists are often involved in assessing a consumer's discharge context. Important barriers to recovery may include the location of the housing in terms of safety, access to public transportation, and other needed community support. Occupational therapists can influence housing policy at the local level through participation on boards or community development associations.

Work and Employment Support

The Ticket to Work and Work Incentives Improvement Act of 1999, or the Ticket to Work and Self-Sufficiency Program (Ticket Program), is an employment program for people with disabilities who are interested in going to work. The Ticket Program is part of the 1999 legislation designed to remove many of the barriers that previously influenced people's decisions about going to work because of concerns over losing health care coverage. "The goal of the Ticket Program is to increase opportunities and choices for Social Security disability beneficiaries to obtain employment, vocational rehabilitation . . . and other support services from public and private providers, employers, and other organizations" (Your Ticket to Work, n.d., para. 1). One of the ways that choice is promoted is through the issuing of "tickets" to consumers. The ticket is accepted by an employment network to assist the consumer in obtaining employment, vocational rehabilitation services, or other services to meet vocational goals. Workshops are offered to SSI and SSDI recipients regarding the choices and process (Social Security Online, 2009). The unemployment rate of people with serious and persistent mental illness remains at 85% to 90%. This population is one of the largest on federal disability rolls. They are more likely to enter the rolls at younger ages and remain on them longer than people with other disabilities (Mental Health America, 2007a).

Each state has a designated vocational rehabilitation agency that provides vocational services for people who meet the criteria. Services are described in the Rehabilitation Act of 1973 Amendments and require, among other things, an individualized plan for employment. It is not necessary to receive SSI or SSDI to qualify, but receipt of either of those benefits can speed up the decision-making process. These programs are chronically underfunded. In addition, many states implement an "order of selection" process that basically requires that people with the most severe disabilities be served first when funding falls short. Often, people with disabilities as a result of mental illness are at the bottom of the list. In addition, because states must balance budgets, limits on new cases and opportunities may also exist during times of fiscal crisis. Occupational therapists need to be knowledgeable about key administrative organization and funding structures to enable participation in employment services for clients with mental illness.

Civil Rights

Policies reflect a society's values. In general, U.S. policies protect individual liberties. Ongoing tension in mental health policy exists around the issue of involuntary care; at one end are people who want to protect the civil liberties of the individual at all costs, and at the other are those who believe that in some circumstances, the state should act to ensure that a person receives necessary care (Mechanic, 2008). Many states have outpatient commitment laws. Implementation, however, has not been consistent because of liability concerns, economic concerns, and challenges of working with an uncooperative individual. Rights to receive treatment exist in hospital settings, but because of the paucity of community services, this is no longer the case once a person is discharged. More attention has been placed on an individual's right to refuse treatment, using a constitutional rather than medical malpractice approach.

Several federal actions have resulted in increased attention to the civil rights of people with disabilities, including those with a disability as a result of a mental health condition. These actions include the Americans With Disabilities Act (ADA) of 1990, the U.S. Supreme Court's *Olmstead* decision in 1999, the Mental Health Parity Act of 1996, and the Fair Housing Act of 1968, all of which specifically support the civil rights of people with disabilities relative to discrimination. The following sections describe several of these actions; readers are encouraged to further exploring this topic using agency Web sites.

The ADA is designed to assist people with disabilities in fully participating in all aspects of daily life in communities of their choosing. According to the Equal Employment Opportunity Commission (EEOC; 2009), the ADA protects people with a disability, people with a history of disability, and people perceived as having a disability. Some observers (e.g., Moss & Burris, 2007) believe that civil rights protections have been eroded in various ADA judicial decisions. The ADA Amendments Act of 2008 was intended to restore such protections. According to Moss and Burris (2007), plaintiffs with psychiatric disabilities have been perceived differently from those with physical disabilities in terms of treatment and satisfaction with outcome. In addition, plaintiffs with psychiatric disabilities received fewer settlements or favorable decisions even when other factors were controlled, raising concerns about discriminatory justice.

The *Olmstead* decision addressed structural barriers to community integration such as lack of funding portability and lack of services that leave some with serious mental illness little option but an institutional setting. In this landmark case, two qualified people with disabilities, whose physicians determined that institutional care was not medically justified, were unable to obtain state Medicaid coverage of community-based services to enable them to live outside of the institutional setting.

The U.S. Supreme Court decided for the plaintiffs and stated that remaining in a state hospital was a violation of the ADA's least-restrictive-environment aspects and constituted discrimination under Title II of the act. This ruling reiterated that people have a right to live in integrated community settings (Day, 2006). States are required to assess all people living in institutional settings to determine the least restrictive environment. Occupational therapists are well suited for leadership of such initiatives (Cottrell, 2003).

Mental Health Parity Laws

Historically, insurance coverage for mental health care has been subject to greater restriction than coverage for general medical care. Among the reasons given include the presence of a public safety net—in effect, private insurers do not have the incentive to cover serious mental illnesses because Medicaid and the state will step in to provide necessary care through the public mental health system. The federal Mental Health Parity Act of 1996 prohibited group health plans of employers with more than 50 employees that offer mental health benefits from imposing more restrictive annual or lifetime limits on spending for mental illness than for physical illness (GAO, 2000a). Mental health advocates accepted this as a first step but believed that the act did not go far enough to ensure full parity between mental health and other medical conditions. Concerns on the part of the insurance industry that parity would produce increased demand and concomitant costs were not borne out. In fact, Goldman et al. (2006) determined that managed care methodologies were more influential than the Mental Health Parity Act in determining mental health costs.

Despite the limits of the Mental Health Parity Act, it did put the issue of inequitable insurance coverage of mental illness and substance abuse at the forefront of policymakers' attention. One of the benefits has been the increase in the number of states that have some type of mental health parity or mandated benefits. To date, 32 states require some form of mental health parity (Mental Health America, 2009). Some state parity legislation is more generous than the federal Mental Health Parity Act; however, state laws do not apply to self-insured employers.

On October 3, 2008, the Paul Wellstone and Pete Domenici Mental Health Parity and Addiction Equity Act of 2008 was enacted. It has similarities to the 1996 Mental Health Parity Act. For example, the new bill does not require coverage for mental health or substance use disorders, continues to apply to all group health plans of employers with 50 or more employees, and provides an exemption for group health plans that incur a certain level of increased cost arising from complying with the law (James Mayhew, personal communication, December 18, 2008). Among the changes are that if mental health coverage is provided, any cost-sharing or treatment limitations for mental health services cannot be more restrictive than the predominant restrictions for medical services, and if out-of-network providers are covered for medical services, the same must be provided for mental health (Mental Health America, 2009).

Private Insurance and Public Mental Health Policy

Private mental health policy is affected by federal and state governments. Federal regulations that affect private mental health insurance include civil rights laws, such as the ADA; portability and privacy requirements, such as those established in the Health Insurance Portability and Accountability Act of 1996; parity require- ments as established by the Paul Wellstone and Pete Domenici Mental Health Parity and Addiction Equity Act of 2008; and compliance with accessibility standards as required by the Rehabilitation Act of 1973 and its amendments. State laws and regu- lations that affect private mental health insurance include state-level mandated ben- efits, such as by diagnosis or procedure, and state-regulated premiums and providers.

In the United States, people who have private mental health and substance abuse insurance typically get it through their employers (Mechanic, 2007). Although more people have private mental health coverage, those benefits have shrunk in terms of depth of coverage (Mechanic, 2002). Behavioral health policies use cost- containment methods to manage care. They tend to be structured like a health maintenance organization (HMO), in which care is prepaid and capitated, or carved out of the basic policy and managed separately.

According to Mechanic, Schlesinger, and McAlpine (1995), *managed care* refers to "a variety of organizational and financial structures, processes and strategies designed to influence treatment decisions and provide care in the most cost effec- tive way" (p.19). Managed care uses various strategies to influence supply and demand of mental health care (Milbank Memorial Fund, 2000). Examples of sup- ply-side incentives that are designed to influence provider behavior include gate keeping, or having a primary care provider referral necessary for all specialty vis- its; provider panels, which involve a credentialing process and contractual arrange- ment in which the panel members agree to accept referrals for a reduced fee; and capitation, in which providers enter into a contractual arrangement for a fixed fee to manage risk. Examples of demand-side incentives designed to influence policy- holder behavior include cost-sharing strategies such as copayments or reduced or no coverage if the holder goes out of network to see a provider who is not part of the approved panel. Utilization management strategies such as precertification, in which the policyholder will not be covered for services that were not authorized by the insurer before their receipt, are also common. Managed care methods encourage other cost-saving mechanisms such as hiring less expensive personnel and develop- ing a variety of less costly, non–inpatient services such as intensive outpatient pro- grams. In managed care environments, occupational therapists theoretically have opportunities to demonstrate value to payers that could improve access to services.

Policy Issues That Affect Occupational Therapists

Occupational therapists are affected by the policy areas described earlier. For example, occupational therapists who want to participate in community practice with adults with serious and persistent mental illness need to be familiar with Med- icaid policy on both the federal and state levels. Being familiar with this policy will provide occuptional therapists with information about what services are covered, how they are organized, and who the key decision makers are relative to influencing change. Occupational therapists working with clients receiving supported employ- ment, supported housing services, or both need to be aware of civil rights policies such as the ADA and the *Olmstead* decision to ensure that clients' rights are not being violated. Occupational therapists interested in expanding into an emerging practice area such as community practice with people who are homeless and who also have mental illness benefit from knowledge about state initiatives that might support occupational therapy services, such as a grant to the state or large nonprofit. Knowledge of the policy process enables occupational therapists to confidently participate in the design of mental health initiatives with key stakeholders.

Summary

This chapter describes several organizational and funding structures and key legislation that affect mental health service delivery in the United States. To effect mental health policy change, occupational therapists need to understand how key decisions are made. Access to occupational therapy services is influenced by how services are defined, organized, and funded. Knowledge of those processes is critical for ongoing and expanded access to occupational therapy services in the evolving mental health care delivery system.

References

ADA Amendments Act of 2008, Pub. L. 110–325.

American heritage dictionary of the English language (4th ed.). (2000). Boston: Houghton Mifflin.

Americans With Disabilities Act of 1990, Pub. L. 101–336, 42 U.S.C. § 12101.

Brown, R. (2001). *Addressing substance abuse and mental health problems under welfare reform: State issues and strategies.* Washington, DC: National Governors Association, Center for Best Practices.

Cottrell, R. P. F. (2003, March 10). The *Olmstead* decision: Fulfilling the promise of the ADA? Implications for occupational therapy. *OT Practice, 8,* 17–21.

Day, S. L. (2006). Issues in Medicaid policy and system transformation: Recommendations from the President's commission. *Psychiatric Services, 57,* 1713–1718.

Equal Employment Opportunity Commission. (2009). *Executive Summary: Compliance manual Section 902, definition of the term "disability."* Retrieved February 2, 2010, from www.eeoc.gov/policy/docs/902sum.html

Fair Housing Act of 1968, Pub. L. 100–420.

Foote, S. M., & Hogan, C. (2001). Disability profile and health care costs of Medicare beneficiaries under age sixty five. *Heath Affairs, 20,* 242–253.

Frank, R. G., & Glied, S. (2006). Changes in mental health financing since 1971: Implications for policymakers and patients. *Health Affairs, 25,* 601–613.

Goldman, H. H., Frank, R. G., Burnham, M. A., Huskamp, H. A., Ridgley, M. S., Normand, S. T., et al. (2006). Behavioral health insurance parity for federal employees. *New England Journal of Medicine, 354,* 1378–1386.

Health Insurance Portability and Accountability Act of 1996, Pub. L. 104–191.

Institute of Medicine. (2007). Health care transitions for young people. In Committee on Disability in America, M. J. Field, & A. M. Jette (Eds.), *The future of disability in America* (pp. 98–135). Washington, DC: National Academies Press.

Jacobson, N., & Greenley, D. (2001). What is recovery? A conceptual model and explication. *Psychiatric Services, 52,* 482–485.

Mashow, J. L., & Reno, V. P. (Eds.). (1996). *The environment of disability income policy: Programs, people, history, and context.* Washington, DC: National Academy of Social Insurance.

Mechanic, D. (2002). Removing barriers to care among persons with psychiatric symptoms. *Health Affairs, 21*(3), 137–147.

Mechanic, D. (2007). Perspective: Mental health services then and now. *Health Affairs, 26,* 1548–1550.

Mechanic, D. (2008). *Mental health and social policy: Beyond managed care* (5th ed.). New York: Allyn & Bacon.

Mechanic, D., Schlesinger, M., & McAlpine, D. (1995). Management of mental health and substance abuse services: State of the art and early results. *Milbank Quarterly, 73,* 19–55.

Mental Health America. (2007a). *Position Statement 31: Employment development of services for adults in recovery for mental illness.* Retrieved January 30, 2008, from www.mentalhealthamerica.net/go/position-statements/31

Mental Health America. (2007b). *State Children's Health Insurance Program (SCHIP).* Retrieved January 30, 2008, from www.mentalhealthamerica.net/go/schip

Mental Health America. (2009). *Fact sheet: Paul Wellstone and Pete Domenici Mental Health Parity and Addiction Equity Act of 2008.* Retrieved September 14, 2009, from http://takeaction.mentalhealthamerica.net/site/PageServer?pagename=Equity_Campaign_detailed_summary

Mental Health Parity Act of 1996, Pub. L. 104–204, 110 Stat. 2944.

Milbank Memorial Fund. (2000). *Effective public management of mental health care: Views from the states on Medicaid reform that enhance integration and accountability.* New York: Author/Bazelon Center for Mental Health Law.

Monahan, J., Swartz, M., & Bonnie, R. J. (2003). Mandated treatment in the community for people with mental disorders. *Health Affairs, 22*(5), 28–38.

Moss, K., & Burris, S. (2007). The employment discrimination provisions of the Americans with Disabilities Act: Implementation and impact. In Committee on Disability in America, M. J. Field, & A. M. Jette (Eds.), *The future of disability in America* (pp. 453–477). Washington, DC: National Academies Press.

National Governors Association. (2001). *Issue Brief—Strengthening the mental health safety net: Issues and innovations.* Washington, DC: Author. Retrieved September 15, 2009, from www.nga.org/files/pdf/mentalhealthib.pdf

Olmstead v. L. C., 527 U.S. 581 (1999).

Paul Wellstone and Pete Domenici Mental Health Parity and Addiction Equity Act of 2008, Pub. L. 110–343. Retrieved December 2, 2008, from http://takeaction.mentalhealthamerica.net/site/PageServer?pagename=Equity_Campaign_detailed_summary

Personal Responsibility and Work Opportunity Reconciliation Act of 1996, Pub. L. 104–193, 110 Stat. 2105.

Rehabilitation Act of 1973, Pub. L. 93–112, 29 U.S.C. § 701 *et seq.*

Rehabilitation Act of 1973 Amendments, Pub. L. 95–602, H.R. 12467, H. Rept. 95–1149.

Semansky, R., & Koyanagi, C. (2001). *Recovery in the community: Funding mental health rehabilitative approaches under Medicaid.* Washington, DC: Bazelon Center for Mental Health Law.

Sharfstein, S., Boronow, J., & Dickerson, F. (1999). Managed care and clinical reality in schizophrenia treatment. *Health Affairs, 18*(5), 66–70.

Smith, G., Kennedy, C., Knipper, S., O'Brien, J., & O'Keeffe, J. (2005). *Using Medicaid to support working age adults with serious mental illness in the community: A handbook.* Washington, DC: U.S. Department of Health and Human Services, Office of the Assistant Secretary for Planning and Evaluation.

Social Security Online. (2009). *About Ticket to Work.* Retrieved April 20, 2008, from www.ssa.gov/work/aboutticket.html

Ticket to Work and Work Incentives Improvement Act of 1999, Pub. L. 106–170, 113 Stat. 1860.

U.S. Department of Health and Human Services. (1999). *Mental health: A report of the Surgeon General.* Rockville, MD: U.S. Department of Health and Human Services, Substance Abuse and Mental Health Services Administration, Center for Mental Health Services & National Institute of Mental Health. Retrieved November 17, 2009, from www.surgeongeneral.gov/library/mentalhealth/home.html

U.S. General Accounting Office. (2000a). *Implementation of HIPAA: Progress slow in enforcing federal standards in nonconforming states* (Report to the Chairman, Committee on Health, Education, Labor, and Pensions, U.S. Senate, GAO/HEHS–00–85). Washington, DC: Author.

U.S. General Accounting Office. (2000b). *Mental health: Community-based care increases for people with serious mental illness* (Report to the Committee on Finance, U.S. Senate, GAO–01–224). Washington, DC: Author.

Whittaker, J. (2005). *Social Security Disability Insurance (SSDI) and Medicare: The 24-month waiting period for SSDI beneficiaries under age 65* (Order Code RS22195). Washington, DC: Library of Congress, Congressional Research Service. Retrieved April 22, 2008, from http://digital.library.unt.edu/govdocs/crs/permalink/meta-crs-7749:1

Wieman, D. A., & Dorwart, R. A. (1999). A comparison of public and privatized approaches to managed behavioral health care for persons with serious mental illness. *Mental Health Services Research, 1,* 159–170.

Your Ticket to Work. (n.d.). *The ticket program.* Retrieved January 27, 2008, from www.yourtickettowork.com/program_info

CHAPTER 18

Collaborative Work With Teams and Policymakers

*Deborah B. Pitts, MBA, OTR/L, CPRP, BCMH,
and Karla W. Gray, OTR/L, LICSW*

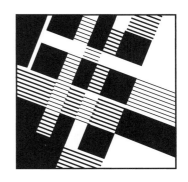

Learning Objectives

After reading this material and completing the examination, readers will be able to

- Identify the specific systems-level mandates creating the opportunity for occupational therapists to collaborate with other mental health professionals and policymakers,

- Identify and delineate the issues around and successful methods for communicating with payers to obtain reimbursement for occupational therapy services in mental health settings,

- Identify and delineate the issues around and successful methods for working effectively with other mental health professionals for systems change, and

- Identify and delineate the issues and possible successful methods for advocating at the public policy level for systems change.

In light of the findings and recommendations of the President's New Freedom Commission on Mental Health (2003) and given the complexities of the mental health system, how can the profession of occupational therapy, as well as individual occupational therapists, help facilitate a well-coordinated and high-quality mental health service system to meet the needs of children and adults at risk for mental illness and those living with the effects of illness? Moreover, how can therapists have an impact on the mental health system to increase occupational therapy's visibility and presence? Cottrell (2007) argued that the President's New Freedom Commission provided particular opportunities for occupational therapy in the areas of practice, advocacy, and research. This chapter considers particular aspects of those questions as they relate to advanced practice—specifically, working effectively with other mental health professionals, communicating with payers of mental health services, and advocating at the public policy level.

Contextualizing the Questions

Historical reviews have noted that the need for well-coordinated mental health services emerged as a result of the deinstitutionalization of the 1950s and 1960s (Mechanic & Rochefort, 1990). Before deinstitutionalization, the mental health system consisted primarily of community and state inpatient psychiatric hospitals, with limited aftercare services. However, by the 1970s a critical need emerged for a coordinated system of care, at least to meet the needs of community-dwelling people with psychiatric disabilities (Carling, 1995; Mechanic, 2007). It was argued that this system of care needed to go beyond a focus on mental health services alone and include health and dental care, housing, income support and entitlements, protection and advocacy, family and community support, peer support, and rehabilitation services (Stroul, 1986, 1989). These early efforts resulted in the emergence of a new type of service provider—the case manager (Floersch, 2002).

Moreover, the landmark Surgeon General's report on mental health (U.S. Department of Health and Human Services, 1999), followed by the final report of the President's New Freedom Commission on Mental Health (2003) and the Substance Abuse and Mental Health Services Administration's (2005) transformation action agenda report, emphasized the fragmented nature of the U.S. mental health system. The Surgeon General's report documented the continued complexity of the system, noting that it contains multiple service sectors and settings and varied durations of care funded by a dual structure of private and public financing.

In addition to these reports, the Institute of Medicine's (2005) Quality Chasm initiative addressed concerns about quality in mental health and substance abuse health care. The report asserted that

> mental health and substance abuse health care—like general health care—is often ineffective, not patient centered, untimely, inefficient, inequitable, and at times unsafe. It, too, requires fundamental redesign. Mental, substance-use, and general illnesses are highly interrelated, especially with respect to chronicity. Improving care delivery and health outcomes for any one of the three depends upon improving care delivery and outcomes for the others. (p. 56)

Further quality concerns focus on the behavioral health workforce, specifically (1) the readiness of new professional program graduates to practice in the current health care environment; (2) the limited access of those already in practice to effective continuing education for emerging evidence-based models of practice; (3) minimal training received by practitioners without graduate degrees, even though they may have the most contact with clients; and (4) the limited access that consumers and family members have to training despite the enormous role that they play as primary caregivers (Hoge, 2002; Hoge, Jacobs, Belitsky, & Migdole, 2002). The Annapolis Coalition on the Behavioral Health Workforce (www.annapoliscoalition.org) has outlined the necessary steps to achieve certain goals and to address quality concerns, including health care coverage, caregiving, and readiness of health professionals. The Annapolis Coalition's report indicates that to address the nation's growing crisis surrounding efforts to recruit, retain, and effectively train a prevention and treatment workforce in the mental health and addiction sectors of this field, the following steps must take place (Hoge et al., 2007):

- Evidence-based practices must be taught.
- Teaching methods must demonstrate effectiveness in building skills.
- Competencies must be identified and the competency of individual trainees assessed.
- Curricula should cover skill development related to clinical, rehabilitative, and recovery approaches to treatment; communication and shared decision making with consumers and families; maximizing patient safety and reducing errors in care; practicing in managed health systems; treating people with co-occurring mental illness and addictions; collaborating with primary (medical) care providers; and providing culturally competent care.
- Training experiences must be interdisciplinary.
- Training sites and experiences should parallel those that trainees will encounter after training completion.
- The diversity of the community should be reflected by those preparing to enter the clinical workforce.
- Consumers and families must have a role as educators in the training program.

Recently, American Occupational Therapy Association (AOTA) Presidents Carolyn Baum and Penelope Moyers Cleveland, partly in response to Representative Assembly motions, appointed ad hoc work groups targeting opportunities and threats to occupational therapy in mental health practice (AOTA President's Ad Hoc Committee on Mental Health Practice in Occupational Therapy, 2006; AOTA Representative Assembly Ad Hoc Workgroup on Policy Barriers and Strategies to Gain QMHP Status for Occupational Therapy, 2006; AOTA Workgroup on Occupational Therapy in Mental Health Systems, 2005). The initial work group report (AOTA Workgroup on Occupational Therapy in Mental Health Systems, 2005) laid the groundwork, recommending specific action strategies (Table 18.1) to counter three broad areas representing threats and opportunities to the promotion of occupational therapy within the mental health system:

1. The readiness of occupational therapists to practice in the current environment informed by evidence-based mental health practices, particularly in leadership roles;
2. Public policy and regulatory issues regarding mental health practice, particularly for adults and children at risk for or with serious and persistent mental illness; and
3. Payment or reimbursement sources for occupational therapy and mental health services.

Working Effectively With Other Mental Health Professionals

Abbott (1988) defined *professions* as "exclusive occupational groups applying somewhat abstract knowledge to particular cases" (p. 8). Moreover, he stated that

Table 18.1. Action Strategies Recommended by the American Occupational Therapy Association's Mental Health Work Group

Strategy	Example
Influence the readiness of occupational therapists to participate in mental health systems.	• Develop, fund, and implement a national initiative that would actively recruit, prepare, and support advanced-practice occupational therapists to take on targeted leadership roles in mental health systems.
	• Conduct evidence-based reviews of occupational therapy practice consistent with outcomes that are meaningful to mental health systems, that is, increased days in community placements, reduction in staff hours, reduction in crisis calls, decreased number of community complaints, sustained work, academic achievements, and decrease in substance misuse in older adults.
	• Develop, fund, and implement a national initiative in partnership with occupational therapy mental health educators, their educational institutions, and coalitions for behavioral health to ensure that current and future entry-level occupational therapists are prepared to implement evidence-based mental health practices.
Influence public policy at the state and federal levels to promote participation of occupational therapy as a core mental health profession.	• Track and analyze public policy issues related to mental health systems for which occupational therapists are well suited to be responsive.
	• Advocate for occupational therapy to be identified as a core mental health profession in all federal documents.
	• Encourage and take a proactive stance with state occupational therapy associations to assist them in their legislative efforts to have occupational therapists identified as qualified mental health providers.
Influence payment for occupational therapy for people at risk for or with psychiatric disorders.	• Advocate with behavioral health managed care organizations to pay for occupational therapy for psychiatric disorders.

Source. American Occupational Therapy Association, Workgroup on Occupational Therapy in Mental Health Systems (2005).

"professions constitute an interdependent system" (p. 86) and that within that system they negotiate and claim particular practice jurisdictions. He argued that internal and external system perturbations, in particular social and cultural change, result in the emergence of practice claims by particular professions seeking to sustain or expand their jurisdictions. Shifts in explanatory models for etiology of mental illness (i.e., biological vs. psychosocial perspectives) and resultant intervention approaches (i.e., deinstitutionalization) and the resultant reorganization of services represents an example of such social and cultural change internal to the mental health system. The civil rights, women's rights, gay rights, and disability rights movements represent external social and cultural changes that have affected the mental health system. As therapists reflect on their own practice contexts, they should consider what other internal and external social and cultural changes have affected their relationship with other mental health providers.

The workplace serves as an arena in which professional groups make jurisdictional claims (Abbott, 1988). Claims made in the workplace focus on who can control and supervise the work and who is qualified to do which parts of it. Although professions use legal and regulatory, as well as public opinion, arenas to establish and support claims, the actual divisions of labor are established through negotiation and custom by the specific providers in a particular practice context. So in some instances, occupational therapists in mental health settings will address all occupational areas, what Meyer (1922) called "the big four—work, rest, play, and

Table 18.2. Three Models of Professional Collaboration

Model	Description
Multidisciplinary	• Each practitioner completes profession-specific evaluation and intervention plan and treats separately. • Practitioners from different professions meet to share information (i.e., case conference), but each profession works separately.
Interdisciplinary	• Each practitioner may evaluate separately or with other professionals. • An integrated plan is developed, but each practitioner treats problems or needs identified in his or her evaluation. • Team members have an increased level of communication before and after their individual interventions and may cotreat.
Transdisciplinary	• Evaluations, treatment plans, and interventions are often carried out jointly. • Intentional role exchange occurs when a practitioner from one profession carries out a program recommended by another professional.

Source. Paul & Peterson (2001).

recreation" (p. 6), whereas in others, they will share evaluation and intervention with nursing, recreational therapy, vocational rehabilitation, or other mental health providers.

Abbott (1988) went on to emphasize that the "real complexity" (p. 65) of professional practices is represented in the workplace, as opposed to the legal or public opinion arenas, because the workplace is not only where the differences between different types of providers must be negotiated but also where the differences among individual providers of a particular profession must be resolved. For example, each occupational therapist builds a unique skill set and perspective regarding his or her practice and brings them to bear in each new setting in which he or she works. As occupational therapists enter and leave jobs within particular workplaces, jurisdictional claims are renegotiated with other providers (i.e., recreational therapy, social work).

The most common structure of service provision in mental health settings is that of the team. The fact that team members bring their individual and professional perspectives to inter-, multi-, and transdisciplinary teamwork may help frame workplace jurisdictional claim negotiation (Table 18.2). These varied perspectives represent to some degree the evolution regarding theoretical and practical ways of working across teams (Paul & Peterson, 2001; Rushmer & Pallis, 2003). The culture of each team is an amalgamation of the respective conceptualizations carried forth by individual team members. Easen, Atkins, and Dyson (2000) found that members of health care teams reported that effective communication was "essential for understanding both differing perspectives and differing expectations of what each could do" (p. 358).

Conditions under which collaboration occurs contribute to the success or failure of the process. As noted previously, the workplace demands and identified responsibilities of the participants therein influence practitioners' physical, cognitive, and emotional availability. The extent to which practitioner responsibilities are determined by regulation or agency policy, the availability of time and other resources, and the perceived status of the various professions represented contributes to the complexity of the process. "Moreover, the conditions of professional work varied significantly between different levels and branches of the same service, and between individuals at the same level working in different contexts, thereby creating difficulties for intra-agency collaboration" (Easen et al., 2000, p. 358).

In addition to these factors, successful interprofessional collaboration appears to require time. As noted by Eason et al. (2000), health care team members reported that a minimum of 3 years was needed to develop the reliable working relationships necessary to support "effective, multi-professional collaboration" (p. 362), especially when working on projects of significance. Outcomes arrived at through a commitment of significant time and resources on the part of participants tended to be more sustainable than those achieved by short-lived work groups. Moreover, whether the level of interprofessional understanding deepened over the extended course of the work or whether time merely allowed exploration of a greater scope of options remains a question.

Consistent with the focus on teamwork and the strong commitment to community-based interventions in the contemporary public mental health system, the community mental health team has become the primary method of service delivery. In the United States and internationally, occupational therapists are members of such teams, along with psychiatrists, psychologists, social workers, psychiatric nurses, mental health consumers, family members, and others. Internationally, occupational therapists have expressed concern regarding the obligation of practicing as generalists on such teams (Lloyd, King, & Bassett, 2002; Parker, 2001), in particular teams following the assertive community treatment philosophy. Other mental health providers have expressed similar concerns regarding role blurring and loss of professional identity when working on such teams (Brown, Crawford, & Darongkamas, 2000). As noted earlier, such dilemmas are not unique to mental health teams. Recommendations regarding teamwork in health care have emphasized the need for a "reflective ethic" (Drinka & Clark, 2000, p. 64). That is, health care providers working in collaborative settings need to become more aware of how their own professional backgrounds, training, work experience, and relationships have shaped who they are and how they think (p. 64).

Although occupational therapists are on publicly funded (i.e., Medicaid and other state revenues) community mental health teams in the United States, their numbers are inconsistent across states and certainly are fewer than those of other mental health professionals. This situation is partially the result of occupational therapists not being identified as core or qualified mental health providers[1] at the federal level (AOTA Representative Assembly Ad Hoc Workgroup on Policy Barriers and Strategies to Gain QMHP Status for Occupational Therapy, 2006; AOTA Workgroup on Occupational Therapy in Mental Health Systems, 2005). Although some states have identified occupational therapists as eligible mental health providers for publicly funded services, including serving as the single fixed point of responsibility, they do not usually have the authority to open a case. In addition, occupational therapists often require a qualified mental health provider to cosign the care, service, or treatment plan, despite occupational therapists' being identified as mental health providers by the U.S. Public Health Service's (PHS; 2004) Office of Force Readiness and Deployment and the presence of occupational therapists on

---

[1]*Qualified mental health providers* include psychiatrists, psychologists, licensed clinical social workers and, in some states, advanced nurse practitioners and licensed professional counselors.

U.S. Army Medical Department Combat Stress Control teams. As a result, in some states, recruitment and retention of occupational therapists in public mental health services has been limited (AOTA Representative Assembly Ad Hoc Workgroup on Policy Barriers and Strategies to Gain QMHP Status for Occupational Therapy, 2006).

Communicating With Payers

Although health (or sickness) insurance has existed in the United States since the mid-1800s, payers may be working with a definition of occupational therapy that is exclusive rather than inclusive of mental or behavioral health diagnoses on the "covered diagnoses list." Inclusion of occupational therapy for behavioral disorders and mental illness is a relatively new but growing phenomenon (Hester, 2009). At the same time, care or benefits managers within various companies may not be aware of occupational therapy's role within behavioral health. On the basis of their understanding of occupational therapy, care managers may deny coverage of services that benefit the consumer. This creates a quagmire for occupational therapists and for the consumer seeking services.

Some insurance systems, such as Medicare, subcontract with third parties to administer the insurance plan. Depending on the agreement with the parent company, the intermediary may have the authority to further refine or restrict the extent of coverage for any condition in its Local Medical Review Policy and Local Coverage Determinations (Centers for Medicare and Medicaid Services [CMS], 2007), thereby creating additional barriers to treatment. Compounding the situation is the employer's or consumer's choice of plan when the insurance is purchased. Some plans are so restrictive that the only treatment covered is emergency medical care.

The restriction of coverage is not a malicious action on the part of insurance companies. It is done through a logical process that seeks to balance cost and benefit to the individual and the company. Discussions with payers must take these factors into consideration. In-the-moment direct benefit negotiation may be called for on a case-by-case basis; however, the education of internal decision makers such as the care manager is the most effective long-term solution to the issue of coverage. A significant amount of preliminary work goes into the educational process.

Along with having the current definition of occupational therapy and descriptors of practice outcomes, the advocate will need to know the parties within the organization and their respective functions in the scope-of-coverage decision process. Initial contact may be at the level of the care manager, a person who may or may not have formulated his or her own definition of occupational therapy. This person can be a strong internal advocate if educated gently and given documents such as the *Occupational Therapy Practice Framework: Domain and Process* (AOTA, 2008) to share or reference in the future. A variety of tools may be used to educate care managers about the scope and role of occupational therapy in mental health. One resource is Cottrell's (2000) *Proactive Approaches in Psychosocial Occupational Therapy*. *Occupational Therapy and Mental Health* (Creek & Lougher, 2008) also contains useful examples of occupational therapy interventions with people with mental illness.

These same documents will be helpful in the educational process throughout the organization, but some people will want hard data to support covering occupational therapy in claims of people with mental illness. Data from the local or state employment office that tell how many workers are unemployed because of mental illness will be helpful in this discussion, as will the national figures of average work days lost because of mental illness. Data are also available regarding the use of emergency rooms or urgent care facilities and the frequency of physician office visits and can be roughly translated into both lost revenue (premiums) and higher benefit cost and used to educate the people who attend to the company's financial aspects.

Concerted efforts of local practitioners or state associations may influence changes in local medical review policies and will open the gates for discussions at the higher regional and corporate levels. In organizations as geographically extended and large as national insurers, policy change will occur slowly, and future generations of practitioners will benefit from the efforts undertaken today. Particularly in situations where intermediaries are used, significant time and resources are invested in tracing local interpretations back to company policy and promoting revision of either.

The same may be true of federal and state programs such as Medicare and Medicaid, although the internal structures of these programs are different from that of private industry. Although CMS administers the programs, it does so on the basis of congressional direction. The formulas used to determine the rates, scope of services covered, and criteria for service provision come from laws passed in Congress and exist until those laws are changed. Grassroots advocacy through the legislative process has been used successfully to modify interpretation of rules and continues to be the most effective strategy for effecting change in any arena. The key to success is to keep all the parties engaged in the process throughout the course of education and negotiation.

Advocating at the Public Policy Level

Occupational therapists practicing in the mental health sector, like other health care professionals, have a responsibility to advocate at the local, state, and federal levels for governmental policy that will support the full participation of people they serve. Moreover, advocacy is needed to optimize occupational therapists' opportunity to facilitate that participation. In response to the AOTA *Centennial Vision* (AOTA, 2007), occupational therapists are concerned with public policy[2] in specific strategic areas—children and youth; health and wellness; mental health; productive aging; rehabilitation, disability, and participation; and work and industry.

Occupational therapists practicing in the mental health sector have focused their policy-monitoring efforts, in particular, on access to health and mental health services (i.e., mental health parity, Medicaid mental health, rehabilitation and recovery), the focus of mental health services (i.e., occupational engagement and recovery), access to federal transfer payments (i.e., Social Security Disability Income and Supplemental Security Income), discrimination in housing (i.e., fair housing laws), and employment and education (i.e., American With Disabilities Act of 1990, Individuals With Disabilities Education Act of 1990).

---

[2] *Public policy* is defined as the set of policies (laws, plans, actions, behaviors) of a government. Because governments claim authority and responsibility (to varying degrees) over a large group of individuals, they see fit to establish plans and methods of action that will govern society. ("Public policy," n.d.)

Successful public policy advocacy in the mental health sector requires occupational therapists and occupational therapy's professional associations to partner and collaborate with advocacy groups such as the National Alliance on Mental Illness (www.nami.org); mental health consumers and their organizations, for example, the National Coalition of Mental Health Consumer/Survivor Organizations (www. ncmhcso.org); other professional associations, including the U.S. Psychiatric Rehabilitation Association (www.uspra.org) and the National Council for Community Behavioral Healthcare (www.thenationalcouncil.org); and other groups that monitor and advocate for access, equity, and nondiscrimination, for example, the Mental Health Liaison Group (www.mhlg.org), the Campaign for Mental Health Reform (www.mhreform.org), the National Association of State Mental Health Program Directors (www.nasmhpd.org), and the Bazelon Center for Mental Health Law (www.bazelon.org).

AOTA has partnered with some of these organizations to advocate for particular public policy initiatives that argue for particular understandings of and approaches to meeting the needs of people at risk for or having psychiatric disabilities, such as mental health parity. Moreover, like AOTA, the organizations have information on their Web sites that serves as a valuable resource to help individual occupational therapists stay up to date on public policy issues of concern to their practice in the mental health sector. In addition, some organizations have local and state chapters in which individual therapists can participate as part of their commitment to public policy advocacy.

Public policy is influenced by myriad factors, only one of which is the individual consumer's needs or opinions. At the national level, forces that affect outcomes include priorities set by the current administration, financial viability, philosophies of the ranking political party, personal values of the law makers and rule makers directly involved, and the extent to which one is able to leverage one's priorities against those of others who are seeking to move in different directions. Similar pressures may be more visible to the constituent at the state or local level because of the greater degree of media coverage and geographic proximity.

The multitude of potential roadblocks to policy change requires a focused and consistent effort over time. Many ideas are put forth in the form of bills that do not become law in their first year: "About 6% of all legislation introduced in Congress actually passes" (Jenks, 2006). One source that offers fairly up-to-date information about the progression of bills through Congress is the Library of Congress Web site (http://thomas.gov).

The identification of something that needs to be changed is often the first step in the process of advocating for a change in public policy. Proceeding in advocacy from the assumption that the status quo is broken or requires fixing sets the stage for conflict and defeat. Reframing the situation as the positive outcome one wants to see lays a platform from which collaborative relationships can grow and develop. People from opposite sides of an issue can come together over a common value to develop collaborative solutions (Easen et al., 2000).

Before approaching an organization's governing body with a proposal for change, it is important to research the background and current state of the issue. In doing so, dissenters and advocates for the desired change can be identified and information regarding the environment of change can be gathered. Few concerns are truly localized, and it is important to evaluate the state of affairs at a macro level rather than at a micro level to ensure consideration of all potential forces for and against the proposed change (Badaracco, 2003).

An environmental analysis will identify sources of support outside the immediately affected group or area. Broadening the base of support by involving many people who support the values on which the change is predicated increases the probability of success. A similar value system will not, however, remove all obstacles. Successful negotiation requires respect, perseverance, and flexibility (Neff, Citrin, & Friedman, 2005). Policy change involves a conscious shift in conceptualization, a process that occurs at different rates for every person involved. Awareness of and appreciation for the constraints within which other members of the coalition are operating is imperative if change is to occur without undue delays.

Many policymakers, consumers and families, professionals, and members of the general public have a consensus in principle in some areas, including alleviation of stigma, access to treatment, individual responsibility and choice, and freedom. These areas of concordance became clear during the hearings held by the President's New Freedom Commission on Mental Health and were incorporated as the overarching principles on which its recommendations for change were based (President's New Freedom Commission on Mental Health, 2003). The commission's report provided a centralizing document around which disparate groups could unite and move forward toward a functional system of service delivery.

Occupational therapists contribute to this process through local organizations, national memberships, and direct advocacy (contact with legislators, payers, providers, families). As noted earlier, familiarity with the President's New Freedom Commission on Mental Health's (2003) final report, as well as other federal reports, AOTA position papers and previous work toward specific policy change, congressional delegates' assignments, and the structure of rule-making bodies is important for therapists who choose to pursue policy change.

Summary

The need for collaboration in mental health practice has been influenced by multiple factors, including the complexity of the life circumstances and illness experience for many people with psychiatric disabilities; the significant growth in the understanding of both the illness experience and the process of recovery; the complexity of and need to work across all service systems to promote recovery (i.e., criminal justice, social services, vocational rehabilitation, primary health care, mental health care); and the call to end the historical "silo" nature of professional education and practice.

The complexity of factors related to successful collaboration requires all practitioners to keep their eye on the prize—that is, to stay focused on the desired outcomes of the people that they serve (Rushmer & Pallis, 2003). Moreover, it demands that each practitioner have clarity regarding his or her particular practice values and role; be open to and respect others' practice perspective; and have a capacity for critical dialogue and reflection when perspectives collide (Rushmer & Pallis, 2003). Without such a focus, professional territoriality can inadvertently prevent consumer recovery.

Compounding the issue is the reality that effective collaboration with other mental health professionals and policymakers requires advanced practice knowledge, reasoning, and performance skill sets. Early in their careers, professionals are quite often more focused on other professional issues. The depth of experiences that advanced practitioners have lends credibility to their statements and recommendations when dealing with policymakers and others who strive to address the big picture.

References

Abbott, A. (1988). *The system of professions: An essay on the division of expert labor.* Chicago: University of Chicago Press.

American Occupational Therapy Association. (2007). AOTA's *Centennial Vision* and executive summary. *American Journal of Occupational Therapy, 61*(6), 613–614.

American Occupational Therapy Association. (2008). Occupational therapy practice framework: Domain and process (2nd ed.). *American Journal of Occupational Therapy, 62,* 625–683.

American Occupational Therapy Association, President's Ad Hoc Committee on Mental Health Practice in Occupational Therapy. (2006, December 18). *Discussion and recommendations of 2006 Ad Hoc Group on Mental Health.* Bethesda, MD: Author. Retrieved December 1, 2009, from www.aota.org/News/Centennial/AdHoc/2006/40406.aspx

American Occupational Therapy Association, Representative Assembly Ad Hoc Workgroup on Policy Barriers and Strategies to Gain QMHP Status for Occupational Therapy. (2006). *Committee report.* Bethesda, MD: Author.

American Occupational Therapy Association, Workgroup on Occupational Therapy in Mental Health Systems. (2005, October 12). *Promotion of OT in mental health systems* (Report to the American Occupational Therapy Association Board of Directors). Bethesda, MD: Author. Retrieved December 1, 2009, from www.aota.org/News/Centennial/AdHoc/41327/41347.aspx

Americans With Disabilities Act of 1990, Pub. L. 101–336, 42 U.S.C. § 12101.

Badaracco, J. L. (2003). *We don't need another hero.* Boston: Harvard Business School.

Brown, B., Crawford, P., & Darongkamas, J. (2000). Blurred roles and permeable boundaries: The experience of multidisciplinary working in community mental health. *Health and Social Care in the Community, 8*(6), 425–435.

Centers for Medicare and Medicaid Services. (2007). *The Medicare Medical Review Program.* Retrieved February 11, 2010, from www.cms.hhs.gov/MLNProducts/downloads/MedReviewProgbroch07.pdf

Carling, P. J. (1995). *Return to community: Building support systems for people with psychiatric disabilities.* New York: Guilford Press.

Cottrell, R. P. F. (2000). *Proactive approaches in psychosocial occupational therapy.* Thorofare, NJ: Slack.

Cottrell, R. P. F. (2007). The New Freedom Initiative—Transforming mental health care: Will OT be at the table? *Occupational Therapy in Mental Health, 23*(2), 1–25.

Creek, J., & Lougher, L. (Eds.). (2008). *Occupational therapy and mental health* (4th ed.) New York: Churchill Livingstone

Drinka, T. J. K., & Clark, P. G. (2000). *Health care teamwork: Interdisciplinary practice and teaching.* Westport, CT: Auburn House.

Easen, P., Atkins, M., & Dyson, A. (2000). Inter-professional collaboration and conceptualisations of practice. *Children and Society, 14*(5), 355–367.

Floersch, J. (2002). *Meds, money, and manners: The case management of severe mental illness.* New York: Columbia University Press.

Hester, T., Sr. (2009). *Legislative panels approve autism health coverage.* Retrieved June 6, 2009, from www.newjerseynewsroom.com/state/legislative-panels-approve-autism-health-coverage

Hoge, M. A. (2002). The training gap: An acute crisis in behavioral health education. *Administration and Policy in Mental Health, 29*(4/5), 305–317.

Hoge, M. A., Jacobs, S., Belitsky, R., & Migdole, S. (2002). Graduate education and training for contemporary behavioral health practice. *Administration and Policy in Mental Health, 29*(4/5), 335–357.

Hoge, M. A., Morris, J. A., Daniels, A. S., Stuart, G. W., Huey, L. Y., & Adams., N. (2007). *An action plan for behavioral health workforce development* (No. 280–02–0302). Rockville, MD: U.S. Department of Health and Human Services, Substance Abuse and Mental Health Services Administration.

Individuals With Disabilities Education Act of 1990, Pub. L. 101–476, 20 U.S.C., Ch. 33.

Institute of Medicine. (2005). *Improving the quality of health care for mental and substance-use conditions.* Washington, DC: National Academies Press.

Jenks, P. (2006, February 7). *CongressLine by GalleryWatch.com: A bill in Congress.* Retrieved February 2, 2010, from www.llrx.com/congress/billincongress.htm

Lloyd, C., King, R., & Bassett, H. (2002). A survey of Australian mental health occupational therapists. *British Journal of Occupational Therapy, 65,* 88–96.

Mechanic, D. (2007). Mental health services then and now. *Health Affairs, 26*(6), 1548–1550.

Mechanic, D., & Rochefort, D. A. (1990). Deinstitutionalization: An appraisal of reform. *Annual Review of Sociology, 16*(1), 301–327.

Meyer, A. (1922). The philosophy of occupation therapy. *Archives of Occupational Therapy, 1*(1), 1–10.

Neff, T. J., Citrin, J. M., & Friedman, C. (2005). *You're in charge—Now what?* New York: Three Rivers Press.

Parker, H. (2001). The role of occupational therapists in community mental health teams: Generic or specialist? *British Journal of Occupational Therapy, 64,* 609–610.

Paul, S., & Peterson, C. Q. (2001). Interprofessional collaboration: Issues for practice and research. *Occupational Therapy in Health Care, 15*(3/4), 1–12.

President's New Freedom Commission on Mental Health. (2003). *Achieving the promise: Transforming mental health care in America* (Final Report; DHHS Pub. SMA–03–3832). Rockville, MD: Author.

Public policy. (n.d.). Retrieved January 19, 2009, from www.allwords.com/word-public+policy.html

Rushmer, R., & Pallis, G. (2003). Interprofessional working: The wisdom of integrated working and the disaster of blurred boundaries. *Public Money and Management, 23*(1), 59–66.

Stroul, B. A. (1986). *Models of community support services: Approaches to helping persons with long-term mental illness.* Washington, DC: National Institute of Mental Health.

Stroul, B. A. (1989). Community support systems for persons with long-term mental illness: A conceptual framework. *Psychosocial Rehabilitation Journal, 12*(3), 9–26.

Substance Abuse and Mental Health Services Administration. (2005). *Transforming mental health care in America—The federal action agenda: First steps.* Rockville, MD: Author.

U.S. Department of Health and Human Services. (1999). *Mental health: A report of the Surgeon General.* Rockville, MD: U.S. Department of Health and Human Services, Substance Abuse and Mental Health Services Administration, Center for Mental Health Services & National Institute of Mental Health. Retrieved November 17, 2009, from www.surgeongeneral.gov/library/mentalhealth/home.html

U.S. Public Health Service. (2004). *A guide for the deployment of therapist officers.* Washington, DC: Author.

CHAPTER 19

Community Resources and Care Management

Karla W. Gray, OTR/L, LICSW

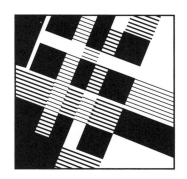

Learning Objectives

After reading this material and completing the examination, readers will be able to

- Recognize the similarities and differences among care management models,

- Recognize considerations that influence the provision of care management services to children and isolated older adults with mental illness,

- Identify circumstances that support implementation of advance planning and directives, and

- Identify community support services.

People with mental illness, regardless of age, often have difficulty successfully performing the complex instrumental activities of daily living (IADLs). Illness creates barriers to effective social participation, work, and even play. Enjoyment of leisure activity is, for many people, an experience associated with a past, more functional stage of life. These same people engage in active treatment, sometimes with supervision from others, taking medication and attending therapies as prescribed. For many of them, however, a disconnect exists that requires further intervention to alleviate. A common strategy used in both public and private mental health service systems to bridge this disconnect is that of care (or case) management. The *care manager* is simultaneously a broker of service, skill instructor, conflict mediator, and cheerleader. The theoretical and evidence base of occupational therapy and its unique perspective on the interaction between the person and the environment make occupational therapists exceptionally qualified to assume this responsibility. This chapter describes various models of care management and their application to occupational therapy.

Scope of Care Management

Care managers form the backbone of formal support within the federally mandated aging and long-term care service and public mental health systems. Other systems, such as private and public child foster care and drug rehabilitation and those providing services to people with developmental delay or medical complications, use care managers with targeted focus areas. In mental health systems, the care manager is the primary contact person for many and facilitates access to a wide range of resources and services (Cottrell, 2000).

A cursory Internet search performed August 30, 2008, using the phrase *community mental health and case manager,* indicated that case management is a key component of service in virtually every community mental health agency nationwide. Exploration on a more detailed level revealed that several private agencies now provide this service as well. The care manager has more contact with the client than any other provider within the system. Depending on the person's needs, the care manager may check with him or her about medication adherence, assist with making a grocery list and guide him or her in selecting products to ensure the person stays within budget during the shopping trip, guide the budgeting to cover the month's expenses, or structure a homemaking routine that is both tolerable and healthy. The care manager is often the one who relays the family's observations and concerns to the larger treatment team and supports the client in the treatment planning process.

The public mental health system tends to treat care management as an entry-level position, but it requires advanced skills and tested clinical judgment (Cottrell, 2000). The care manager is essentially the service recipient's life coach, and it is essential that the guidance provided be supported by a planned, deliberate, sequential process that enables the person to develop skills and increase independence to the extent that she or he desires (Summers, 2006). Occupational therapists have a framework and skill set that is uniquely suited to providing comprehensive care management.

Occupational therapists look at not only performance and client factors but also the demands of the activity and the contexts within which clients must operate (American Occupational Therapy Association, 2008). Disconnects can occur at the junctures of these aspects of participation. The community, including treatment providers, may have expectations of a client that are in direct conflict with his or her abilities or interests. Occupational therapists, in the role of care manager, are perfectly situated to assess and mediate that dialectic as the client develops skills or compensatory strategies.

Models of Care Management

Within the realm of human services, various case or care management models are used. Woodside and McClam (2006) divided care management into three primary categories: (1) responsibility based, (2) role based, and (3) organization based. Each type of care management is used at various points within the mental health system.

Responsibility-Based Care Management

When a client is transitioning from acute, intensive mental health services to a less formal support system, he or she moves to *responsibility-based care management*

(Woodside & McClam, 2006). The client's informal support system assumes care management, and the care manager provides support but few direct services to that informal system. The core of the informal support system is often the immediate family of the person with mental illness along with others with whom he or she comes in regular contact. In this situation, the care manager may have minimal contact with the identified client unless she or he or the support system identifies a need for greater involvement.

Case Example: Susan

Susan is 26 years old and striving to develop autonomy from her family, with whom she has lived her entire life. She was recently discharged from the psychiatric unit of a general hospital and moved to her own apartment, where a member of her family checks on her daily, asking her about her diet, medication regime, leisure pursuits, and so forth. Susan is not happy with this arrangement and is refusing to open the door to her family or return their calls. A care manager meets with Susan and her parents and siblings weekly to clarify the difference between actions that support Susan's independence and those that undermine their relationship with her. The care manager assists the family with identifying alternative activities they can use as vehicles to interact with Susan while respecting her desire for autonomy. The care manager also routinely speaks with Susan's apartment manager to ensure that he has no concerns about Susan's safety, behavior, or rental payments. When concerns do arise, the care manager coaches the landlord on communication strategies that clearly articulate the landlord's concerns and support Susan's development.

Role-Based Care Management

Role-based care management, as Woodside and McClam (2006) described it, is consistent with that which is commonly provided to clients with mental illness who have greater needs for support. The care manager assumes a variety of responsibilities that are directed toward maintaining the person in the community at the highest level of functioning. Care managers often have large caseloads and act as broker, counselor, problem solver, record keeper, or planner–coordinator as their clients' needs change, connecting them to the various community entities that can best meet their needs at the time. The goal of this process is to meet the client's needs through a single point of access and prevent service fragmentation, which could result in decompensation or deterioration of function. Kanter (1989) referred to this type of care management as *clinical case management.*

Case Example: Mike

Mike is a client of the local community mental health agency. His care manager meets with him individually at least monthly to help him plan how to meet his commitments for the next 2 weeks. The care manager provides transportation for Mike to attend appointments with his psychiatrist and outpatient therapist, and he drives Mike to the pharmacy to pick up his medication. When Mike's therapist suggested that Mike apply for vocational rehabilitation services, the care manager assisted him in filling out the application and making the appointment. The care manager also addresses Mike's friends' concerns (with Mike's written permission) by educating them about Mike's mental illness and how they can support him.

Organization-Based Care Management

The most global model, the organization-based model, serves as a framework for programs such as assertive community treatment (ACT; or program of assertive community treatment [PACT]), which consists of professionals from several disciplines within the same organization who are available to provide support and services to the client 24 hours a day, 7 days a week, as needed.

Case Example: Donna

The PACT team has received a referral of a consumer, Donna, who is new to the area, has recently been released from a psychiatric hospital after a stay of 20 days, and is ambivalent about whether she will take her medication. On meeting with the team, Donna voices her fear that medication will prevent her from working and that she will be a mental patient for the rest of her life. This particular PACT team consists of a registered nurse, a licensed clinical social worker, a licensed occupational therapist, and a psychiatrist, each of whom is available to assist the client in their respective areas of expertise at any time. Donna is able to identify areas of employment that interest her, and time is set aside in the next day for her to meet with the occupational therapist to further explore areas of strength and any factors that may affect her goals and develop a plan for moving forward. She meets with the psychiatrist and nurse to discuss medication options and is given the nurse's telephone number and instructions to call at any time if she has untoward side effects or questions or concerns. The social worker starts to identify the scope of Donna's support system for the purpose of helping her identify how to fill the voids in her social network and strengthen healthy alliances. By the end of the first week, Donna has met with all members of the PACT team individually and with the team collectively, and she now believes that she is supported in her recovery. She knows that that her future holds relapses but also is assured that she has the resources of the entire team at her disposal should she need them.

Other Care Management Frameworks

The title *case manager* or *care manager* can also describe a person who monitors the financial implications of treatment provided and assists the client in obtaining the most cost-effective services, although this role is gradually being redefined as *utilization management.* Some state Medicaid programs (e.g., Washington) have adopted this model for managing inpatient utilization costs and are effectively using it to encourage the development of less restrictive services in the community.

The traditional model of public mental health care management involves a caseload of consumers, often with varying levels of functional impairment as a result of mental illness. The care manager is employed by an agency to assist the client with meeting any needs that have been unmet as a result of his or her mental illness. The specific model of care management used within an agency is dependent on the agency's mission, fiscal and human resources, catchment area, and clientele. Cottrell (2000) identified variations on the three categories of care management noted previously. In the Single Case Manager Model, Cottrell (2000) noted, one person "works individually with clients maintaining responsibility for all aspects of the client's case" (p. 268), which may mean monitoring medication consumption, taking the person to mental and physical health appointments, and assisting with shopping and other IADLs. Additional common activities include acting as a protective payee[1] for the person, being the liaison between the person and any financial or medical assistance programs, and assisting with applications for housing, Social Security, or other resources.

In the Sequential Case Manager Model (Cottrell, 2000), these duties are transferred from one care manager to another as he or she moves through a system of care, for example, from a residential treatment facility to semi-independent living to independent living.

In contrast to the Single Case Manager and Sequential Case Manager Models is the Cluster Case Management Model, which is arranged around occupations rather than people, similar to how education is designed around topics. When applying this model to mental health, for example, a cluster of people who needed to apply for entitlements would be assigned to one care manager who would facilitate that activity.

Team case management, in which a team of professionals supports a person, in conjunction with intensive case management (24-hour, on call) and assertive case management (the focus of which is rehabilitation and recovery; Cottrell, 2000), have been integrated into what is now the ACT model, described earlier. Services are "wrapped around" a small group of consumers in a concerted fashion. People who are unable to maintain a stable level of function or who require a high level of support or treatment to stabilize at a new functional level are offered ACT programs more frequently as the use of this model spreads. Details on implementing this model, including an evidence-based tool kit, can be obtained online from the Substance Abuse and Mental Health Services Administration (SAMHSA; n.d.) and through the ACT Association (www.actassociation.org).

Systems of Support in the Community

Clinicians in community mental health centers and in private practice are the most common form of formal support in the area of mental health. Typically, traditional settings provide outpatient group or individual therapy and medication management services. Some mental health providers may offer day treatment, sheltered employment, clubhouses, 24-hour case management, crisis response or outreach, and transportation to and from appointments. Although the identified formal system may include only the direct or assigned treatment providers, in reality everyone within the agency who comes in contact with the person is a part of the support system. Understanding this phenomenon allows the care manager to integrate the formal provider system with community-based supports to develop the most effective network for the person.

Federally Supported Programs

SAMHSA provides grants to all 50 states, the District of Columbia, Puerto Rico, and four U.S. territories through the Projects for Assistance in Transition From

---

[1]A *payee* is a person who receives funds (e.g., from Social Security) for someone who is unable to manage or direct the management of his or her money. The payee is responsible for using or guiding the use of the funds for the beneficiary's current and foreseeable needs.

Homelessness (PATH) program to engage many people who are mentally ill and homeless in treatment or recovery services and, as a by-product, identify the scope of informal services available in communities (see www.pathprogram.samhsa.gov/ for a list of communities operating these programs). Another SAMHSA project that has evolved from PATH is called SSI/SSDI Outreach Access and Recovery (www. prainc.com/soar/). This program helps identify homeless people in 34 states who are potentially eligible for Supplemental Security Income (SSI) or Social Security Disability Insurance (SSDI) and helps them apply for and obtain the examinations for disability determination and, if needed, appeal a decision.

Peer Support Programs

Structured programs such as Alcoholics Anonymous (AA), which describes itself as a fellowship (Alcoholics Anonymous World Services, 1972), the Depression and Bipolar Support Alliance (DBSA; www.ndmda.org/), and the National Alliance on Mental Illness (NAMI) Connection (NAMI, n.d.) are three examples of peer support systems that are available in many areas. Many of the local affiliates of these groups are periodically listed in local newspapers or are posted on community bulletin boards.

Finding Other Community Supports and Resources

Conversations with treatment providers, advocacy groups, consumers, and family members will identify many options available in an area. Local newspapers or Internet networking sites or blogs will also be a resource (Cottrell, 2000). Checking the calendars and public service announcements of local hospitals and community centers may prove successful because they often provide meeting space for groups. Faith and fraternal organizations (e.g., Veterans of Foreign Wars) may be a resource that, if not already providing a support group, can be encouraged and assisted in doing so (McConchie, 2000).

Accessing Financial or In-Kind Services on Behalf of Others

People without means may not be able to access formalized support systems in the community, so a significant function of care managers is the initiation and maintenance of a source of funding and other benefits. Although state and federal funding sources are available, the application process is often cumbersome, and the award may not be made for several months after the application is submitted. Because of existing relationships and interests, communities may be able to tap local fiscal and in-kind resources. The community agency that began a pilot program, operated it for a year, and then used the data on its success to garner governmental support on a larger scale is but one example of using more than one funding stream to support a needed service.

Most communities have a chapter of the Red Cross that can help in times of true environmental emergency (e.g., displacement resulting from fire or flood) and has access to information on a variety of other resources. Local branches of the Salvation Army, Goodwill Industries, and the Society of St. Vincent De Paul provide, within their respective abilities, clothing to people in need. Local YWCA and YMCA chapters may have emergency housing or food banks that can be accessed if needed. Many cities have an organized shelter for people who are homeless that posts addresses of local food banks, 12-step meetings, including Friends of Bill W and Alano Clubs, parenting support groups, and free clinics. Do not overlook community service groups and education centers. The people in these groups may have access to resources that consumers need but are not able to access independently.

Some communities have established their own community service resource centers to serve in a "one-stop shopping" manner. These services operate in a System Case Management Model (Cottrell, 2000) that merely refers people to services to treat or otherwise mitigate identified needs. If this service is not available, people may still be able to turn to local offices of state or national Aging and Disability Resource Centers (ADRCs). ADRCs, created by the Older Americans Act of 1965 (amended in 2006; Administration on Aging, n.d.) and called *aging and long-term care facilities* in some locales,

> provide information and assistance to individuals needing either public or private resources, professionals seeking assistance on behalf of their clients, and individuals planning for their future long-term care needs. ADRC programs also serve as the entry point to publicly administered long term supports including those funded under Medicaid, the Older Americans Act and state revenue programs. (Eldercare Locator, n.d., para. 2)

State and Federal Benefit Programs

Many people with mental illness qualify for state or federal disability benefits, or both. Negotiating the various systems can be time consuming and frustrating for people not familiar with the jargon and procedures. Each has specific criteria for eligibility and formats in which the material must be submitted. Attempting to speed the process by using a generic form or attaching information in a nonstandard format may only result in a denial and delay the process for the client. A common reason for denial is clerical error, which can often be easily corrected. Another reason for denial is failure to prove disability. Putting together the necessary documentation to submit an effective appeal may take more effort on the part of the care manager and the client. An appeal of a failure-to-prove-disability decision may have a financial impact for the client if copies of medical records are needed or additional evaluations have to be performed.

Social Security

The federal Social Security Administration provides two forms of financial support for which people with mental illness may be eligible: SSDI and SSI. The primary determining factors are the level of disability resulting from the mental illness, the age at onset, and the person's work history (see the Social Security Disability Planner available at www.socialsecurity.gov/dibplan/index.htm).

SSDI is available to people who have contributed individual social security taxes for a designated length of time before being determined to be disabled. Children may be eligible for SSDI on the basis of a parent's work history if the child's disability occurred before age 22 or if the parent is deceased or has started to draw SSDI him- or herself.

SSI is paid to adults and children who meet the federally established low-income threshold, are age 65 or older, or are determined to be disabled but have not worked to the level of SSDI eligibility (Social Security Adminstration, n.d.-c). Application for

SSI and SSDI can be made in person at a local Social Security office. Field office locations can be determined by accessing https://secure.ssa.gov/apps6z/FOLO/fo001.jsp for locations in the United States or www.socialsecurity.gov/foreign/ for locations in other countries.

Before submitting an application, it may be helpful to use the Benefits Eligibility Screening Tool (BEST; http://connections.govbenefits.gov/ssa_en.portal). This tool does not access Social Security records or make predictions of the amount of funds one might receive. It uses the data entered by the person to identify whether the potential for benefits exists and suggests next steps. A medical and job worksheet is available at www.socialsecurity.gov/disability/Adult_StarterKit_Worksheet.pdf to help the applicant prepare for the personal interview, which may take place over the telephone or in person. Applicants are allowed to have someone present to act as their advocate in this process. This person can be a care manager, family member, friend, or another person who knows the client's circumstances.

Medicare

People who are age 65, have end-stage renal disease, or have received SSI or SSDI because of a disability for 24 months are eligible to apply for Medicare, a federal medical insurance program (Social Security Administration, n.d.-c; U.S. Department of Health and Human Services, n.d.). Medicare has four different plan components:

1. *Part A* covers hospitalization, long-term care, hospice, and home health if specific criteria are met, up to the allowable limit for the service.
2. *Part B* covers outpatient medically necessary services such as doctor visits and some preventive care using similar allowable limits. Part B is an optional component and has a monthly premium attached.
3. *Part C,* also known as Medicare Advantage Plans, is a combination of Parts A, B, and D that is administered by private organizations (i.e., health maintenance organizations, preferred provider organizations) through contracts with the Centers for Medicare and Medicaid Services (CMS) and often entails a copayment on the part of the client at the time of service.
4. *Part D* covers prescription medication and differs from other Medicare components by having a gap in coverage after a set threshold of spending has been met. In other words, when one has spent the designated amount for covered medications, a period of time exists during which limited or no insurance coverage for medications is available and the full expense must be paid out of pocket until the total amount paid reaches another predetermined threshold. The scope of prescriptions covered varies widely because CMS contracts with many entities to provide this coverage.

The "Medicare and You" section of Medicare.gov has detailed information about the scope of Medicare benefits, including the details of available prescription plans, organized by ZIP code for easy access. This information is available for download in PDF format at www.medicare.gov/Publications/Pubs/pdf/10050.pdf. Applying for Medicare is done through either www.medicare.gov or the local Social Security Administration field office. The Medicare Web site has a Medicare Eligibility Tool to help clarify the application process and includes clear instructions for appealing an unacceptable decision.

Medicaid

Medicaid is a health insurance program jointly funded by federal and state funds intended to provide assistance with the cost of medical care to people who meet specific income and other eligibility requirements. The CMS brochure *Medicaid at a Glance* (CMS, 2005) explains the main components of the Medicaid program (see also CMS, n.d.-a). Medicaid applications can be obtained from the state department of social or health services, through its Web site, by picking one up in person at a local office, or by calling the state Medicaid office and asking that one be mailed. People who have income may be eligible for Medicaid if they have significant medical expenses (e.g., recent hospitalization, expensive medication) or other mitigating factors. After submission of the written or electronic application, the applicant will be notified of an interview time, the place, and the types of documentation to bring. During this interview, the applicant is required to provide a valid Social Security card, picture identification, and validation of the claims made on the application. Written verification of residence can be through landlord statement or mortgage payment record. Utility bills, cancelled checks, or money order duplicates provide verification of housing expenses. A maximum limit is allowed for utility expenses, depending on the number of people in the household. Financial status is verified through bank statements, Social Security award letter, pay stubs, and the like. Failure to provide this information will result in the delay, and eventual closure, of the application. During the interview, any mitigating factors that may influence eligibility can be discussed. Even when some financial resources are available, the applicant may be determined to be eligible for a program that covers any medical expenses after he or she pays a preset amount (spend down) or a copay may have to be paid at the time of service. After the interview, the applicant will get an award or determination of benefits letter. If the application was denied, instructions for appealing an unfavorable decision and the reasons for any denial will be included.

Medicaid service providers contract either directly with the state or indirectly through another entity such as the county or township government. Independent providers (e.g., physicians, nurse practitioners, dentists) typically receive a designated amount of money for each service provided (i.e., fee for service) to the consumer. This amount may be much less than is recovered from patients with other payers, causing some providers to limit the number of people with Medicaid insurance they treat. Agency-based providers (i.e., mental health agencies) may be excluded from fee-for-service reimbursement and receive funding on a per capita basis. Under this type of agreement, the agency receives a specified amount of money to provide all the designated services needed by people residing within the specified catchment area. The details of this type of agreement or contract are the result of much interplay and discussion between federal and state agencies, and the local agency may have little input into the final agreement (Jacobson, Marsh, & Winston, 2005).

Accessing Employment Resources

Productive use of self and time are basic human needs. Individual consumers may be eligible for publicly funded programs to enable them to gain and keep employment, including the evidence-based practice of supported employment.

Federal Programs

Ticket to Work is a federal program offered through the Social Security Administration that provides both support to the employee and incentives to the employer. Changes made in 2008 are designed "to promote more partnering between organizations and expand the range of services offered to beneficiaries" (Social Security Administration, n.d.-a, para 3). Whereas participation had been restricted before July 2008, the revisions made anyone between ages 18 and 64 eligible. The program is designed to allow the person to gradually increase his or her work skills over a 60-month period without losing Social Security benefits. After sustaining a designated level of employment, benefits are pro rated on the basis of income level. SSI recipients also have the option of participating in a Plan to Achieve Self Support (PASS; Social Security Administration, n.d.-b) with individualized coaching and other supports.

State Programs

The Workforce Investment Act of 1998 required the establishment of "one-stop delivery systems" within states "to consolidate, coordinate, and improve employment, training, literacy, and vocational rehabilitation programs in the United States." Because each state is free to develop the plan for administering the program, it requires some searching to determine which department of state government is responsible. Some states (e.g., Oklahoma) have designated responsibility to the Department of Vocational Rehabilitation, others (e.g., Washington) have located it within the Division of Employment and Assistance, and still others (e.g., Pennsylvania) manage these services through the Department of Labor and Industry.

Local Resources

Some communities have created local work development programs through public–private partnerships that are specific to the needs of a particular geographic area. These partnerships are reminiscent of journeyman programs familiar to public utilities and the fishing and logging industries that are designed to continually develop the next generation of knowledgeable and skilled employees. Chambers of Commerce, community colleges, public and private high schools, and local business development organizations are common partners in these relationships. Within communities, businesses may exist that focus on employment development and have contracts with employers who allow job shadowing or other opportunities such as job coaching, job sharing, or structured employment reentry.

Housing

As much as people need to be productive, it is almost imperative to have a safe base from which to go forth. For many people with mental illness, obtaining and maintaining adequate housing is a challenge. Lack of a place to sleep and bathe safely creates sequelae that ripple throughout the client's world, often with negative rebounds ("Hearings Before the Senate Appropriations Subcommittee," 2009).

Perhaps the most well-known housing support is Section 8 housing, so named because it is authorized by Section 8 of the Housing Act of 1937 (U.S. Department of Housing and Urban Development [HUD], n.d.). This program is administered by HUD's Office of Public and Indian Housing, which has delegated the daily operations to local offices of the housing authority or similarly named branch of local government. Income level is the basis for qualification, and the HUD USER Web site (www.huduser.org) has geographically adjusted tables available to reference. The number of qualified applicants far outreaches the supply in many areas of the country, but that should not prevent one from being placed on a waiting list. Because a variety of programs are available, care managers should review the *Voucher Program Guidebook: Housing Choice* (HUD, 2001) before talking with local housing authorities. The guide is available online at www.hud.gov/offices/pih/programs/hcv/forms/guidebook.cfm.

Within most communities is a group of people concerned about the lack of affordable or suitable housing for people with limited means. Coalitions of mental health providers, law enforcement, and landlords have been successful ways to develop safer housing. Becoming involved in such a group can be extremely important to developing the relationships that will eventually open doors for people with mental illness and inadequate housing. These groups are most visible when a crisis such as flooding, tornado or hurricane damage, or severe winter weather needs to be resolved. Although those are opportune times to join the work, such groups are often planning and working throughout the year, and many would welcome a care manager's involvement. Local governments have an office of human or community services that would be most likely to know the key people to contact. Depending on the manner in which mental health services are funded within the state, an opportunity may exist to work with treatment providers to develop supported housing programs. The support provided may range from purely financial (with the person attending work or treatment activities elsewhere) to structured life skills training with situational coaching throughout the day, several days a week. Occupational therapists are experts at both designing and implementing such a program (Cottrell, 2000).

Care Management With Specific Populations

Heretofore, the focus has been on the application of care management models to the needs of adults. Children and older adults, and the systems with which they interact, have different needs, as described in the sections that follow.

Care Management and Children

Care managers involved with children who have a mental illness find themselves actively negotiating a variety of complex systems with and on behalf of their clients (Zeitz, 2000). Many children with mental illness have fragile, if not compromised, relationships with their families (Torrey, 2001) and may be in foster care, residential treatment, supported home placement, or some combination thereof. Concerns may exist regarding blended or single-parent families and common developmental processes such as sibling conflicts and individuation. All of these factors compound the complexity of life for the child with mental illness and can create chaos within the family.

It is important that the care manager have advanced training in child development, family dynamics, and family interventions because of the many and competing demands at any given time. This type of training is available through a variety of reputable providers including some states' mental health service administration. The role of the care manager, and that of others involved in care, should be clearly defined (preferably in writing) to avoid compounding any confusion on the part of the child, the family, or others. Working in a multifaceted arena such as this one involves inherent risks. The care manager is wise to seek regular professional supervision and personal support to repair the effects of vicarious trauma (Saakvitne & Pearlman, 1996).

Care Management and the Isolated Older Adult

The needs of older adults with mental illness are much different from those of other age groups. Effective care management requires an acute appreciation of the person's culture of origin; life experiences; reactions and results; medical conditions, including the symptoms thereof; and medication interaction. Within the traditional community, families and friends rally to support the older adult through the aging process whether he or she needs 24-hour nursing care or cognitive supervision. Older adults who do not have family or friends nearby may choose to join senior centers, social clubs of one form or another, or retirement communities to obtain support as they age. In addition to providing an emotional support system, these groups informally provide information, recommendations, and referrals on the basis of participants' life experiences, thus serving as informal care managers.

Older adults with mental illness, however, may have limited options in terms of natural supports and may be extremely isolated. It is not uncommon for families to become alienated from consumers during times of symptom exacerbation and have difficulty reestablishing rapport once the crisis passes (Torrey, 2001). Without intervention, older people tend to remain in their home unless an activity (e.g., grocery shopping) is necessary. Care managers can be instrumental in breaking this pattern of self-imposed isolation. Older consumers may have a hard time breaking into and connecting within formal support groups as a result of symptoms of the illness that inhibit their confidence (e.g., inattention to subtle social cues) or behaviors that make them stand out from those who are not ill. The care manager can ease the integration of older adults with mental illness into a community social group by having first established a relationship with the people who coordinate the group or center staff and gained the trust of the informal leadership. Care should be taken to ensure that the consumer wants engagement in the group and that group participation is not a means to an identified agency or provider goal. Lack of consumer investment and potential exacerbation of symptomatology in a new situation guarantee failure.

Advance Planning as a Function of Care Management

Regardless of age, the person with mental illness and his or her family often need assistance in planning for the time when parents will no longer be able to provide guidance and support. This topic is seldom a concern of people without illness, and when an illness is present, the realities of day-to-day life often push future planning to a back burner. Although the care manager cannot insist that future planning occur, it can gently be broached repeatedly and assistance offered.

Each state has specific parameters that must be heeded for trusts and endowments to be valid and legal. Attorneys in the field of disabilities law are knowledgeable in the process of establishing and administering such accounts and can ensure that all necessary details are attended to. Families may want to consult a financial advisor to ascertain the relative values and risks of the different types of trusts and endowments available within the state in which the recipient of the trust resides.

The NAMI Web site contains links on its Web site to the Special Needs Estate Planning Guidance System and the Planned Lifetime Assistance Network (www. nami.org/Content/NavigationMenu/Find_Support/Legal_Support/NAMI_Legal_ Support.htm). Other resources are available through the National Institute of Mental Health (www.nimh.nih.gov).

Another form of advance planning is the mental health advance directive. Advance directives enable a person to identify, at a time of stability, his or her wishes in writing regarding such topics as medications, power of attorney, restraint, and other treatment issues. Such directives are used, to the extent possible, to guide care at a time of crisis or hospitalization. Although relatively new, mental health advance directives are recognized in several states (New York, North Carolina, Washington, Texas, California, Oregon, Ohio). Advance directives are a valuable resource for shared decision making with and empowerment of consumers (Schauer, Everett, del Vecchio, & Anderson, 2007). In addition to the respective states' Office of the Attorney General, the Bazelon Center for Mental Health Law (n.d.) is a resource for information on this document and the process involved.

Conclusion

The need for care management is not limited to one age group or aspect of life. People with mental illness have many needs that can be ameliorated through use of competent care management over time. The literature describes various models of care management, some of which are more easily implemented than others. Regardless of the model used to construct the delivery system, effective care management engages the client as the driver of everything that occurs and enlists both formal and informal supports to effect change. The unique awareness of the interaction of person and context that occupational therapy brings to the field of care management allows for a planned, scientific approach to problem resolution that enables the client to move forward in the recovery process.

References

Administration on Aging. (n.d.). *Unofficial compilation of the Older Americans Act of 1965 as amended in 2006 (Public Law 109–365)*. Retrieved September 11, 2009, from www.aoa. gov/AoAroot/AoA_Programs/OAA/oaa_full.asp#_Toc153957631

Alcoholics Anonymous World Services. (1972). *A brief guide to Alcoholics Anonymous*. New York: Author. Retrieved August 20, 2008, from www.aa.org/pdf/ products/p-42_abriefguidetoaa1.pdf

American Occupational Therapy Association. (2008). Occupational therapy practice framework: Domain and process (2nd ed.). *American Journal of Occupational Therapy, 62,* 625–683.

Bazelon Center for Mental Health Law. (n.d.). *Advance psychiatric directives*. Retrieved September 16, 2008, from www.bazelon.org/issues/advancedirectives/index.htm

Centers for Medicare and Medicaid Services. (2005). *Medicaid at-a-glance 2005: A Medicaid information source*. Retrieved December 2, 2009, from www.cms.hhs.gov/Medicaid Eligibility/Downloads/MedicaidataGlance05.pdf

Centers for Medicare and Medicaid Services. (n.d.-a). *Medicaid eligibility: Are you eligible?* Retrieved September 11, 2009, from www.cms.hhs.gov/Medicaid Eligibility/02_AreYouEligible_.asp

Centers for Medicare and Medicaid Services. (n.d.-b). *Methodology for estimates by sponsor.* Retrieved August 31, 2008, from www.cms.hhs.gov/NationalHealthExpendData/downloads/bhg-methodology-07.pdf

Cottrell, R. P. F. (2000). Clinical case management: Expanding the role of the occupational therapist in mental health practice. In R. P. F. Cottrell (Ed.), *Proactive approaches in psychosocial occupational therapy* (pp. 266–279). Thorofare, NJ: Slack.

Eldercare Locator. (n.d.). *Aging and disability resource centers.* Retrieved August 30, 2008, from www.eldercare.gov/Eldercare.NET/Public/Network/ARC.aspx

Hearings before the Senate Appropriations Subcommittee on Labor, Health and Human Services, and Education Concerning Programs in the United States Departments of Labor, Health and Human Services, and Education, 111th Congr. (2009). (Written testimony of National Alliance to End Homelessness, Nan Roman, President). Available at www.endhomelessness.org/content/article/detail/2348

Housing Act of 1937, Pub. L. 93–383, 88 Stat. 653, 42 U.S.C. 1437 et seq.

Jacobson, J., Marsh, S., & Winston, P. (2005). *State and local contracting for social services under Charitable Choice: Final report.* Washington, DC: U.S. Department of Health and Human Services, Office of the Assistant Secretary for Planning and Evaluation. Retrieved February 11, 2010, from http://aspe.hhs.gov/hsp/05/contracting/charitablechoice.pdf

Kanter, J. (1989). Clinical case management: Definition, principles, components. *Hospital and Community Psychiatry, 40,* 361–368

McConchie, S. D. (2000). Establishing support and advocacy groups. In R. P. F. Cottrell (Ed.), *Proactive approaches in psychosocial occupational therapy* (pp. 451–454). Thorofare, NJ: Slack.

National Alliance on Mental Illness. (n.d.). *NAMI Connection* [Brochure]. Retrieved August 30, 2008, from www.nami.org/Content/NavigationMenu/Find_Support/Education_and_Training/Education_Training_and_Peer_Support_Center/NAMI_Connection/NAMI_Connection_Brochure.pdf

Older Americans Act Amendments of 2006, Pub. L. 109–365, 120 Stat. 2522.

Older Americans Act of 1965, Pub. L. 89–73, 79 Stat. 218, 42 U.S.C. § 3001 et seq.

Saakvitne, K., & Pearlman, L. A. (1996). *Transforming the pain: A workbook on vicarious traumatization.* New York: W. W. Norton.

Schauer, C., Everett, A., del Vecchio, P., & Anderson, L. (2007). Promoting the values and practice of shared decision making in health care. *Psychiatric Rehabilitation Journal, 31*(1), 54–61.

Social Security Administration. (n.d.-a). *About Ticket to Work.* Retrieved September 11 2009, from www.socialsecurity.gov/work/documents/SSA-63-024%20Overview%20of%20Final%20Regs.pdf

Social Security Administration. (n.d.-b). *Plan to Achieve Self-Support (PASS).* Retrieved September 11, 2009, from www.socialsecurity.gov/disabilityresearch/wi/pass.htm

Social Security Administration. (n.d.-c). *Understanding Supplemental Security Income Social Security entitlement 2009 edition.* Retrieved September 13, 2009, from www.socialsecurity.gov/ssi/text-entitle-ussi.htm

Substance Abuse and Mental Health Services Administration. (n.d.). *Evidence-based practices: Shaping mental health services toward recovery—Assertive community treatment: Information for mental health program leaders.* Retrieved December 2, 2009, from http://mentalhealth.samhsa.gov/cmhs/communitysupport/toolkits/community/ACTprogleadinfo.asp

Summers, N. (2006). *Fundamentals of case management practice: Skills for the human services* (2nd ed.). Belmont, CA: Thomson Higher Education.

Torrey, E. F. (2001). *Surviving schizophrenia: A manual for families, consumers, and providers.* New York: HarperCollins.

U.S. Department of Health and Human Services. (n.d.). *Medicare eligibility tool.* Retrieved September 11, 2009, from www.medicare.gov/MedicareEligibility/Home.asp?dest=NAV/Home/GeneralEnrollment#TabTop

U.S. Department of Housing and Urban Development. (n.d.). *Section 8 rental voucher program.* Retrieved August 31, 2008, from www.hud.gov/progdesc/voucher.cfm

U.S. Department of Housing and Urban Development. (2001). *Voucher program guidebook: Housing choice.* Washington, DC: Author.

Woodside, M., & McClam, T. (2006). *Generalist case management: A method of human service delivery.* Belmont, CA: Thomson Higher Education.

Workforce Investment Act of 1998, Pub. L. 105–220, 112 Stat. 936. Retrieved September 11, 2009, from http://frwebgate.access.gpo.gov/cgi-bin/getdoc.cgi?dbname=105_cong_public_laws&docid=f:publ220.105

Zeitz, M. (2000). The mother's project: A clinical case management system. In R. P. F. Cottrell (Ed.), *Proactive approaches in psychosocial occupational therapy* (pp. 443–449). Thorofare, NJ: Slack.

Advocacy

CHAPTER 20

Advocacy for Occupational Therapy and Mental Health Issues

M. Beth Merryman, PhD, OTR/L

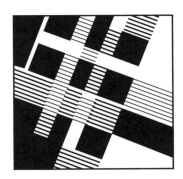

Learning Objectives

After reading this material and completing the examination, readers will be able to

- Identify different types of advocacy, including when each is indicated;

- Delineate sociopolitical trends relative to mental health that influence people, professions, and public policy;

- Identify key stakeholders with whom occupational therapists collaborate to affect public policy;

- Delineate effective empowerment strategies to support advocacy efforts; and

- Recognize the steps to developing and implementing an advocacy plan to benefit the person, the profession, and public policy.

Historically, mental health services have been underfunded at the federal, state, and local levels. This underfunding has had serious consequences for consumers of services in both the private and the public sectors. With the shift of care from institutions to the community and the emerging embrace of a public health model for community mental health, it is clear that well-being includes a person's total health status, including mental health. Health politics has been identified as an emerging trend; therefore, to continue to serve client needs, occupational therapists need to be aware of how to effect change.

This chapter discusses advocacy in terms of the sociopolitical aspects of mental health policy and service delivery. First, it defines advocacy and presents a model of intervention. Then, the chapter describes sociopolitical trends relative to mental health policy and service delivery and identifies key stakeholders relative to mental health policy and decision making. It next discusses social influences that affect successful advocacy, such as poverty, stigma and discrimination. Finally, the ethical challenges inherent in this practice area are presented in case vignettes that readers may use to develop an advocacy plan.

Historical Overview

The shift to community-oriented mental health services as embraced by the recovery movement began as society decided on a philosophy of inclusion for people with disabilities, including mental illness (Lewis, Shadish, & Lurigio, 1989). The deinstitutionalization movement began in the 1950s with the advent of effective medications and progressed through the belief that a change in the environment—from the hospital to the community—was possible for many people with mental illness (Geller, 2000). In the 1960s and 1970s, civil rights legislation was enacted that benefited people with disabilities, including those with mental illness, and that supported individual rights to treatment and treatment refusal. These decades also saw the development of key social policies—Medicare and Medicaid in 1965 and Supplemental Security Income and Social Security Disability Insurance and modifications to the Rehabilitation Act in the 1970s—that supported the right of people with disabilities to live in the community (a list of Web resources for advocacy is provided at the end of the chapter).

The 1980s brought the recognition of the skyrocketing cost of all health care and attempts to rein it in through various managed care methodologies. The consumer movement in mental health also grew, similarly to the independent living movement of people with disabilities in the 1970s. The growth of advocacy groups such as the National Alliance on Mental Illness (NAMI) and the development of peer-run services and centers have progressed since this time.

The 1990s, labeled by the administration of President George H. W. Bush as the "Decade of the Brain," saw funds for basic biological research that supported the interests of mental health advocates. The Institute of Medicine produced a report addressing quality and the need to embrace evidence-based interventions in routine practice (Olsen, Aisner, & McGinnis, 2007). Managed care methodologies were adopted by both private and public providers of mental health services. In 1999, the Supreme Court ruled in the *Olmstead* decision that continuing to institutionalize people who were deemed capable of receiving treatment in the community was a violation of the Americans With Disabilities Act (Mechanic, 2008). The U.S. Surgeon General issued a report on mental health that emphasized the need to adopt evidence-based practices and recovery-oriented delivery of services and to combat stigma (U.S. Department of Health and Human Services, 1999). In 2001, President George W. Bush created the New Freedom Initiative, declaring, among other things, the need for a transformation of the mental health delivery system (President's New Freedom Commission on Mental Health, 2003). Three main obstacles to mental health care were identified, including (1) the stigma of mental illness, (2) a lack of fairness in private insurance health benefits for mental illness, and (3) the fragmentation of the mental health service delivery system.

Advocacy Defined

Advocacy is defined as "active support of a cause or course of action" (*Collins Essential English Dictionary,* 2006). It involves direct involvement with clients, such as advising

Table 20.1. Types of Advocacy

Type	Example
Individual	Referring a client for services and making a call on his or her behalf
Professional	Participating in Hill Day at the American Occupational Therapy Association to educate policymakers about the occupational therapy profession
Program policy	Meeting with the psychosocial rehabilitation program executive director to educate him or her about the cost and benefits of occupational therapy services
Public policy	Joining a task force on affordable housing to address access needs for people with disabilities on a limited income

them of resources and rights, and indirect involvement, such as petitioning for a change in legislation or public policy. The rehabilitation literature examining therapists' perception of advocacy identifies one of three types: (1) therapists viewing themselves as protecting clients' rights, (2) therapists presenting client functional status to various agencies to support acceptance, and (3) therapists being involved on the treatment team. Different types of advocacy are described in Table 20.1.

Many descriptions of how to prepare for advocacy activity are available. When evaluating state-level initiatives, such as proposed legislation, NAMI (2007) describes four basic steps:

1. Gathering information on various proposals that are being put forth
2. Analyzing the content in terms of what is included and excluded; means of access; degree of choice; how it will be funded; and the specifics of each proposal in terms of benefits, who can provide them, and where
3. Completing an analysis of pluses and minuses for each proposal from the occupational therapy perspective
4. Being prepared with fact sheets and educational materials on the value of occupational therapy intervention for this population for visits to key stakeholders, such as legislators or representatives of advocacy groups.

These four steps are described here as an example of public policy advocacy; however, they are relevant for each of the types of advocacy identified in Table 20.1. In each instance, the occupational therapist first gathers information to understand and define the presenting issue or problem. The second step involves an analysis of potential solutions or alternatives and listing the criteria or features of each. The third step involves assessing the pluses and minuses of each alternative, and the fourth step involves decision making and an action plan in which the presentation to key stakeholders occurs with targeted information based on Steps 1 through 3.

Professional Ethics and Advocacy

The professional behavior of occupational therapists is guided by the Occupational Therapy Code of Ethics (Crepeau, Cohn, & Boyt Schell, 2003), in which therapists agree to "demonstrate a concern for the well being of the recipients of their services" and "respect the rights of [their] clients" (pp. 1008–1009). In addition, occupational therapists adhere to identified core values of the profession, including altruism, dignity, equality, freedom of choice, justice, prudence, and truth (Crepeau et al., 2003). Mental health occupational therapy practice produces ethical challenges on a daily basis. In terms of individual-level advocacy, occupational therapists are often the key team members to assess client safety for discharge from an inpatient setting. Has the client been discharged to whatever setting was available and approved for payment rather than one that the client was involved in choosing and that was indicated from the results of the functional assessment? In terms of professional advocacy, how many occupational therapists are on staff in psychosocial rehabilitation programs (PRPs), despite the client-centeredness that is congruent with their recovery philosophy and skill at matching environments to skill sets? In terms of program policy, are clients being denied occupational therapy services in lieu of other therapies that—although they do not harm clients, are less costly, and keep them busy during the day—may not be actively assisting them to build a life in recovery? In terms of public policy, are occupational therapists restricted from practice because of state definitions of *qualified mental health provider,* and if so, how might this restriction affect client success in recovery?

Occupational therapists practicing in mental health engage in advocacy on the individual level—to get a referral, provide feedback in rounds, or join a family education meeting to discuss client discharge needs. The skills that enable a therapist to be successful in advocating on an individual level are similar to those needed at all other levels of advocacy. Those skills include

- Becoming knowledgeable about the issue and system in which key decisions get made;
- Developing necessary skills of assertiveness, presentation, and influence;
- Identifying key stakeholders and collaborating with them toward a mutual goal;
- Adhering to the Occupational Therapy Code of Ethics; and
- Developing the plan, implementing it, and evaluating its outcome.

Sociopolitical Trends in Mental Health

All types of health policy are guided by the "three-legged stool" of cost, quality, and access. The goal is to develop the policy that will provide the highest quality at the lowest cost to the most people. It is no secret that over the past 25 years, the cost of health care has grown exponentially. As of 2008, health care represents 15% of the U.S. gross domestic product (Organization for Economic Cooperation and Development, 2008). This means that many people have a stake in the economics of health care—from health systems, providers, and insurers to equipment vendors and pharmaceutical companies. Health care is big business and a large part of the U.S. economy. Like any policy area, there are limits to what can be provided. As costs grew, various economic solutions were designed to attempt to rein them in, theoretically without negatively affecting quality or access. Managed care strategies have been the preferred form of cost containment for the past 20 years. Managed care methodologies typically include limits on access in the form of necessary referral from a gatekeeper, adherence to strict medical necessity criteria for service through preauthorization and ongoing utilization review, and contracting arrangements with providers that ensure client volume for discounted rates. Some feel that although managed care arrangements are designed with the three-legged stool in mind, the cost leg is most influential in care decisions, which has implications for all involved with the mental health delivery system.

Private Insurers

People seeking mental health care who have private insurance are typically guided by managed care methodologies that are designed to reduce costs and influence health-seeking behavior. These methods include need for preauthorization, use of provider lists, limits on days of care or number of outpatient sessions per year, and a limited medication formulary. For mental health issues, insurers typically cover hospital-based care, outpatient hospital-based care, or private provider care but limit services such as residential treatment or psychiatric rehabilitation. Access to specialized services, such as occupational therapy, is typically limited.

Public Mental Health System

The public mental health system includes federal, state, and local involvement. Medicare is a federal health care entitlement for people ages 65 and older, but people with a documented long-term disability can apply for consideration. Medicaid is a joint, federal- and state-funded entitlement that involves state-specific criteria based on income and disability status. People with serious and persistent mental illness often meet the criteria for Medicaid, and in fact, knowledge of state Medicaid policy is increasingly critical to effectively plan state public mental health policy. Over the past 10 years, virtually all states have adopted some form of Medicaid managed care. Knowledge of managed care methods, therefore, is critical for occupational therapists regardless of the population or setting in which they provide mental health services.

Access

Access is an ongoing issue in the United States because health care is not a guaranteed right. Whether a person has private, public, or no insurance, they are likely to face access issues if they have a serious mental illness. *Access* is defined as the ability to obtain appropriate health care when needed, and it has several dimensions. Those dimensions include predisposing factors, need factors, and enabling factors (Barton, 1999).

- *Predisposing factors* are those inherent to the person, such as age, sex, race, and socioeconomic status. An example of how predisposing factors affect access to care might include the fact that youth typically do not self-refer or that adults of color may have cultural or trust barriers to access because of historically discriminatory health care practices. Adherence to the time or scheduling needs of parents or caregivers, then, is an example of examining relevant predisposing factors in providing mental health services to children or adolescents. Outreach may be needed to educate and encourage people to engage in services.
- *Need factors* include the person's perception of his or her health status. An example of how need factors affect access might be a person experiencing a manic episode with psychosis who does not see a need for care. He or she will not benefit from access services designed only for those who can self-refer.
- *Enabling factors* include features that affect access such as convenience of setting of care, characteristics of the system such as having a full

continuum of services and continuity of providers, personal income, and insurance type. Limited income or restrictive insurance policies are examples of enabling factors that may prevent a person from receiving recommended services because they are unable to pay out of pocket for care (Barton, 1999).

Poverty

Although the federal government is able to run a deficit, state governments must produce and adhere to a balanced annual budget, which has serious ramifications for populations who are dependent on services supported by the state-funded safety net. In efforts to balance state budgets, it is not uncommon to freeze admissions to programs that support recovery such as vocational services, therapeutic after-school programs, or supported housing. Other cost-saving strategies may include redefining the medical necessity criteria for current services so that only the patients who are sickest may be served. Such strategies leave patients who are unable to pay for services out of pocket to fend for themselves in terms of daily structure and support, a situation that negatively affects recovery.

People who receive federal disability payments, which includes people with serious mental illness, receive an annual cost-of-living adjustment. It is noteworthy that the 2008 increase of 2.3% was the smallest adjustment since 2003. The cost of daily life for people with disabilities is often greater than the cost-of-living adjustment because they typically experience higher health and medication costs, and these costs have been rising faster than other costs (Crutsinger, 2007).

Research has shown that people with serious and persistent mental illness have a life expectancy of 25 years less than those without this challenge (Power, 2007). This problem is certainly complex; however, the challenges of navigating the physical health system and gaining access continue to be factors for people with public insurance. In addition, if people must use their limited income for daily survival, as people with serious and persistent mental illness often do, basic prevention such as annual physicals, Pap smears, or dental checkups becomes an additional challenge that is not likely to be easily met.

Social Stigma

A key factor in public policy success is how a problem is viewed by the general public. Although survey results are promising, in that people report increased knowledge about mental illness as a treatable biological disease, most would agree that stigma is still attached to these conditions (Rusch, Angermyer, & Corrigan, 2005). *Stigma* is described as a "negative and erroneous attitude" that may lead to prejudice and discrimination (Corrigan & Penn, 1999, p. 765). In the case of mental illness, stigma includes perceptions that the person with the illness or his or her family may in some way be responsible for the illness (Smart, 2001). Social stigma has several potentially negative consequences, including decreased community participation because of discriminatory practices by landlords, employers, and health care providers or reduced socialization opportunities as a result of attempts to avoid self-disclosure (Corrigan, 2004). These experiences may lead to marginalization and self-restricting activities in the community (Miller Polgar & Landry, 2004).

Research has shown three main types of intervention to address stigma: education, contact, and protest. Education methods might include distributing public service announcements, in-services, or written materials with facts about mental illness. The Contact Theory (Allport, 1954) posits that attitude change is possible with exposure to mental illness in which social status is equal—in a social or work setting, for example, rather than a provider–consumer relationship. Protest methods might involve, for example, an organized letter-writing campaign threatening to boycott a television station or product to protest an offensive advertisement.

Parity

Parity has to do with fairness. Although the federal Mental Health Parity Act of 1996 was enacted in 1998, advocates agree that it was quite modest and only a first step toward parity between mental health and physical health insurance. The act required private employers of 50 or more who provided mental health coverage to ensure that the lifetime limits on coverage for mental illnesses be removed. The law did not require small businesses, people who experienced a hardship by covering mental health conditions, or those who chose not to cover mental health at all to change their practices. The law also excluded substance abuse from the mental health conditions covered by the act. As of this writing, 32 states have some type of mandatory mental health coverage, in the form of either a state parity law or a mandated benefit (Robinson, Connolly, Whitter, & Magana, 2007). Coverage varies in terms of what is covered.

On October 3, 2008, the Paul Wellstone and Pete Domenici Mental Health Parity and Addiction Equity Act of 2008 was enacted. The act builds on the 1996 parity law and contains the following provisions:

- The act continues to apply to all group health plans of 51 or more employees;
- The act does not require coverage for mental health or substance use disorders;
- The act does require that if coverage for mental health is provided, cost sharing and treatment limitations for mental health services must be no more restrictive than those for medical services;
- State mental health parity laws that are stronger are not preempted by this law; and
- A cost exemption can occur if there is a substantial increase as a result of parity, but additional criteria apply (Mental Health America, 2009).

The lack of full, universal mental health parity negatively affects people with conditions that are not covered, those who live in states with weak laws, and those with chronic conditions. The lack of a comprehensive parity law leaves people and families vulnerable to additional financial and psychosocial stress because of the unpredictable nature of these illnesses and the burden of planning without a safety net—which, ironically, is the purpose of insurance.

Political Stakeholders

Many stakeholders are involved in mental health service and delivery, each with a unique view of an issue (see Table 20.2). Some have a formal role, such as elected

Occupational Therapy in Mental Health: Considerations for Advanced Practice

officials or political appointees at the federal, state, and local levels. Others come to the issue with a personal investment and may include consumers and family members. Many have a professional interest, including agencies or organizations that provide care, professional and provider groups, and private and public insurance leadership. Mental health advocates often have similar goals, such as recovery for consumers, but varying agendas have undermined fragile coalitions and made change difficult to achieve. Examples include passage of the Americans With Disabilities Act by compromising coverage of substance abuse, states sacrificing outpatient commitment laws because of the concerns of civil liberties advocates, and unions fighting closure of state hospitals that might shift needed funds to the community. Admittedly, one of the issues underlying each of these challenges is that mental health has historically had too little funding, so change is viewed with mistrust that reduced services will not come along with the change. Further fragmentation because of stakeholder partisanship has negatively affected mental health reforms.

Self-Determination and Choice

Historically, the mental health delivery system has not provided consumers of services much involvement in the design or implementation of their care. Cook and Jonikas (2002) detailed the history of self-determination and the consumer movement in mental health by emphasizing its grassroots nature. *Self-determination* refers to the "right of individuals to have power over their own lives" (Cook & Jonikas, 2002, p. 87) and includes such concepts as freedom of choice, civil rights, independence, and self-direction. Consumers of mental health services experience discrimination as a result of a widespread lack of knowledge about mental illness, resulting in false assumptions about dangerousness. In addition, the tendency of

Table 20.2. Key Stakeholders

Stakeholder	Example
Formal elected leadership—many on state level	Governor, state representatives
Formal program leadership—local	CEO of local psychiatric rehabilitation program
Advocacy groups supporting mental health	National Alliance on Mental Illness
Federal stakeholders	Leadership at Medicaid, Social Security, U.S. Department of Health and Human Services
Insurance leadership	Leadership at Blue Cross/Blue Shield, other private payers
State Medicaid leadership	State Medicaid director
State mental health leadership	State mental health program director
Disease group organizations	Autism Speaks, Depression and Related Affective Disorders Association
Advocates for older Americans	AARP
Child advocates	School system; pediatricians
Clients	
Families	
Professional colleagues	American Occupational Therapy Association, state occupational therapy association, state Board of Practice; professional associations of social workers, psychosocial rehabilitation providers, home health agencies

such conditions to exacerbate and remit can lead to misunderstanding about both the gravity of the condition when the person is ill and his or her potential when not symptomatic. Finally, society continues to demonstrate a lack of understanding about such conditions through stigmatizing language and media portrayals that emphasize the drama of acute illness rather than the more common challenges of everyday life.

Self-determination is based on the American value of individualism; however, recent research has demonstrated the worth of social support and participation in valued social activities as factors in longevity and quality of life. In this emerging view, therefore, interdependence is the valued goal of recovery. The emerging paradigm of disability emphasizes the person's interaction with a supportive environment rather than focusing solely on the person. Of interest are the barriers to full participation in environments of choice for people with serious mental illness, including basic resources such as finances and safe affordable housing and aspects of the environment such as opportunities for social connectedness.

Laugharne and Priebe (2006) reviewed the literature on mental health choice and empowerment. They found that the shift from paternalism to autonomy occurred along a continuum and included areas such as informed consent, desire for information, and treatment choice. Researchers have explored consumer decision making and mental health treatment and found that although consumers want information about their care, they have less consensus decision making about their care. Greater desire for participation was seen in younger consumers, those who were employed, and those with a less positive attitude about treatment (Hamman, Cohen, Leucht, Busch, & Kissling, 2005; Hill & Laugharne, 2006). Wareing and Newell (2002) cautioned that providers often envision themselves as supporting a recovery framework that involves choice but that consumers view their only choice as one of refusal. An example might include declining a recommendation for an increase in medication recommended by a psychiatrist. Wareing and Newell emphasized that choice and self-determination imply that a choice is there to be made.

Consumer and provider perspectives on various community mental health services have been explored. Salem (1990) stated that services need to be developed from the consumer perspective and by definition need to meet diverse individual needs. Wolf-Branigan and Daeschlein (2000) found that consumers and providers ranked different service priorities and stated that these differences have serious implications for advocates of recovery-oriented systems.

Occupational therapists believe that engagement in occupation affects health. Inherent in this process is the active engagement of the client, reflected through occupational choice. Occupational therapy researchers have examined the role of occupational engagement in mental health practice. Haertl and Minato (2006) examined the daily occupations of people with mental illness and found that engagement in occupations was normalizing for participants and that occupational choice and structure was valued as well. Minato and Zemke (2004) examined the occupational choices of people with schizophrenia in their study of occupation and health. They found that participants chose occupations for different reasons— as stress reduction or to provide structure and influence life satisfaction, even if the choice increased stress. Mee, Sumsion, and Craik (2004) conducted a qualitative study of mental health consumers to examine occupation and health. Results revealed that occupation supported health by enabling participants to acquire needed skills and have experiences that demonstrated to them that they were capable of success. Additional studies are needed to demonstrate the value of occupational engagement and quality of life.

Consumer Choice and Empowerment

Several initiatives supporting consumer choice have emerged since the President's New Freedom Commission on Mental Health (2003), including increased peer support and peer-run services and increased involvement of consumers in what services are offered and who provides them. For example, the Centers for Medicare and Medicaid Services sponsored 1115 waivers for some states to enable consumers to hire or purchase services for personal assistance or a recovery coach (Smith, Kennedy, Knipper, & O'Brien, 2005). Other trends in consumer choice include mental health advance directives—legal documents based on state laws that enable consumers to determine how their care should be addressed should they be unable to participate in decisions because of the severity of their illness. Clark and Krupa (2002) described empowerment as dealing with "power, control, and struggle" (p. 343). They discussed consumer empowerment as involving partnerships with professionals, involvement in decision making, program development and evaluation, and engaging in self-help and economic development. Empowerment in community mental health has been embraced in the Social Model of Disability, in which the roles of the environment and policies are targeted for change, as in the growth and development of consumer-controlled organizations.

For example, the state of Maryland used some funds from a 5-year Mental Health Systems Transformation Grant from the Substance Abuse and Mental Health Services Administration to launch two important initiatives—the Network of Care and the wellness recovery action plan (Copeland, 1997). The Network of Care (www.networkofcare.org) is a Web site that provides numerous links to services, resources, an article library, and a message board and legislative bill tracking page. Wellness recovery action plans are self-management tool kits to enable people to develop personal plans to manage stress and enlist support.

Empowerment and Participatory Action Research

In line with the President's New Freedom Commission on Mental Health and demand for transformation of the mental health delivery system, the increase in self-help and mutual aid organizations for psychiatric consumers has been dramatic (Nelson, Ochocka, Griffin, & Lord, 1998). One method that has been used to empower marginalized populations is participatory action research. According to Nelson et al. (1998), *participatory action research* is "a research approach that consists of the maximum participation of stakeholders, those whose lives are affected by the problem under study, in the systematic collection and analysis of information for the purpose of taking action and making change" (p. 885). This method is congruent with empowerment theories. Stringer (1996) identified the main tenets of participatory action research as choice, participation, inclusion, and communication. These tenets are congruent with the collaboration and empowerment inherent in the client-centered practice of occupational therapy. Rappaport (1987) conceptualized empowerment as a complex construct occurring on multiple levels. Segal,

Silverman, and Temkin (1995) identified three levels of empowerment for consumers of psychiatric services: (1) *personal empowerment,* in which a person experiences the ability to exercise control; (2) *organizational empowerment,* in which self-determination of the people participating in the organization increases; and (3) *community empowerment,* a broader influence including political change activity.

Self-help and mutual aid organizations, through various types of participatory approaches, empower consumers of mental health services. These approaches include participatory action research that is conducted by consumers themselves and research that is a partnership between professionals and members of self-help organizations. Examples in the occupational therapy literature include the work of Townsend, Birch, Langley, and Langille (2000), who examined data from an institutional ethnography of a mental health clubhouse and likened the research process to a form of client-centered practice. Cockburn and Trentham (2002) articulated the similarities of community-based, client-centered occupational therapy practice and participatory action research in a project involving mental health consumers. Taylor (2003) used participatory action research methodology to analyze three case studies of people with chronic fatigue syndrome and examine the effects of participating in an empowerment-oriented program. Suarez-Balcazar, Martinez, and Casas-Byots (2005) used participatory action research methods to engage an underserved Hispanic population in articulating health and community needs and concerns. The value of this methodology in engaging the community in identifying and solving problems is emphasized as a core tenet of client-centered practice beyond the individual level, which is congruent with support for the shift from a medical model of mental health care to a community or population public health model that emphasizes prevention.

Quantitative outcomes of such interventions include the extent to which consumers of mental health services reduce reliance on formal mental health structures, such as reduction of inpatient hospitalization. Qualitative measures are just as critical and include perception of control over daily decision making, degree of participation in community of choice, and quality of life. These methods hold promise to move the mental health delivery system toward the goal of recovery. The scope and practice of occupational therapy is a good fit for leadership of such initiatives.

Case Studies

This section uses the steps of advocacy as outlined earlier to problem solve and generate a plan of action, including advocacy as described by Sandstrom, Lohman, and Bramble (2009). Each case addresses the following five statements:

1. Gather data to define the problem.
2. Define and analyze criteria, including generating possible alternative solutions.
3. Weigh the pros and cons of each alternative.
4. Choose a plan of action, including the type of advocacy action.
5. Evaluate outcomes of actions.

Case Example 1

A service recipient must be dependent on taking medication to be eligible for supported housing. The service recipient has other deficits in skills for instrumental activities of daily living but could likely learn to take daily medications with rehearsal, color coding, and a weeklong medication dispensing system. On the basis of your knowledge of the recipient, you believe that he can become more independent in administering his medication but will still need supported housing to remain in the community.

Types of Advocacy

The types of advocacy will be determined after following the four-step process.

Steps

1. Gather information about the issue, including identifying key stakeholders and their position on the issue, which might include examining eligibility and medical necessity criteria for supported housing services and contact with team members who are involved with the service recipient. Engage other providers at this organization or agency to discuss the effects of this policy on the recovery goals of the population they serve. If the issue can be resolved at the individual level, it is much less complicated.
2. Define and analyze criteria to determine whether this issue is an individual one, affects a small portion of the population, or impedes many service recipients. Once the affected population has been determined, discuss alternatives and their features, such as not addressing medication at all (to maintain dependence and supported housing) or fully addressing medication administration (realizing that some may lose housing supports).
3. Weigh pluses and minuses of each alternative on the basis of the data generated in Steps 1 and 2.
4. Determine a plan of action and prepare to meet with key stakeholders. If the issue is individual, it will involve the client and treatment coordinator or case manager of housing or PRP. If it involves a small group of clients, PRP leadership would be involved in determining whether increased independence in one area might not penalize a person's living arrangement. If it involves a significant population served by the agency, then the leadership of the PRP and other professional groups, such as state associations and advocacy groups, would be included in planning for appropriate state action via a coalition of interested parties.

Depending on the level of advocacy, the strategy could be one of the following:

- *Individual:* If the service recipient is eligible for services because of another medical issue, then obtaining approval to continue services might be indicated.
- *Profession:* If the issue is that medication is the turf of another discipline, then approaching that discipline to collaborate on a protocol to assist service recipients in recovery, including an occupational therapy approach, might be indicated.
- *Programmatic:* If the issue is one of program philosophy, discussing concerns with the CEO of the program and proposing a medication self-management protocol might be indicated.

- *Public policy:* If the issue is the way in which services are defined, organized, and funded by the state, a more comprehensive approach might be indicated. Accessing resources from the professional association at the state or national level would help to determine whether there are other states in which this is not policy and what effects on service recipients have been. In addition, examining whether other groups besides the state occupational therapy association might be interested in building a coalition to support this type of intervention is indicated. The greater the number of concerned stakeholders is, the greater is the potential to influence policy. This strategy would involve a longer period of time, several meetings with coalition group members, and contacts with key decision makers, among others (Sandstrom et al., 2009).

Case Example 2

The literature shows that only 10% to 15% of people with serious and persistent mental illness are gainfully employed. The state in which you work has received word that the focus of employment funding will be on people with serious illness. You work with a population of young adults who could benefit from minimal supported education and skill training. Make a plan of action to advocate for funding this population.

Types of Advocacy

The types of advocacy will be determined following the four-step process.

Steps

1. Gather information on the criteria for the decision to focus on the people who are most ill. This information would include key decision makers, their point of view, and the level at which the decision was made. This information will inform the occupational therapist of where to focus efforts. For example, was the decision made at the state level on the basis of a philosophy or because of limited funding, or do regions, local agencies, or specific populations have some degree of flexibility in terms of access to vocational preparation? If there is flexibility, what criteria are used in decision making?
2. Define and analyze criteria on the basis of the results of Step 1.
3. Weigh pluses and minuses of each alternative, from accepting the situation as it is and offering limited vocational preparation activities for the client population to proceeding with an educational plan of action for the key decision makers.
4. Determine a plan of action and prepare for meeting with key stakeholders on the basis of the analysis of Steps 2 and 3.

Case Example 3

You believe that people with mental health needs in the community are limited in access to occupational therapy because of your state's definition of who is a qualified mental health provider. Discuss an advocacy plan of action in which you collaborate with key stakeholders and resources to address this challenge.

Types of Advocacy

The type of advocacy is public policy.

Steps

1. Gather information from the state mental health office about how the plan defines a mental health provider. Contact the American Occupational Therapy Association (AOTA) for information about other states in which occupational therapists are addressing this issue, including therapists who have been successful and those who have not. Involve other interested occupational therapists in the state association, and consider other potential collaborators, which might include client advocacy groups, specific disease advocacy groups, or other professional provider group associations.
2. Define and analyze the criteria that the state uses to determine who is a qualified mental health provider and work with the occupational therapy practitioner group and with AOTA to address each one with evidence from the state practice act or other relevant information.
3. Weigh pluses and minuses of each alternative, including accepting things as they are and approaching the issue in another way, such as consultation services, to prepare to propose the consideration of occupational therapists as qualified mental health providers.
4. Determine a plan of action and prepare for meeting with key stakeholders on the basis of the decisions made after Steps 2 and 3.

Summary

Occupational therapists are familiar with individual-level advocacy in which resources are recommended for a particular client or family. This chapter describes advocacy in greater detail and includes several ways in which occupational therapists might become involved in advocating for broader access to services. Issues include those that exist because of public or private mental health policy as well as social factors, such as poverty or stigma, that require advocacy relative to program or public policy. Another key aspect of advocacy includes supporting individual recovery through services and policies that empower service recipients. The ways in which occupational therapists are involved include participatory action research and supporting services that are directed by the recipient. This chapter describes a four-step process to analyze and chart a course of advocacy action. This process can assist occupational therapists in developing advocacy skills beyond the individual level to the program, profession, and public policy levels.

References

Allport, G. (1954). *The nature of prejudice.* Cambridge, MA: Addison-Wesley.

Barton, P. B. (1999). *Understanding the U.S. health services system.* Chicago: Health Administration Press.

Clark, C. C., & Krupa, T. (2002). Reflections on empowerment in community mental health: Giving shape to an elusive idea. *Psychiatric Rehabilitation Journal, 25,* 341–349.

Cockburn, L., & Trentham, B. (2002). Participatory action research: Integrating community occupational therapy practice and research. *Canadian Journal of Occupational Therapy, 69*(1), 20–30.

Collins essential English dictionary (2nd ed.). (2006). New York: HarperCollins.

Cook, J. A., & Jonikas, J. A. (2002). Self-determination among mental health consumers/ survivors: Using lessons from the past to guide the future. *Journal of Disability Policy Studies, 13,* 87–95.

Copeland, M. A. (1997). *Wellness recovery action plan.* Dummerston, VT: Peach Press.

Corrigan, P. W. (2004). Target-specific stigma change: A strategy for impacting mental illness stigma. *Psychiatric Rehabilitation Journal, 28,* 113–121.

Corrigan, P. W., & Penn, D. L. (1999). Lessons from social psychology on discrediting psychiatric stigma. *American Psychologist, 54,* 765–776.

Crepeau, E., Cohn, E., & Boyt Schell, B. A. (Eds.). (2003). *Willard and Spackman's occupational therapy* (10th ed.). Philadelphia: Lippincott Williams & Wilkins.

Crutsinger, M. (2007, October 17). Social security only going up 2.3 percent. *The Washington Post.* Retrieved January 30, 2008, from www.washingtonpost.com/wp-dyn/content/article/2007/10/17/AR2007101701057.html

Decade of the brain. (1990, July 17). *Presidential Proclamation 6158.* Retrieved February 2, 2010, from www.loc.gov/loc/brain/proclaim.html

Geller, J. L. (2000). The last half century of psychiatric services as reflected in *Psychiatric Services. Psychiatric Services, 51,* 41–67.

Haertl, K., & Minato, M. (2006). Daily occupations of persons with mental illness: Themes from Japan and America. *Occupational Therapy in Mental Health, 22,* 19–32.

Hamann, J., Cohen, R., Leucht, S., Busch, R., & Kissling, W. (2005). Do patients with schizophrenia wish to be involved in decisions about their medical treatment? *American Journal of Psychiatry, 162,* 2382–2384.

Hill, S. A., & Laugharne, R. (2006). Decision making and information seeking preferences among psychiatric patients. *Journal of Mental Health, 15,* 75–84.

Laugharne, R., & Priebe, S. (2006). Trust, choice, and power in mental health. *Social Psychiatry and Psychiatric Epidemiology, 41,* 843–852.

Lewis, D. A., Shadish, W. R., & Lurigio, A. J. (1989). Policies of inclusion and the mentally ill: Long-term care in a new environment. *Journal of Social Issues, 45,* 173–186.

Mechanic, D. (2008). *Mental health and social policy: Beyond managed care* (5th ed.). New York: Allyn & Bacon.

Mee, J., Sumsion, T., & Craik, C. (2004). Mental health clients confirm the value of occupation in building competence and self-identity. *British Journal of Occupational Therapy, 67,* 225–233.

Mental Health America. (2009). *Fact sheet—Paul Wellstone and Pete Domenici Mental Health Parity and Addiction Equity Act of 2008.* Retrieved September 14, 2009, from http://takeaction.mentalhealthamerica.net/site/PageServer?pagename=Equity_Campaign_detailed_summary

Mental Health Parity Act of 1996, Pub. L. 104–204, Title VII, 110 Stat. 2944.

Miller Polgar, J., & Landry, J. E. (2004). Occupations as a means for individual and group participation in life. In C. H. Christiansen & E. A. Townsend (Eds.), *Introduction to occupation: The art and science of living* (pp. 197–220). Upper Saddle River, NJ: Prentice Hall.

Minato, M., & Zemke, R. (2004). Time use of people with schizophrenia living in the community. *Occupational Therapy International, 11*(3), 177–191.

National Alliance for Mental Illness (2007). *Fact sheet—The uninsured: Five steps to advocate for individuals with serious mental illnesses.* Alexandria, VA: Author.

Nelson, G., Ochocka, J., Griffin, K., & Lord, J. (1998). "Nothing about me, without me": Participatory action research with self-help/mutual aid organizations for psychiatric consumers/survivors. *American Journal of Community Psychology, 26*(6), 881–912.

Olmstead v. L. C. 527 U.S. 581 (1999).

Olsen, L., Aisner, D., & McGinnis, J. M. (Eds.). (2007). *The learning healthcare system: Workshop summary* (IOM Roundtable on Evidence-Based Medicine). Washington, DC: National Academy of Sciences.

Organization for Economic Cooperation and Development. (2008). *Policy Brief—Economic survey of the United States 2008.* Retrieved September 14, 2009, from www.oecd.org/dataoecd/60/54/41812368.pdf

Paul Wellstone and Pete Domenici Mental Health Parity and Addiction Equity Act of 2008, Pub. L. 110–343.

Power, A. K. (2007). *Putting consumers at the center of care: Remarks.* Rockville, MD: Center for Mental Health Services National Advisory Council Subcommittee on Consumer Survivor

Issues. Retrieved February 6, 2008, from http://mentalhealth.samhsa.gov/newsroom/speeches/061407.asp

President's New Freedom Commission on Mental Health. (2003). *Achieving the promise: Transforming mental health care in America* (Final Report, DHHS Pub. No. SMA–03–3832). Rockville, MD: Author. Retrieved February 14, 2008, from www.mentalhealthcommission.gov/reports/reports.htm

Rappaport, J. (1987). Terms of empowerment/exemplars of prevention: Toward a theory for community psychology. *American Journal of Community Psychology, 15,* 121–144.

Rehabilitation Act of 1973 Amendments, Pub. L. 95–602, H.R. 12467, H. Rept. 95–1149.

Robinson, G. K., Connolly, J. B., Whitter, M., & Magana, C. A. (2007). *State mandates for treatment for mental illness and substance abuse disorders.* Washington, DC: U.S. Department of Health and Human Services, Substance Abuse and Mental Health Services Administration, Center for Mental Health Services.

Rusch, N., Angermeyer, M. C., & Corrigan, P. W. (2005). Mental illness stigma: Concepts, consequences, and initiatives to reduce stigma. *European Psychiatry, 20,* 529–539.

Salem, D. A. (1990). Community-based services and resources: The significance of choice and diversity. *American Journal of Community Psychology, 18,* 909–915.

Sandstrom, R. W., Lohman, H., & Bramble, J. D. (2009). *Health services: Policy and systems for therapists.* Upper Saddle River, NJ: Prentice Hall.

Segal, P., Silverman, C., & Temkin, T. (1995). Measuring empowerment in client-run self-help agencies. *Community Mental Health Journal, 31,* 215–227.

Smart, J. (2001). *Disability, society, and the individual.* Austin, TX: Pro-Ed.

Smith, G., Kennedy, C., Knipper, S., & O'Brien, J. (2005). *Using Medicaid to support working age adults with serious mental illness in the community: A handbook.* Washington, DC: U.S. Department of Health and Human Services, Office of the Assistant Secretary for Planning and Evaluation.

Stringer, E. T. (1996). *Action research: A handbook for practitioners.* Thousand Oaks, CA: Sage.

Suarez-Balcazar, Y., Martinez, L. J, & Casas-Byots, C. (2005). A participatory action research approach for identifying health service needs of Hispanic immigrants: Implications for occupational therapy. *Occupational Therapy in Health Care, 19*(1/2), 145–163.

Taylor, R. R. (2003). Extending client-centered practice: The use of participatory methods to empower clients. *Occupational Therapy in Mental Health, 19*(2), 57–75.

Townsend, E., Birch, D. E., Langley, J., & Langille, L. (2000). Participatory research in a mental health clubhouse. *OTJR: Occupation, Participation and Health, 20*(1), 18–44.

U.S. Department of Health and Human Services. (1999*). Mental health: A report of the Surgeon General.* Rockville, MD: U.S. Department of Health and Human Services, Substance Abuse and Mental Health Services Administration, Center for Mental Health Services & National Institutes of Health, National Institute of Mental Health.

Wareing, D., & Newell, C. (2002). Responsible choice: The choice between no choice. *Disability and Society, 17,* 419–434.

Wolf-Branigan, M., & Daeschlein, M. (2000). Differing priorities of counselors and customers to a consumer choice model in rehabilitation. *Journal of Rehabilitation, 66,* 18–22.

Advocacy Web Sites

Centers for Medicaid and Medicare Services: www.cms.hhs.gov

Medicaid (Pub. L. 89–97): www.cms.hhs.gov/home/Medicaid.asp

Medicare (Pub. L. 89–97): www.Medicare.gov

Social Security Online (Social Security Administration): www.ssa.gov

Supplemental Security Income (Pub. L. 92–603): www.ssa.gov/pgm/links_ssi.htm

Social Security Disability Insurance Program (Pub. L. 96–265): www.ssa.gov/pgm/links_disability.htm

National Alliance on Mental Illness: www.nami.org

Olmstead decision (Olmstead v. L. C. 527 U.S. 581 (1999)): www.cms.hhs.gov/smdl/downloads/smd072500b.pdf

Rehabilitation Act of 1973 (Pub. L. 93–112): www.ada.gov/cguide.htm#anchor65610

CHAPTER 21

Leadership in Occupational Therapy and Mental Health

Rondalyn V. Whitney, MOT, OTR/L, and
Elizabeth Cara, PhD, OTR/L

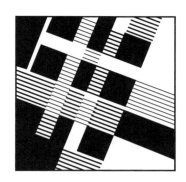

Learning Objectives

After reading this material and completing the examination, readers will be able to

- Identify differences and similarities in occupational therapists and business leaders;

- Identify differences and similarities of managers and leaders;

- Identify the skills and attributes of leaders;

- Recognize leadership as agency;

- Identify the tools and strategies needed to develop leadership in teams, organizations, and fieldwork;

- Recognize the important role of fieldwork supervision in cultivating future leaders; and

- Identify one's own leadership style and one's individual style in one's own particular organization.

Senior occupational therapists have identified the need to improve clinical reasoning, problem-solving, management, and leadership skills and to increase understanding of leadership skills as they relate to occupational therapy practice (Brachtesende, 2004). However, occupational therapists who have just a few years of clinical experience are being asked to step into management roles because of their skills in organizing, controlling, directing, and planning their own professional craft. Although personal management skills do not necessarily transfer smoothly to the leadership of others, management should not be viewed as a new job with new skills. Both leadership and management practices call for a new perspective, a unique application of familiar skills. As such, this sometimes subtle transformation within a work environment requires a critical shift in thought, introspection, and self-assessment and developmental skills that are central to committed professionals. Moreover, learning new ways of being in a professional context can be a profound yet invisible cognitive shift.

This shift is a transformation by any definition, and it requires the energy and regard due a change of such magnitude. One must acknowledge and understand the relationship between managerial styles and behaviors related to those styles within the work culture and address both the innate skills and the absent traits of management characteristics. Leaders, in contrast to managers, inspire others; followers want to emulate their example. Good leaders energize and intellectually stimulate their followers (Ray & Myers, 1996).

This chapter, then, introduces a way of conceptualizing a harmonious coexistence between the context of business management and leadership in the professional practice of occupational therapy. The chapter defines the concepts of manager and leader and distinguished to help occupational therapists solidify their identity in an administrative context. It also presents problem-solving tools and strategies for successfully navigating the stress that accompanies rapid change. Occupational therapy's role in leading and contributing within teams is identified to help therapists as they orchestrate ethical commitments, student mentoring, and occupational behaviors. Ultimately, this chapter will help therapists work productively by demonstrating care for themselves and others with whom they work and develop the agency needed for leadership or management. Appendix 21A provides a short self-assessment activity to aid readers in self-reflection and help them gain a better understanding of their own leadership and management style.

Concepts of Leadership

The obscure we see eventually.
The completely apparent takes longer.

—Edward R. Murrow
(cited in Jones, 1999)

Models used to guide business leadership align with occupational therapy's core values. Occupational therapists are in the business of occupation and, as such, are engaged with a specific concern of interest. The word *business* comes from the Middle English root *busy* and implies the state of being in action, having industry, and producing. So the profession of occupational therapy arguably has the same roots as business, the art and science of being engaged in meaningful and purposeful actions.

Business leaders in all fields are indicating that they have come to the end of an old paradigm (Wheatley, 1992), with conceptual models that are impotent to create change in the world. A new paradigm is needed if occupational therapy is to help people become as effective as they want to be and resolve many of the pertinent central issues of the time: mental health disparity, meaningful participation for people with chronic disability, and health care disparity. Some leaders in the business realm have been designated *futurists*. Futurists synthesize multidisciplinary, quantitative data to track relevant trends, analyze them, and think creatively about their direction and meaning. They do not predict the future insomuch as they project the future as many as 50 years in advance (van der Werff, 2008).

One could argue that the founders of occupational therapy were futurists, people who looked into the future and saw the waning attention to people's psychospiritual needs as they encountered the stress of disability. They intuitively assessed the need for vital occupations that would serve as a protection against the imminent stressors of increasing societal demands. They responded to their growing intuition that something was wrong in the way in which people who were dispirited were cared for. They formed not only a profession but a new body of thought, a new paradigm, and assembled an organization of conversationalists who could create cohesive patterns of thought in anticipation of future problems.

In the profession of occupational therapy, a renewed commitment to mental health concerns has been reestablished as an essential component of all areas of practice. Thus, a revitalization of occupational therapy's core value has been announced, and therapists are charged by leadership to stop at nothing short of rehabilitating life so that it can be lived to its fullest. This edict is in response to a growing global intuition that something more than greater range of motion or temporary reduction of acute symptoms is required if the promise of occupational science—and even human potential—is to be realized.

Scholars of leadership today have come to the same conclusion about business and management styles as did the founders of occupational therapy almost a century ago—that seeing organizations (or human beings) as machines is a bankrupt perspective that will not resolve complex presenting problems. Instead, occupational therapy must begin to conceptualize organizations and human beings as dynamic, complex living systems acting within environments. Leaders must seek to understand how living systems grow and thrive, develop resilience, and transform into new entities that go around environmentally imposed barriers. Moreover, leaders must access wisdom through cross-pollination of bodies of knowledge previously housed in distinctly bounded fields. According to Wheatley (1992), leaders encourage conversations, and through these active, chaotic interchanges, real solutions to complex problems beyond predictable lines of linear thought can emerge.

Thus, both occupational therapists and business professionals have a great deal to offer one another when leadership topics are explored (Whitney, 1996). Both communities of practice are engaged in facilitating change, working to achieve goals, and making themselves known to markets looking, sometimes in dispirited frustration, for services that provide real solutions to these problems. Traditional business models have felt inflexible and ill fitting to therapists attempting to emulate their principles. However, visionaries in business communities are advancing new paradigms of leadership much aligned with occupational therapy's core values. New paradigms include cross-fertilization among specialists, embracing change, incorporation of spiritual values, and the essential need to understand the whole before locating and resolving any underlying disharmonies (Ray & Myers, 1996).

The new American Occupational Therapy Association (AOTA) brand for occupational therapy is "Living Life to the Fullest" (www.aota.org). Mental health practitioners were perhaps the first to realize the bankruptcy in clinical practice that sought to reduce symptoms without restoring meaningful engagement. Perhaps mental health practitioners are to the profession of occupational therapy what the canary was once to the coal miners—when the canary stopped singing, only moments were left before the environment was without air. One might assert that the leaders and steadfast practitioners in mental health were the first to sing out about the suffocation they felt under a medical model controlled by third-party payers (Howard, 1991). Today in business, the phrase "a canary in a coal mine" is used to describe people who are willing to experience threats without concession. Anyone who thwarts his or her own nature when working in an environment in which he or she feels no deep connection to coworkers is a caged canary, waiting to be overwhelmed by invisible toxins. The leaders in mental health practice continued to work toward holistic outcomes with integrity and without compromise, and in so doing transformed the people around them to consider health to be something that indeed, at times, escaped finite measure. Transformational leadership is a call to future practice that will be an epiphany for some, a challenge for others, and an avalanche of change to perhaps a few. For any who have stayed attentive to their clients' mental health, regardless of practice setting, transformational leadership will be an opportunity to release a long-held breath of hope. Regardless of where a practitioner, manager, or leader stands, it is clear now that the job is not done until people are actively engaged in the lives they long to live. Work must be meaningful, spirit must be valued and able to replenish itself, and leaders must have vision. Therapists' efforts to be purposeful must ultimately engage them in socially responsible actions (Moyers, 2008; Ray & Myers, 1996; Wheatley, 1992), or we are lost in the mire of assembly line construction and not occupational creation—or, as in the canary in the mine analogy, we will wither from a loss of vital air.

Management and Leadership

Leaders and managers in occupational therapy are clinicians with clinical frameworks for resolving problems and organizing constructs. "OT practitioners are frequently thrust into management positions within their first few years of professional practice" (Snodgrass, Douthitt, Ellis, Wade, & Plemons, 2008, p. 38), primarily on the basis of their technical abilities. This thrust is made both without regard to the unique skills required to manage oneself or others and the professional commitment inherent in successful managers. In addition, little attention has been given to distinguishing management from leadership and ensuring a good fit between occupational therapists' skills and the tasks associated with the job. Competent therapists seek access to models of management and leadership that align with and expand on their internal working models of meeting goals, motivating others, and solving complex problems. However, skills of management and skills of leadership, although complementary systems of action and both necessary in the business environment, are distinct (Kotter, 2001). When the strengths of individual leaders and individual managers are not acknowledged and cultivated, the organization risks being overmanaged and simultaneously underled. Some people are good at managing themselves but not others. Some manage others but not themselves and experience stress and burnout. Management skills can be directed at the self, others, the profession, and even society. Managerial models based in old paradigms of competition, product-oriented goals, and rigid alignment with a preexisting culture seem in conflict with occupational therapy's core values: altruism, equality, freedom, justice, dignity, truth, and prudence (AOTA, 1993).

Occupational therapists have a duty to explore examples of leadership in the profession of occupational therapy, to find models of management that can guide what we want to achieve while continually maintaining the higher standards of competence that moved us into management. Therapists feel obligated to embody fidelity in their interactions with others, which can seem incompatible with the business of business. Perhaps it would be best, then, to consider the new paradigms being advanced in business today by the leaders in that profession (Ray & Meyers, 1996; Wheatley, 1992).

The United States has seen a similar transformative process. Before industrialization, people worked alone honing their unique crafts. When the United States entered the industrial age, many workers were brought together, and as a means of managing the new collective resources, some were reclassified as managers. This reclassification was not meant to be an elevation but rather a reutilization of demonstrated skills (Drafke, 1994). Management requires organizational skills, the ability to control the time and movement of the day's work, and the ability to direct others to accomplish tasks and to plan one's own direction to increase competency as a way to follow the recommended practice of professional intervention. Good clinicians are natural performers of these skills, and it is easy to see how they, even early in their clinical practice, could be tapped for a management position although they are not always leaders. However, managers can learn to be leaders. They can learn how to inspire, they can grow to be admired and respected, and they can, through daily relationship building, gain their peers' trust.

Leaders, instead, are people who can inspire others and who may or may not have the additional skills necessary to manage others. They are admired, respected, and trusted by those with whom they interact, and their followers wish to emulate them. Leaders consider their followers' needs, share risks with them, and perform in ways that are consistent with underlying ethics within teams. Good leaders both energize and intellectually stimulate their followers (Ray & Myers, 1996) while ensuring they are leading them toward a future that considers their followers' needs above their own (Snodgrass, 2006) with flexibility and compassion (Ray & Myers, 1996). However, even though they are inspiring, admired, and followed, leaders are not always good at organizing or directing others. They can, then, lead others into chaos and disorganization and the messy business of seeking the future without any evidence other than their own charismatic curiosity. Sheep farmers identify the one sheep that others follow and hang a bell from its neck so they can harness the natural ability of this one sheep to lead the flock. The sheep leads, however, unconsciously. Some leaders are natural bellwethers and serve as leading indicators of future trends, but they can do so either consciously or unconsciously.

Of course, leaders can learn to be conscious in their directions, can become aware that others are following and emulating them, and can learn to be good managers. However, to learn the complementary skills of management, they must seek out the partnership of a manager or honor and cultivate the unique skills of management, just as managers would need to learn skills from leaders.

Anyone who works can behave professionally, but professionals have both the honor and the responsibility to work autonomously, with integrity, dedication, and an ongoing commitment to critical appraisal and self-improvement (Higgs, 2003).

Leadership is a dynamic interaction between the needs of society, the professional organization, the individual self, and the activities associated with managing others, as illustrated in Figure 21.1. *Autonomy* is the ability to have self-determination and

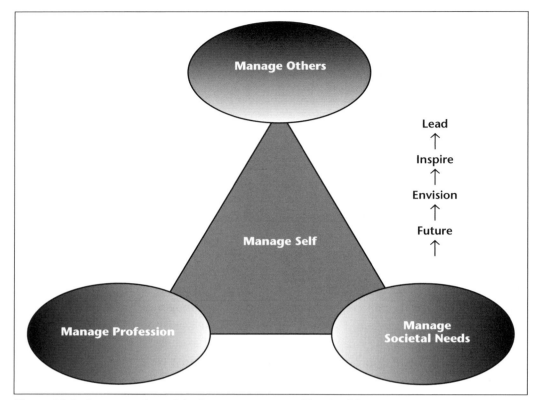

Figure 21.1. Conceptual model of management and leadership.
Source. Author.

independence. Managers plan, control, organize, and direct resources as well as perform the work within an organization (Drafke, 1994) autonomously. Leaders set the vision and the direction using a decision-making process and keep their sights fixed on the future. They work independently. They are distinguished by their ability to inspire others, envision the future and orient to it and, to state the obvious, have others follow them as they build bridges to new horizons. No one body of knowledge or expertise can transfer intact from one system to another, and great leaders who can manage and great managers who can lead are frequently hybrids who have grown as a result of cross-pollination.

A paradigm shift is under way—one that insists on meaningful work, socially responsible occupational behaviors, and visionary leadership (Renesch, 1993). These new paradigms of leadership are more aligned with occupational therapy's core identity, but others have not been trained to see occupational therapy professionals as leaders. Perhaps more important, occupational therapists and occupational therapy assistants often do not have a personal identity as leaders. Leadership activity has been seen as incongruous with the prioritized value of caring for others (Scott, 1985), and such people are prone to resist being singled out as leaders. People who are new to practice can be thrust into management roles before they have time to integrate the new learning, resulting in a struggle to reconcile the roles of practitioner, manager, and leader that later results in burnout. Those of us who mentor newer therapists need to plan the growth and development of leadership and management skills and insist that leaders and managers manage their internal resources to create sustainability in both the profession and the professionals leading the profession.

Occupational therapists have the opportunity to integrate their clinical practice and management skills and become leaders. For example, if one finds oneself controlling outcomes without vision, one can establish a self-assessment mechanism to acquire new habits and routines that foster greater autonomy in the people one manages. Alternatively, one needs to learn to manage occupational behaviors so that one's leadership is conscious, for example, by making sure one has strong evidence, beyond tacit knowledge, when implementing a new procedure or protocol in practice, thus being conscious that others are watching and following one's lead. Therapists must do this work if they are to become leaders of programs that ensure participation, active engagement, and living life to its fullest. How, then, does one gain essential skills for such transformational leadership? The answer to this question is embedded in occupational therapy practice—one looks for ways to ensure the client's simultaneous growth and wellness and makes a plan that takes the client beyond what he or she can attain alone. In her presidential address, Baum (2005) asked members to "hold your leadership to a high level of accountability" (p. 249). She acknowledged the leaders within the profession, from the reconstructive aides of 1918 to the leaders in the membership today. These leaders are actively enlightening policymakers, relentlessly agitating for the relationship between occupation and health, and creating collaborative and productive teams that are transforming practice to create strong evidentiary measures of achieved outcomes.

Table 21.1 captures the distinctions between leaders and managers and how these roles overlap within the occupational therapy profession.

Strategies to Deal With Change and Tools for Problem Solving

According to Jaffe-Epstein (1999), noticing and orienting one's attention to stressors is a "key adaptive mechanism and occurs when new information has not yet been processed by the body" (p. 398). Adaptation and improved function occur in the environment of change when the orientation response triggers this short burst of

Table 21.1. Critical Analysis of Occupational Therapists, Managers, and Leaders

Occupational Therapists	Managers	Leaders
Write down a clinical question.	Plan by setting strategic goals and establish routines and standard procedures.	Set the vision; feel they have a calling; encourage others to envision the future.
Gather current published evidence that might answer the question.	Control the discipline's methods and evaluate change as a way to guide the organization toward stated goals.	Inspire others to admire them, to trust them, and to follow them; others want to emulate them.
Evaluate the gathered evidence to determine what is the "best" evidence for answering the question.	Organize operations within the department by forming task groups and allocating resources to accomplish goals.	Stimulate innovation; embrace and welcome change; find novelty refreshing.
Communicate with clients and colleagues about the evidence as evaluation and intervention decisions are being made during occupational therapy.	Direct other workers by building consensus; doing so through inspiration distinguishes a manager who is also a good leader.	Profess their beliefs; arouse team spirit; create supportive environments that are conducive to growth.
Evaluate the chosen evidence-based evaluation and intervention procedures as they are implemented with clients and revise and individualize them as appropriate.	Use the decision-making process and are responsive to team's needs to manage stress associated with change.	Use decision-making process; encourage others to question assumptions, reframe problems, and attack known obstacles in novel, creative ways; agitate for change.

Sources. Hendrix (2004); Kotter, (2001); Snodgrass, Douthitt, Ellis, Wade, and Plemons (2008); Tickle-Degnen (2000).

energy, resulting in adaptive reaction. This adaptive reaction, or stress, can be a positive energizer. When overstimulated, people and the teams they work within can become disorganized and ineffective at best and distressed at worse.

In addition to commonly practiced stress management techniques focused on relaxation and time management, good problem solving can provide a mechanism for managing stress by introducing a systematic approach to address problems. Occupational therapists need to inspire an attitude that embraces or even agitates for change and help others understand that perspective makes a difference. Whereas it was once sufficient to merely cope with change, over time the requirement has escalated to manage change, embrace change, lead change, activate change, and, now, agitate for change. When therapists begin to extrapolate the philosophical principles of occupational therapy, these essential ideas and values merge into principles of leadership with a muted simplicity.

Robert Sapolsky's (n.d.) Third Law of Science stated, "Often, the biggest impediment to scientific progress is not what we don't know, but what we know" (para. 1). "Self-esteem, self-knowledge, and caring for oneself are prerequisites in effective supervision" (Jaffe-Epstein, 1999, p. 65). Developing this insight can make the difference between approaching change as unwelcome or devastating or as exhilarating. One can be frightened by the ever-rising waves, one can make the waves, or one can dive in and ride the naturally occurring waves. Ideally, one would stand poised, weathered surfboard at the ready, for the exhilarating, ever-changing sea before one. To lead, one must first know oneself before asking another to follow. Veracity in practice, or self-knowing, is one of occupational therapy's ethical principles. First, one needs to know how one manages or handles change and how effective one's adaptive skills are. How does one build teams that are resilient in the face of change?

Occupational therapists are principally reliable and hold solid convictions that give them unwavering ideas, and they use these ideologies to formulate ideas, personal plans, and client interventions (Soles & Moller, 2001; Washburn, 1991). They use their sensing judgment in their inner life and their thinking judgment in their outer life. They respect science and facts, yet trust their tacit knowledge, and they use this holistic picture to help them take calculated risks. Although they enter situations with caution, once in, they persevere (Soles & Moller, 2001).

The idea that overcoming obstacles or adversity makes great leaders is consistent throughout the literature (Wheatley, 1992). Thus, the key to winning is to face change head on, not wait for it to be imposed. "A proactive approach to change enables it to become our ally rather than our adversary" (Jacobs & Logigian, 1999, p. 1). Personal adaptation to change requires strong problem-solving skills.

Problem solving as a way to approach critical reasoning and evidence-based practice follows identifiable steps that have been outlined by many fields (Buysse & Wesley, 2006; Polya, 1957; Tickle-Degnen, 2000). These steps can be represented by a four-letter acronym, WISE: identifying first and foremost, *what* seems to be the problem, *isolating* what is known yet still needs to be known, attempting an informed *solution,* and then *evaluating* the outcome (see Table 21.2).

On the one hand, the chemicals that stress releases can be energizing and help people persist with challenges that are joyful such as crossing the finish line after a hard-fought 26th mile. On the other hand, prolonged, persistent stress, or distress, depletes people's reserves and makes one more step look and feel like a marathon.

Table 21.2. Comparing and Contrasting Evidence-Based Practice and Problem Solving

Evidence-Based Practice	WISE Approach to Problem Solving
Write down a clinical question.	*W:* What are you being asked to find, solve, or resolve?
Gather current published evidence that might answer the question.	
Evaluate the gathered evidence to determine the best evidence for answering the question.	*I:* Isolate what you know from what you need to know to understand the problem.
Communicate with clients and colleagues about the evidence as evaluation and intervention decisions are being made during occupational therapy.	*S:* Make a strategy and start to carry out your plan. Be thorough and methodical.
Evaluate the chosen evidence-based assessment and intervention procedures as they are implemented with clients and revise and individualize as appropriate.	*E:* Evaluate and reflect on whether you solved the problem.

It's all about people's perception of the situation, how they label the environmental stressor, and how long they have to travel before they rest. Stress is an adaptive response to change. Distress, by contrast, is the state of being faced with stressors that are unmitigated and protracted and that diminish vitality and wellness. People need to reduce distress because it impedes the immune function and robs them of their vitality. Stress, however, is people's natural response to novelty and surprise, and it occurs in response to both positive and negative situations.

Although therapists are busy with the day-to-day living skills, from personal activities of daily living to the work habits of the people they manage and lead, they must take time to attend to the deeper and more restorative processes of self-making, which will enable them to focus on the core of the organization, the service, and to remember, always, that all change originates when one changes one's perception of who one is. Leaders from the businesses that promote wellness have underscored the importance of stress reduction within organizations. Table 21.3 is a synthesis of recommended practices for teams and will sound quite familiar to any clinician who practices in the mental health area but who might not have evolved in his or her leadership style to organize team-building and group cohesion activities.

Lancaster (2004) proposed, "[S]o much of what is going on in our lives is seen through our own generational lens" and "generational collisions are among the key management issues being faced by leaders of today's organizations" (para. 1). People are living longer and staying in the workforce longer. The research of Lancaster and Stillman (2003) identified the many problems ascribed by senior occupational therapists to loss of employee loyalty and work ethic as instead being generational. Poorly handled generational issues are creating distress for managers and leaders in occupational therapy. Lack of communication and rising tensions between generational values are attenuating the vital exchange between old and new ways of doing and causing significant, unresolved burnout (Brachtesende, 2004). For example, according to Lancaster (2004), although traditionalists (people born from 1925 through 1945) seek stability in the workforce, Baby Boomers (those born from 1946 through 1964) want a personal challenge, and Gen Xers (those born from 1965 through 1980) avoid close supervision but require a great deal of feedback. These generational values can create stressful relationships between and among managers. Managers and leaders who understand

Table 21.3. Stress Management for Teams

Action	Example
Provide activities that facilitate adequate coping behaviors.	Encourage healthy eating by facilitating group lunches or daily brisk walks during afternoon breaks.
Help people be more playful; creativity and purpose need to be infused into all "doing"; act in ways that model occupational engagement.	Consider a weekly award during staff meetings for the most creative problem-solving strategy that week.
Laugh; historically and evolutionarily, laughter is an adaptive response to moments of rest between actions needed for survival.	Model fun, provide a joke board in a common area, give monthly fun awards, use the Creative Whack Pack[a] and similar games for problem solving to encourage a light-hearted approach.
Information is only valued when given in relationship to a current need; life is a fluid, not a solid. This philosophy needs to be implanted in therapists' leadership philosophy as it is in their practice.	Use the principle of the "just-right" challenge for the people you lead and manage, giving information judiciously and making sure you have built a strong rapport with anyone to whom you deliver correction ("I like your independence, but in the future I need you to check with me before you order more office supplies—we're going to be moving our offices over the holiday while they move the workstations and make room for a new position they're opening up in the new year.").
Pay attention to what is working, what good is coming of habits and routines, growth, and your own and others' capacities, and celebrate when you see the "goodness" occurring.	When you see someone practicing a new habit, call it to their and others' attention ("Mary, thank you for putting the charts back after you finished—that makes it easier to get the team meetings completed").
Engage the people you lead in creating an identity—a vital, living entity—and engage others in contributing in meaningful ways to the well-being of this commonly named, newly birthed possibility.	Naming your project can inspire a common purpose; for example, a "Light'n'Up" campaign for enhanced wellness might include nutrition classes, getting pedometers donated, and other inspired acts from team members.
Invite contributions that have and build integrity and inspire and orchestrate service from others in the community who care about what they do, and share your goals to realize the possibility of the organization.	For the "Light'n'Up" campaign, local businesses might donate prizes, host a brunch after a group walk, and so forth.
Remember the root of the word *integrity* means to be intact and to act with tact and tactfully in relationship with others.	Turnover in an organization is expensive, but everyone wants to work in an environment where they feel known, accepted, and encouraged to realize their own greatest selves.

[a]The Creative Whack Pack is an illustrated deck of cards used by NASA and other organizations; it is designed to "whack" participants out of habitual thought patterns (von Oech, 1998).

this and become culturally sensitive to the unique values of each generation can proactively create intact teams and develop work environments that are creative and engaging and foster a sense of integrity for therapists and, in return, the clients they serve.

Occupational Therapists in a Team

Group behaviors are organized around unwritten rules and develop in four organized stages—forming, storming, norming, and performing—and three models—psychoanalytic, humanistic, and behavioral (Cara & Macrae, 1998). Managers orchestrate initial group entry, facilitate people's need to find status and a role within the group, direct the formation of relationships and task norms, and, once norms are set, challenge the group to develop a cohesive, organized entity that can accomplish meaningful work within the organization. Group norms guide the group members' behavior, and management style defines the group leader's role, the techniques used, and the goals for the group's work. Mental health practitioners have the skills to help others plan and achieve goals, calm out-of-control people, use effective communication skills, and use the therapeutic self—just a few examples of harnessed principles of group dynamics easily applicable to managing teams. Others might include the need for greater coping skills among the staff, practitioners who need enhanced skills in direct communication styles, or those who model effective balance in the face of life's challenges.

Occupational therapists need management philosophies that incorporate humanistic components while considering both the client's and society's well-being. Such an approach helps develop an organization that is decidedly responsive and able to promptly adapt to change and to the changes in today's mental health environment (Jaffe-Epstein, 1999). Societal marketing concepts, as one example, focus on integrating client well-being by conducting market analyses, collecting multi-level input from stakeholders, and using future-oriented strategic frameworks and a continuous self-monitoring mechanism to ensure that the organization is operating in a cost-effective, sustainable manner. A *market* is simply the group of people who have either an identified need or a potential need for specified services. Occupational therapists can apply a problem-solving approach to a community and from there identify the tools of occupational science that can resolve those problems. One such market could be foster parents of children who were exposed to drugs during gestation. Another such market might be families dealing with children with early-onset bipolar disorder both at home and in the school setting.

This strategy for marketing is not a hierarchy but an act of community engagement, an interrelated network that serves to move the organization and community forward in the symbiotic dance of life. Occupational therapy needs to inspire the formation of successful communities of practice that can provide new levels of professional wisdom not available to one isolated discipline. A community of practice might include first responders in emergency mental health care, occupational therapists, and local staff at community homeless shelters. Another might be occupational therapy leaders working in mental health settings, area school personnel, and school-based occupational therapists for whom treatment of early-onset mental health concerns are not an area of competence. Through active, engaging, creative, life-affirming conversations, across disciplines, new solutions can be created.

Of course, to accomplish this, occupational therapists who are leaders, who can view solutions through the unique lens of occupational science, need to be present at many tables: school board meetings, parent groups, interdisciplinary community teams, law enforcement task forces, and so forth. Once present at the table, they can then demonstrate their problem-solving skills, offer their clinical reasoning to solve complex problems, and harness their skills of observation, born of long practice. As professionals, occupational therapists can keep their cool when others get overwhelmed by the sensations stirred by imminent change, and they can, as professionals, step up to the challenge and get to work building evidence-based, ethical solutions. As managers, therapists can organize and identify goals, direct others to complete their tasks, control conflicting interests, and appropriately create plans that will execute the vision.

Acquiring Leadership Skills Through Fieldwork

The same concepts of transformational leadership that occupational therapists gain in practice support them in embracing the job of fieldwork educator. Some of the responsibilities of the fieldwork educator are those of a manager. However, a good fieldwork supervisor will also take on the qualities of a leader. As a manager, the fieldwork educator directs and organizes fieldwork students in their journey to acquire the skills necessary to be occupational therapists. In managing, the supervisor follows AOTA-recommended guidelines for the fieldwork educator.

The fieldwork educator is integral for students who are in the process of assuming the identity of a professional occupational therapist. As a transformational leader, the fieldwork supervisor energizes students to embrace their roles and responsibilities and stimulates them to learn their tasks and professional roles and to assume the ethical identity of a professional who embraces the profession's values.

To accomplish these tasks, a transformational fieldwork educator takes on several distinct roles. First, the supervisor is a mentor, whether explicitly or implicitly, to the novice. As a mentor, she or he guides and advocates for her or his students. Second, in the mentor role, the educator is a role model. As a role model, he or she models whom the professional occupational therapist is and whom the student wants to become. Third, as a role model, she or he inspires the student to accomplish the goals of the fieldwork and achieve success; indeed, research has indicated that successful fieldwork experiences include inspiring role models (Lew, Cara, & Richardson 2007). Fourth, inspirational fieldwork educators maintain a "super-vision" and support their students in their integration into a department or organization. That is, the educator has in mind a picture of what the student can become and of the cases with whom the student works. The educator then oversees all student tasks, whether interpersonal or intrapersonal, and all student interactions with clients.

The fieldwork educator has the courage to confront students regarding weaknesses or strengths in these tasks or the nature of the supervisor–student relationship, and he or she provides an atmosphere of trust in which students can confront their own selves. This last quality then leads to personal growth and awareness, which are necessary in the process of becoming a professional. In all of these roles, the fieldwork educator has in mind increasing students' self-efficacy and ability to handle whatever obstacles may occur in their fieldwork.

The fieldwork supervisor's roles are not too different from his or her qualities. Research has indicated that students prefer a fieldwork educator who is warm, encouraging, open, not defensive, trustworthy, and knowledgeable about the field (Lew et al., 2007). Students want a supervisor to whom they can look up and respect and who they sense genuinely likes their work and their students. So it is imperative that a fieldwork educator lead and develop students into professionals who will learn to know themselves. That is, fieldwork educators should consistently examine themselves and their values, their fieldwork supervisory style, and their fieldwork relationship with students and always maintain their personal and professional integrity when working with students.

Fieldwork educators are leaders who are responsible for guiding occupational therapy students in their transition from students to professionals. Their role includes being a supportive mentor and an inspirational model with both the courage to confront a challenge and the ability to sustain students' professional growth. This act of "super-vision" requires knowledge of oneself and a deep commitment to a greater vision for the profession, the student, and the organization. The fieldwork educator's work will increase the self-efficacy and success rate of students who are engaged in the occupations associated with becoming a successful professional. These skills and qualities will eventually facilitate successful fieldwork experiences and the development of future leaders.

Leadership as Agency

Agency is the action, medium, or means by which something is accomplished. If occupational therapists are to lead, if they are to manage teams that are both agents of change and resilient in the face of change, they must engage most people within the organization. Therapists must act with agency if they are to lead others. To conceptualize leadership is this way is a fundamental but essential challenge to any organization (Wheatley, 1992). For occupational therapists, it is a strong argument for the need to belong to AOTA. AOTA houses occupational therapy's most admired leaders and its managers; those who profess the discipline to community stakeholders before the members know they need advocacy and those who plan to realize those optimistic promises. They look to the future and gather people who can organize, control, direct, and plan the craft of the profession while ensuring that the supply closet is restocked in time for groups to meet and get the work done. There is a difference between belonging to a profession and having a professional-level job. Being a professional means one assumes the honor and privilege of practicing with integrity. Being a leader within a profession is to ensure the honor and autonomy of practice.

Organizations are full of people who do not want a hero to come in and tell them what to do. They want, instead, for someone to help them make sense of their own process and to empower them to be more engaged, more alive, and more activated as they engage in the occupations of their own lives. They want leaders who can tolerate the discomfort of watching someone struggle to don a sock again and again until he or she experiences a personal "Eureka!" moment, when the process of self-organization is realized. Occupational therapists know that the other side of struggle is adaptation, function, and newly realized independence. Therapists intentionally use stress and struggle in the therapeutic process, and they have enormous capacity to wait alongside those who are thrashing through their personal struggles, knowing the powerful epiphany of discovering their own feet below them in a shallow pool and needing to be beside them, without judgment, to applaud their victory. "Watchful waiting," when used consciously, is a scientific procedure, a medical intervention and, ultimately, an authentic expression of both caring leadership and management.

Conclusion

Many kernels of wisdom are crystallized in fairy tales and stories. In *Alice in Wonderland*, Lewis Carroll provided a wonderful vignette to help one conceptualize leadership. When Alice came to a fork in the road, she asked the Cheshire Cat which road to take. The cat replied, "That depends a good deal on where you want to go." Alice then confessed, "I don't much care where." The cat remarked, "Then it doesn't matter which way you go" (Gardner, 2000, p. 65).

Alice in Wonderland is a fantasy crafted to explain mathematical logic and problem solving at its essential core, and it provides one of the most lasting reminders of the importance of leadership. Responsible leaders know where they are going and who will be in front of, alongside, and behind them. They are future oriented. To lead, they must keep their sights over the hill and partner with great managers and engaged followers. They must take turns when others know the way better than

Table 21.4. Occupational Therapy Code of Ethics for Managers and Leaders

Principle	Example
1. Beneficence	Demonstrate a concern for the well-being of the people who follow us on the path we are creating.
2. Nonmaleficence	Treat those we lead with care, on behalf of both their growth and well-being.
3. Autonomy	Be a professional, one who respects the honor and privilege to ensure others' success while enjoying the freedom of independence.
4. Duty	Make sure we are walking on a path we would want others to follow.
5. Procedural justice	Be fair, like a parent has to be with his or her children.
6. Veracity	Participate in the profession through continuing education, membership, and mentoring. Follow best practices in all endeavors. Have the integrity to admit when you are wrong and move on.
7. Fidelity	Model integrity or wholeness and faithfulness to people and organizations.

Source. American Occupational Therapy Association (2005).

they. If a leader has not prepared the path, he or she can trip over debris and tumble down a rabbit hole, taking with them any who dared to follow. The practice of occupational therapy embodies key lessons for leaders to use as a protection against the distress of change. These skills of coping are a talisman when change is imminent. We are standing on a precipice of future horizons, held in balance by the profession's ethics and depth of wisdom. Leaders and managers express values, and that expression establishes the organization's intention. Values guide actions, and these actions are then based on a specific ethical code. Occupational therapy leaders are guided by the profession's core values (AOTA, 1993). These leaders put occupational therapists in a strong position to lead and manage in times of change when they set the Occupational Therapy Code of Ethics, which outlines seven principles to guide occupational therapists in their practice: beneficence, nonmaleficence, autonomy, duty, procedural justice, veracity, and fidelity (AOTA, 2005). Table 21.4 suggests an expansion of the profession's code of ethics into the domains of managers and leaders.

References

American Occupational Therapy Association. (1993). Core values and attitudes of occupational therapy practice. *American Journal of Occupational Therapy, 47,* 1085–1086.

American Occupational Therapy Association. (2005). Occupational therapy code of ethics (2005). *American Journal of Occupational Therapy, 59,* 639–642.

Baum, M. C. (2005). Presidential Address, 2005—Harnessing opportunities and taking responsibility for our future. *American Journal of Occupational Therapy, 60*(3), 249–257.

Brachtesende, A. (2004, December 20) Coping with burnout. *OT Practice, 9,* 14.

Buysse, V., & Wesley, P. W. (2006). *Evidence-based practice in the early childhood field.* Washington, DC: Zero to Three.

Cara, E., & Macrae, A. (2005). *Psychosocial occupational therapy: A clinical practice.* Albany, NY: Delmar.

Drafke, M. W. (1994). *Working in health care: What you need to know to succeed.* Philadelphia: F. A. Davis.

Gardner, M. (2000). *The annotated Alice: The definitive edition.* New York: W. W. Norton & Co.

Hendrix, D. (2004, September). *Transition during reorganization of an association.* Presentation at the board of director's meeting of the Occupational Therapy Association of California, San Jose.

Higgs, J. (2003). Do you reason like a (health) professional? In G. Browns, S. A. Esdaile, & S. E. Ryan (Eds.), *Becoming an advanced healthcare practitioner* (pp. 145–160). New York: Butterworth & Heinemann.

Howard, B. S. (1991). How high do we jump? The effect of reimbursement on occupational therapy. *American Journal of Occupational Therapy, 45*(10), 875–881.

Jacobs, K., & Logigian, M. K. (1999). *Change management in functions of a manager in occupational therapy* (3rd ed.). Thorofare, NJ: Slack.

Jaffe-Epstein, E. (1999). A systems approach to community health promotion consultation: The occupational therapist as a change agent. In *Occupational therapy consultation: Theory principles and practice* (pp. 259–283). Baltimore: Mosby.

Jones, N. (1999). *Performance management in the 21st century: Solutions for business, education, and family.* Boca Raton, FL: CRC Press.

Kotter, J. P. (2001). What leaders do. *Harvard Business Review, 79*(11), 85–91

Lancaster, L. C. (2004). *When generations collide: How to solve the generational puzzle at work* (Management Forum Series). Retrieved May 19, 2008 from www.executiveforum.com/PDFs/LancasterSynopsis.pdf

Lancaster, L. C., & Stillman, D. (2003). *When generations collide: Who they are. Why they clash. How to solve the generational puzzle at work.* New York: HarperCollins.

Lew, N., Cara., E., & Richardson, P. (2007). When fieldwork takes a detour. *Occupational Therapy in Health Care, 21*(1/2), 105–122.

Mupinga, D. M., Nora, R. T., & Yaw, D. C. (2006). The learning styles, expectations, and needs of online students. *College Teaching, 54*(1), *185–189*

Polya, G. (1957). *How to solve it* (2nd ed.). Princeton, NJ: Princeton University Press.

Ray, M., & Myers, R. (1996). *Creativity in business.* New York: Doubleday.

Renesch, J. (1993). *New traditions in business and leadership in the 21st century.* San Francisco: Sterling & Stone.

Sapolsky, R. (n.d.) *What's your law?* Retrieved May 18, 2008, from www.edge.org/q2004/q04_print.html

Scott, W. E. (1985). Variables that contribute to leadership among female occupational therapists. *American Journal of Occupational Therapy, 39*(6), 379–385.

Snodgrass, J. E. (2006). *Faculty perceptions of occupational therapy program directors' leadership styles and outcomes of leadership.* Doctoral dissertation, TUI University, Cypress, CA.

Snodgrass, J., Douthitt, S., Ellis, R., Wade, S., & Plemons, J. (2008). Occupational therapy practitioners' perceptions of rehabilitation managers' leadership styles and the outcomes of leadership. *Journal of Allied Health, 37*(1), 38–44.

Soles, C., & Moller, L. (2001). *Myers Briggs type preferences in distance learning education.* Retrieved December 7, 2009, from www.ed.uiuc.edu/ijet/v2n2/soles/index.html

Tickle-Degnen, L. (2000). Evidence-based practice forum—Gathering current research evidence to enhance clinical reasoning. *American Journal of Occupational Therapy, 54*(1), 102–105.

Van der Werff, T. (2008). *What is a futurist, exactly?* Retrieved May 18, 2008, from www.globalfuture.com/futurist-nsane.htm

von Oech, R. (1998). *Creative whack pack* [Cards]. New York: U.S. Games Systems.

Washburn, C. A. (1991). *Comparison of characteristics of occupational therapists in traditional and private practice.* Retrieved November 3, 2007

Weisinger, H. (1998). *Emotional intelligence at work.* San Francisco: Jossey-Bass.

Wheatley, M. (1992). *Leadership and the new science: Learning about organization from an orderly universe.* San Francisco: Berrett-Koehler.

Whitney, R. (1996). Caring: An essential element. In K. Gozdz (Ed.), *Community building— Renewing spirit and learning in leadership* (pp. 199–207). San Francisco: Sterling & Stone.

Appendix 21A. Self-Assessment Activity

The following assessment is not meant to be a definitive indicator of one's innate skills or abilities and is offered for self-reflection only. Questions were synthesized from multiple sources, including Snodgrass, Douthitt, Ellis, Wade, and Plemons (2008) and Kotter (2001).

Part I. Management and Leadership

For the following statements, indicate how often each item is true regarding your REGULAR performance.

1. I'm a role model for those I lead, and they feel inspired around me, maybe because I'm passionate about what I do.
NEVER · · · · · · · · · SOMETIMES · · · · · · · · · REGULARLY

2. I take a rational approach to daily situations.
NEVER · · · · · · · · · SOMETIMES · · · · · · · · · REGULARLY

3. I have a clear vision mapped out in my mind and use it to guide my daily work routines.
NEVER · · · · · · · · · SOMETIMES · · · · · · · · · REGULARLY

4. I am persistent and tough minded when it comes to getting my work done.
NEVER · · · · · · · · · SOMETIMES · · · · · · · · · REGULARLY

5. I am creative and flexible; as long as I'm moving toward my mission, I'm not concerned with the details.
NEVER · · · · · · · · · SOMETIMES · · · · · · · · · REGULARLY

6. No matter what happens, my staff know I am a stable, reliable force in the organization.
NEVER · · · · · · · · · SOMETIMES · · · · · · · · · REGULARLY

7. I am imaginative.
NEVER · · · · · · · · · SOMETIMES · · · · · · · · · REGULARLY

8. I am structured.
NEVER · · · · · · · · · SOMETIMES · · · · · · · · · REGULARLY

9. I like to experiment and take risks when I'm coming up with solutions.
NEVER · · · · · · · · · SOMETIMES · · · · · · · · · REGULARLY

10. I use an analytical approach to solving real-world problems.
NEVER · · · · · · · · · SOMETIMES · · · · · · · · · REGULARLY

Part II. What Is Your Leadership Style?

In this section, you can select only one of each pair. Once you choose which of the two *most closely* matches you, circle your choice and move on to the next pair.

A	B
I do what is needed.	I go the extra mile.
I use rewards to motivate others.	People follow me even without rewards.
I look for and correct deviations in staff performance and guide others toward their commitments.	I look for ways to inspire others' ideas and visions.
I like it when everyone is working as a team, following the procedures and through that, gaining competence.	I like a challenge; I like to stir it up and feel intellectually stimulated, and I appreciate when others work outside of the box.
I use a more laissez faire style of leadership.	I consider each individual in my management style.

Part II: If you selected more items in the A column, you are expressing the characteristics of a manager and tend toward a Transactional Leadership style; if you scored more B items, you have the characteristics of a leader and tend toward a more Transformational Leadership style. The more items, the stronger your tendency.

Subject Index

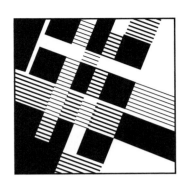

Citation Index

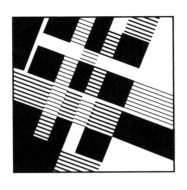